MCQs in
Sports Physiotherapy
(With Explanatory Answers)

Disclaimer Statement

The concepts included in this book are based on the most current research and recommendations of responsible medical and physiotherapeutic sources. Any changes and topics left out will be improved in the future. However, the authors and publisher disclaim responsibility for any adverse effects or consequences resulting from the misapplication or injudicious use of material.

MCQs in
Sports Physiotherapy
(With Explanatory Answers)

Second Edition

Author
S Arun Vijay MPT (Sports PT) PhD (Physiotherapy)
Assistant Professor, Department of Physiotherapy
Chairman, Department of Quality Measurement and Evaluation
Deanship of Quality and Academic Accreditation
Imam Abdulrahman Bin Faisal University
Dammam, Kingdom of Saudi Arabia

Co-Authors
P Shahul Hameed PT PhD MBA (TQM)
Assistant Professor and Program Coordinator
Department of Physical Therapy
Faculty of Applied Medical Sciences
University of Tabuk, Tabuk, Kingdom of Saudi Arabia

P Sivasankar MPT (Ortho) PhD (Physiotherapy)
Lecturer, Studies and Research Unit
Department of Quality Measurement and Evaluation
Deanship of Quality and Academic Accreditation
Imam Abdulrahman Bin Faisal University
Dammam, Kingdom of Saudi Arabia

Forewords
Qassim Al Muaidi
Saad Mohammed Alsaadi

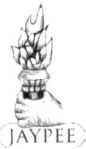

JAYPEE BROTHERS MEDICAL PUBLISHERS
The Health Sciences Publisher
New Delhi | London

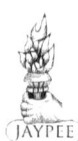 **Jaypee Brothers Medical Publishers (P) Ltd**

Headquarters
EMCA House
23/23-B, Ansari Road, Daryaganj
New Delhi 110 002, India
Landline: +91-11-23272143, +91-11-23272703
+91-11-23282021, +91-11-23245672
E-mail: jaypee@jaypeebrothers.com

Corporate Office
Jaypee Brothers Medical Publishers (P) Ltd.
4838/24, Ansari Road, Daryaganj
New Delhi 110 002, India
Phone: +91-11-43574357
Fax: +91-11-43574314
E-mail: jaypee@jaypeebrothers.com

Website: www.jaypeebrothers.com
Website: www.jaypeedigital.com

Overseas Office
JP Medical Ltd.
83, Victoria Street, London
SW1H 0HW (UK)
Phone: +44-20 3170 8910
Fax: +44(0)20 3008 6180
E-mail: info@jpmedpub.com

© 2022, Jaypee Brothers Medical Publishers

The views and opinions expressed in this book are solely those of the original contributor(s)/author(s) and do not necessarily represent those of editor(s) of the book.

All rights reserved. No part of this publication may be reproduced, stored or transmitted in any form or by any means, electronic, mechanical, photocopying, recording or otherwise, without the prior permission in writing of the publishers.

All brand names and product names used in this book are trade names, service marks, trademarks or registered trademarks of their respective owners. The publisher is not associated with any product or vendor mentioned in this book.

Medical knowledge and practice change constantly. This book is designed to provide accurate, authoritative information about the subject matter in question. However, readers are advised to check the most current information available on procedures included and check information from the manufacturer of each product to be administered, to verify the recommended dose, formula, method and duration of administration, adverse effects and contraindications. It is the responsibility of the practitioner to take all appropriate safety precautions. Neither the publisher nor the author(s)/editor(s) assume any liability for any injury and/or damage to persons or property arising from or related to use of material in this book.

This book is sold on the understanding that the publisher is not engaged in providing professional medical services. If such advice or services are required, the services of a competent medical professional should be sought.

Every effort has been made where necessary to contact holders of copyright to obtain permission to reproduce copyright material. If any have been inadvertently overlooked, the publisher will be pleased to make the necessary arrangements at the first opportunity.

Inquiries for bulk sales may be solicited at: jaypee@jaypeebrothers.com

MCQs in Sports Physiotherapy (With Explanatory Answers)
First Edition: 2010
Second Edition: **2022**
ISBN 978-93-5465-348-3

Foreword

Over the past decades, sports physiotherapy has turned into an appreciated profession and is globally recognized within sports and exercise medicine. Physiotherapists serve with other experts and trainers to train the sportspersons and manage their sports injuries. A sports physiotherapist needs enough knowledge and skills in sports medicine and expertise to assess, diagnose, prevent and manage sports injuries.

In my view, this second edition book of *MCQs in Sports Physiotherapy (With Explanatory Answers)* has managed to provide enough knowledge over the array of sports injuries. The contents of this book have been wisely amassed to cover the essential concepts of sports physiotherapy by a team of contributors with expertise in physiotherapy. Accordingly, the contributors focused their book content with potential MCQs to meet the needs of the students and physiotherapists, who are preparing for various licensure examinations worldwide. This second edition has been updated from the previous one by adding new chapters and more significant MCQs both in quality and quantity. Notably, it embraced the chapters dealing with robotics in sports rehabilitation and the basics of imaging in sports injuries, which gives an extensive understanding to sports physiotherapists. Such updates surely satisfy the readers' desires and become a valuable asset to anyone serving in sports physiotherapy. The authors have also proposed further progression in the form of a second edition to enhance the credibility of the book content. I believe that this book would be a valuable addition to the emerging sports physiotherapy books. Hence, I welcome this book titled, *MCQs in Sports Physiotherapy (With Explanatory Answers)*, and I am eager to look into its progression in the future alongside the exciting career that it ropes.

Overall, Dr S Arun Vijay and his co-authors must be praised and credited for their sincere efforts in evolving this valuable edition.

Prof. Qassim Al Muaidi
President, Saudi Federation of Sports Medicine
Executive Board Member, Asian Federation of Sports Medicine (AFSM)
Member, Development Commission of International Federation of Sport Medicine (IFSM)
Professor and Dean, College of Applied Medical Sciences
Imam Abdulrahman Bin Faisal University
Dammam, Kingdom of Saudi Arabia

Foreword

It is a privilege and honor to write a foreword for the second edition of the *MCQs in Sports Physiotherapy (With Explanatory Answers)*.

The first edition of this textbook reflects a set of MCQs on various topics of sports rehabilitation and therapeutic interventions used in both prevention and treatment of sports injuries, and it was made possible by the joint effort of Dr S Arun Vijay and his co-authors in 2010. Since 2010, the textbook has turned into a familiar one for learning and reference for physiotherapists across the globe. In this state, the progress to the second edition becomes essential to cover the time gap and all recent advances in sports physiotherapy to update the book contents accordingly.

The textbook has excellent relevance as sports injuries are rising worldwide, particularly in developing nations. Moreover, the book covers the entire range of sports physiotherapy briefly and specifically with contributions from several sports physiotherapists. I am sure that this book is an excellent resource for physiotherapy students and helps practicing physiotherapists take licensure and competitive examinations effectively.

I congratulate Dr S Arun Vijay and his co-authors for their drive, passion, commitment, and perseverance to bring out this book in its complete form.

Dr Saad Mohammed Alsaadi
Consultant-Physiotherapy
Chairman, Department of Physiotherapy
King Fahd Hospital of the University
Dean, Graduate Studies
Imam Abdulrahman Bin Faisal University
Dammam, Kingdom of Saudi Arabia

Preface to the Second Edition

The publication of the second edition of the *MCQs in Sports Physiotherapy (With Explanatory Answers)* in 2022 includes five new chapters focusing on various aspects of sports injures and rehabilitation. Among those chapters, principles of athletic conditioning have been updated with additional content on preventing sports injuries. Subsequently, stress fracture and the role of physiotherapy in the surgical management of sports injuries are included to enrich students' and physiotherapists' knowledge. Further, this edition contains MCQs on the essential radiological imaging of sports injuries, giving a new mileage to physiotherapists to understand the utility of imaging in sports assessment. Besides, this book covers the current trends in sports physiotherapy, especially Robotics in Sports Rehabilitation, where the required number of multiple choice questions (MCQs) are added. I hope all these new chapters will add value to the body of knowledge of sports physiotherapy. Furthermore, in addition to the newly added chapters, all previous chapters have been updated with potential new MCQs, considering the changes that happened during the last ten years in the sports physiotherapy field and preparing the physical therapist to take competitive exams worldwide.

S Arun Vijay
P Shahul Hameed
P Sivasankar

Preface to the First Edition

Sports physiotherapy is a branch of physiotherapeutic medicine which mainly deals with prevention, management, and rehabilitation of injuries. There are a large number of books on sports physiotherapy, but a very few multiple choice questions books are available on this topic. In the current scenario, the MCQ patterns are very popular and essential for all the physiotherapists to take up their licensure examinations both in India and abroad.

We sincerely hope that this book, the first of its kind, would provide useful guidance not only to the students of physiotherapy but also to the practicing physiotherapists and others engaged in the sports injury rehabilitation.

S Arun Vijay
V Arthi
Mithun Kuriakose

Acknowledgments

First and foremost, I would like to thank God, the Almighty, for having showered his blessings on me and providing me with physical strength and mental courage throughout the preparation of this book. My sincere thanks to the co-authors, **Dr P Shahul Hameed** and **Dr P Sivasankar**, for their constant support and dedication to completing the book.

A special thanks and gratitude to my institution "Imam Abdulrahman Bin Faisal University (IAU)" where I used its resources in preparing this book. I am also thankful to Shri Jitendar P Vij (Group Chairman), Mr Ankit Vij (Managing Director), Mr MS Mani (Group President), Dr Madhu Choudhary (Publishing Head-Education), Ms Pooja Bhandari (Production Head), Ms Sunita Katla (Executive Assistant to Group Chairman and Publishing Manager), Mr Rajesh Sharma (Production Coordinator), Ms Seema Dogra (Cover Visualizer), Ms Geeta Rani (Proofreader), Mr Ajeet Rathor (Typesetter), Mr Pappu Kumar (Graphic Designer) and team members of M/s Jaypee Brothers Medical Publisher (P) Ltd, New Delhi, India, for their constant cooperation and assistance.

My special thanks to my mother, wife, and daughters, who tolerated my passion for this book and supported and assisted me while working on this project.

S Arun Vijay

Contents

1. Preparticipation Physical Examination — 1
2. Emergency Sports Assessment and First Aid — 13
3. Principles of Athletic Conditioning and Prevention of Sports Injuries — 32
4. Therapeutic Exercise in Injury Rehabilitation — 48
   - A. Stretching and Warm-up 48
   - B. Resistance Training 56
   - C. Plyometric Training 72
5. Basic Concepts in Injury Rehabilitation — 80
6. Shoulder and Arm Injuries — 96
7. Elbow Injuries — 121
8. Wrist and Hand Injuries — 142
9. Injuries to the Groin and Hip — 169
10. Thigh and Leg Injuries — 184
11. Ankle and Foot Injury — 220
12. Spine and Chest Injuries — 243
    - A. Cervical Spine Injuries 243
    - B. Chest and Thoracic Spine Injuries 257
    - C. Lumbar Spine Injuries 270
13. Stress Fracture — 284
14. Basics of Imaging in Sport injuries for Physical Therapist — 293
15. Postsurgical Physiotherapy for Sports Injuries — 320
16. Robotics in Sports Rehabilitation — 337
17. Sports Nutrition — 346
18. Sports Psychology — 359

Bibliography — *367*
- List of Textbooks 367
- List of Journals 369

Preparticipation Physical Examination

CHAPTER 1

1. **The preparticipation physical examination is conducted for the purpose of what?**
   A. Determine any defects or conditions exists which might place the athlete at risk
   B. Bring to the athlete's attention of any muscle weakness or imbalance
   C. Determine whether an athlete may participate safely in the event.
   D. All of the above

2. **When the preparticipation physical examination is conducted ideally?**
   A. One month before the beginning of the season
   B. 15 days before the beginning of the season
   C. One week before the beginning of the season
   D. Six months before the beginning of the season

3. **Which somatotype of an individual has large, efficient abdominal viscera, and tends to be obese?**
   A. Endomorphs
   B. Mesomorphs
   C. Ectomorphs
   D. None of the above

4. **Which somatotypes of an athlete is suitable for marathon running?**
   A. Endomorphs
   B. Viscerotonic
   C. Mesomorphs
   D. Ectomorphs

5. **Following are the extrinsic risk factors in sports injuries, *except*:**
   A. Sports equipment used
   B. Sporting environmental conditions
   C. Type of sporting activity
   D. Physical characteristics of an athlete

6. The lack of which muscle strength is considered as a risk factor in overuse injuries?
   A. Isometric muscle strength
   B. Dynamic muscle strength
   C. Ballistic muscle strength
   D. All of the above

7. Which one of the following is a significant risk factor causing acute sports injuries?
   A. Increased dynamic muscle strength
   B. Decreased dynamic muscle strength
   C. Increased static muscle strength
   D. Decreased ballistic strength

8. Anecdotally, fatigue affects the physical and mental performance of the player during which time of the game?
   A. First quarter
   B. Second quarter
   C. Towards the end of game
   D. Middle of second quarter

9. Which intrinsic feedback mechanism is used by the sports persons to monitor their own ability to maintain stability of a functionally unstable joint?
   A. Biofeed and feedback technique
   B. Proprioceptive retraining
   C. Sensory re-education
   D. Motor re-education

10. A collegiate basketball physical training specialist would like to know which of his players has the most muscular power. Which of the following is the most valid test for monitoring a basketball player's muscular power?
    A. Vertical jump test
    B. 1RM bench press
    C. 100 m sprint
    D. 15 RM squat

11. According to the body mass index (BMI), which of the following athletes are considered obese?
    A. Body builder with BMI of 32.9
    B. Shot-putter with BMI of 28.0
    C. Basketball player with BMI of 25.0
    D. Power lifter with BMI of 29.4

12. Which of the following is an early adjustment to acclimatizing to high altitude?
    A. Decreased tidal volume
    B. Decreased respiratory rate
    C. Increased resting cardiac output
    D. Increased stroke volume
13. The level of strength can be determined by using the following devices, *except:*
    A. Cable tensiometer
    B. Cybex isokinetic dynamometer
    C. Nautilus machine
    D. Dynamometer
14. The highest duration of training should be performed during which of the following sports season?
    A. Post season
    B. Pre-season
    C. In-season
    D. Off-season
15. A sports physical therapist prepares a presentation on presession conditioning for a group of high school athletes. To maximize the effectiveness of the presentation the therapist should:
    A. Develop specific learning objectives
    B. Utilize a variety of audio-visual equipment
    C. Assess the needs of the target audience
    D. Provide an outline
16. Typically, which one of the following information is gathered during the preparticipation physical examination of an athlete?
    A. Athlete's general health
    B. Maturity level
    C. Level of physical fitness
    D. All of the above
17. During preparticipation physical examination, the physical therapist records the individual's baseline physiologic parameters and vital statistics. Following parameters are included as vital statistics, *except:*
    A. Heart rate
    B. Blood pressure
    C. Body mass index
    D. Body temperature

18. Which one of the following measurements technique is the most reliable one to determine the athlete's body fat?
    A. Hydrostatic weighting   B. Skinfold measurement
    C. Girth measurement   D. Tanner scale
19. The purpose of Tanner Scale during preparticipation physical examination of athletes is to measure the:
    A. Physical maturity   B. Body weight
    C. Body composition   D. Psychological status
20. The type of (skin) pinch and standardized skinfold measurement site at the abdominal region is:
    A. Vertical fold; 2 cm on the right side of the umbilicus
    B. Horizontal fold; 2 cm on the right side of the umbilicus
    C. Vertical fold; 2 cm on the left side of the umbilicus
    D. Horizontal fold; 2 cm on the right side of the umbilicus
21. Flexibility is the total range of motion at a joint that occurs pain-free in each of the planes of motion. Which one of the following factors limits flexibility and range of motion in a 26-year-old male athlete who does not sustain any injury or pathological issues?
    A. Gender   B. Age
    C. Dominate limb   D. All of the above
22. The ability of a muscle or group of muscles to produce force in one maximal resistance (1 RM) effort, either statically or dynamically, is known as?
    A. Power   B. Speed
    C. Strength   D. Agility
23. During preparticipation physical examination of sprinters, which of the following on-field tests used to measure agility, balance, and reaction time?
    A. Run-and-cut drills   B. Figure-eight running drills
    C. Shuttle runs   D. All of the above
24. The purpose of conducting a Harvard step test in an athlete is to measure:
    A. The aerobic fitness   B. Strength
    C. Flexibility   D. Agility

Chapter 1: Preparticipation Physical Examination

25. The participant is graded as 'Good' following the Harvard step test. Which one of the following fitness index scores is the most accurate description for this category?
    A. >90
    B. 80–89
    C. 65–79
    D. 55–64

26. The purpose of revealing past medical history of an athlete during the preparticipation examination is to:
    A. Identify any recent weight loss, dizziness or general malaise.
    B. Ascertain relevant medical history (investigations; interventions; trauma)
    C. Review general health of body systems (e.g., digestive, respiratory systems)
    D. All of the above

27. The gold-standard method that works on Archimedes' principle to assess body composition is known as?
    A. Hydrodensitometry
    B. Air displacement plethysmography
    C. Absorptiometry
    D. Surface anthropometry

28. From the following options, identify medical conditions that are contraindicated for sports participation?
    A. Active myocarditis or pericarditis
    B. Hypertrophic cardiomyopathy
    C. Poorly controlled convulsive disorder
    D. All of the above

29. If a collegiate student displays a maximum voluntary contraction (MVC) of less than 20% while increasing a static muscle component during preparticipation physical examination, the participation in which one of the following sports is contraindicated?
    A. Cricket
    B. Gulf
    C. Gymnastics
    D. Billiards

30. During the cardiovascular examination of an individual who is 6.2 feet tall, the sports physiotherapy suspects Marfan's syndrome. Which one of the following symptoms is indicative of Marfan's syndrome?

A. Arm span greater than height and has long fingers and toes
B. Presence of pectus excavatum chest-wall deformity
C. High arched palate
D. All of the above

31. After eliciting the deep tendon patellar reflex testing on an 18-year-old collegiate football player, which one of the following responses considered normal?
    A. Knee flexion
    B. Knee extension
    C. Plant flexion with inversion
    D. Knee flexion with medical rotation

32. The preparticipation examination of a Rifle Shooter's eyes reveals that he can see objects near to him clearly, but objects farther away are blurry. This condition is termed as:
    A. Myopia   B. Hypermetropia
    C. Anisocoria   D. Emmetropia

33. Among the following sports, which one of them warrants excessive flexibility for displaying better performance?
    A. Badminton   B. Volley ball
    C. Gymnastics   D. Tennis

34. The clinical condition where the musculotendinous unit has adaptively shortened and there is a significant loss of range of motion with no specific muscle pathology is known as?
    A. Myostatic contracture
    B. Pseudomyostatic contracture
    C. Fibrotic contracture
    D. Periarticular contractures

35. The periarticular contracture occurs due to:
    A. Hypertonicity associated with a central nervous system lesion, such as a cerebral vascular accident, a spinal cord injury, or traumatic brain injury.
    B. Result of intra-articular pathology which may include adhesions, synovial proliferation, joint effusion, irregularities in articular cartilage, or osteophyte formation.
    C. Connective tissues that cross or attach to a joint or the joint capsule lose mobility, thus restricting normal arthrokinematic motion.

D. Fibrous changes in the connective tissue of muscle and periarticular structures can cause adherence of these tissues and subsequent development of a fibrotic contracture.

36. The palpation of the skin and subcutaneous tissue reveals the following, *except*:
    A. Temperature
    B. Edema
    C. Texture
    D. Trigger points

37. A sports physical therapist positions the football player prone on a plinth and passively flexes his knee. As the knee flexes, the players' hip on the same side also begins to flex. This clinical presentation is most indicative of a:
    A. Tight iliopsoas
    B. Tight rectus femoris
    C. Tight tensor fasciae latae
    D. Tight hamstrings

38. A physical therapist observes the electrocardiogram of a marathon runner during exercise testing prior to his participation in sports. Which of the following ECG changes would be considered abnormal during exercise?
    A. Increase in amplitude of P wave
    B. Shortening of PR interval
    C. ST segment depression of greater than 1 mm
    D. Decrease in amplitude of T wave

39. A sports physical therapist conducts a goniometric assessment of the wrist and hand. When determining the available range of motion for thumb flexion, the therapist should align the axis of the goniometer over the:
    A. Dorsal aspect of the first interphalangeal joint
    B. Palmar aspect of the first carpometacarpal joint
    C. Midway between the dorsal aspect of the first and second carpometacarpal joints
    D. Midway between the palmar aspect of the first and second carpometacarpal joints

40. A physical therapist records grip strength measurement on a 21-year-old tennis player as a part of a preparticipation physical examination. Which description does not accurately illustrate typical results when using a handheld dynamometer?

A. A bell curve is seen when charting multiple recordings from adjustable hand spacings in consecutive order.
B. 20-25% differences in grip strength may be observed between the dominant and nondominant hand.
C. Discrepancies of more than 25% are a test-retest situation may indicate the patient is not exerting maximal force.
D. An individual who does not exert maximal force for each test will not show the typical bell curve.

Chapter 1: Preparticipation Physical Examination

ANSWERS

1. **D.**
2. **A.** Preparticipation physical examination should ideally be conducted approximately one month before the beginning of the season in order to give sufficient time to correct problems, such as muscle weakness, infections and other conditions.
3. **A.** Endomorphs are having large efficient abdominal viscera and digest, absorb and store food efficiently therefore tending to become obese. They are not very muscular and active physically.
4. **D.** The ectomorphs has a high proportion of skin and nerves on a small skeletal frame, with very little subcutaneous fat and tend to make good marathon runners.
5. **D.** The extrinsic risk factors are the exposure to the sporting activity, the manner in which preparation for the activity is undertaken, the equipment used and the prevailing environmental conditions.
6. **A.** Lack of static muscle strength is implicated as a risk factor in overuse injuries. Static strength has been identified as a protective factor because of its stabilizing effect on a joint.
7. **A.** Increased dynamic muscle strength is a risk factor in acute injury. Increased forces generated by individuals with greater strength were significant in producing acute injuries in sports.
8. **B.** Anecdotally, the time of game when the players would be most at risk is after a break in the game (due to injury or scheduled interval) or towards the end of the game when fatigue affects physical and mental performance.
9. **B.** Proprioceptive retraining is the intrinsic feed back mechanism used by the participants to monitor their own ability to maintain stability of a structurally or functionally unstable joint.
10. **A.** Vertical jump is very specific to basketball, which involves vertical jumping during play, and it is the best test to stimulate the physical movements and energy demands of a real game.

11. **A.** BMI is calculated as weight in kilograms divided by height squared in meters. Up to the BMI value of 29.9, the athlete is put under the classification 'Overweight'. If the BMI is between 30 and 34.9, it is classified as class I obesity.
12. **C.** Submaximal heart rate and cardiac output can increase by 30–50% above sea-level values, whereas stroke volume remains constant or slightly reduced. Further, there will be great increase in pulmonary ventilation at rest and during exercise occur early in the acclimatization process.
13. **C.**
14. **D.** Off-season training (base-training) should be composed of long duration and low intensity workouts used to develop a base of cardiorespiratory fitness.
15. **C.** To maximize the effectiveness of the presentation, it is essential to assess the needs of the target audience prior to designing a formal or informal presentation.
16. **D.**
17. **C.** Sport performance is highly dependent on the health- and skill-related components of fitness (power, speed, agility, reaction time, balance, and body composition coordination. Body mass index (BMI) is a useful screening tool for diagnosing overweight and obese individuals involved in sports and fitness.
18. **A.** Hydrostatic weighting and skinfold measurements often are used to determine body fat measurements. Hydrostatic weighting is more accurate, but skinfold measurement is easier, faster, and nearly as reliable.
19. **A.** Tanner scale is a common method of measuring maturation in males and females. There are five stages in this scale and are based on pictorial standards of breast development and pubic hair for females and of genitalia and pubic hair for males.
20. **A.** All skinfold measurement measurements should be made on the right side of the body. According to the standard skinfold assessment protocol of the International Society for the Advancement of Kinanthropometry, the right side of the body is used for unilateral measurements irrespective of the preferred side of the subject, unless impractical to use due

Chapter 1: Preparticipation Physical Examination

to injury or similar cause. For measuring the abdominal skin folder measurement, a vertical pinch should be maintained while reading the caliper 2 cm on the right side of the umbilicus.
21. D. Several factors limit flexibility and range of motion viz. (i) Gender (females tend to be more flexible than males); (ii) Age (flexibility decreases with age) and (iii) Dominant limb tends to be less mobile than the nondominant limb.
22. C
23. D. The examples of agility, balance, and reaction tests include run-and-cut drills, carioca steps, shuttle runs, pivoting drills, front-to-back and side-to-side hops, figure-eight running drills, kicking a stationary or moving target, and beam-walking tests.
24. A. The athlete is instructed to step up onto an 18-inch platform using a four-step cadence "up-up-down-down" at a rate of about 30 times per minute (a metronome is used for cadence). Following 3.5 minutes at a pace of 2 seconds per step, the individual moves as fast as possible for 30 seconds (total time, 4 minutes). The individual then immediately sits down in a chair and relaxes for 3 minutes while the pulse is determined. The pulse is taken at 30, 60, 120, and 180 seconds after the exercise. The index formula for the pulse is:
$$\text{Fitness index} = \frac{(\text{duration of exercise in seconds} \times 100)}{(2 \times \text{sum of any three pulse counts})}$$
The higher the index, the better the person's aerobic fitness.
25. B. The higher the fitness index score, the better the person's aerobic fitness. The fitness index score falling between 80 to 89 is graded as 'good' following the Harvard step test.
26. D.
27. A. Hydrodensitometry, or underwater weighing (UWW), has been considered the gold-standard method for assessing body composition. The technique is based on Archimedes' principle that body mass in air compared to body mass when totally submerged in water is directly related to the density of the water displaced.
28. D.
29. C.

30. **D.** Marfan's syndrome should be suspected in an individual who is tall and has an arm span greater than height, long fingers and toes, pectus excavatum chest-wall deformity, and a high arched palate.
31. **B.**
32. **A.** Myopia, or near-sightedness, occurs when the light rays are focused in front of the retina, making only those objects close to the eyes distinguishable; but objects farther away are blurry. This condition occurs when the eyeball is too long, or the cornea—the protective outer layer of your eye is too curved, the light that enters the eye won't focus correctly. Images focus in front of the retina instead of directly on the retina. This causes blurred vision.
33. **C.** Flexibility is the total range of motion at a joint that occurs pain-free in each of the planes of motion. In most cases, less flexibility is better than too much; however, in certain activities (e.g., gymnastics or wrestling), excessive flexibility is a necessity.
34. **A.**
35. **C.**
36. **D.** A trigger point (TrP) is a hyperirritable spot, a palpable nodule in the taut bands of the skeletal muscles' fascia. Direct compression or muscle contraction is required and can elicit jump sign, local tenderness, local twitch response and referred pain which usually responds with a pain pattern distant from the trigger point.
37. **B.** This scenario describes Ely's test which, if positive, is indicative of tightness of the rectus femoris (two joint hip flexor).
38. **C.** ST segment depression of less than 1 mm may occur in a healthy individual during exercise, however, changes of greater than 1 mm would be considered abnormal.
39. **B.** Carpometacarpal flexion occurs in a frontal plane around an anterior-posterior axis with the patient in the anatomical position.
40. **B.** Grip strength may vary by 5-10% when comparing the dominant and nondominant hands.

Emergency Sports Assessment and First Aid

CHAPTER 2

1. A therapist examines a patient diagnosed with an Achilles tendon injury. Which clinical finding is not indicative of a ruptured Achilles tendon?
   A. Negative Thompson test
   B. Absent Achilles reflex
   C. Lack of toe off during gait
   D. A palpable defect in the musculotendinous units

2. A sports physiotherapist designs an exercise program for an athlete recovering from a lower extremity injury. A single most important factor in an exercise program designed to increase muscle strength is:
   A. The recovery time between exercise sets
   B. The number of repetitions per set
   C. The duration of exercise session
   D. The intensity of the exercise

3. During shock, the optimal position for which the athlete to be placed is:
   A. Reclining with the feet at the same level of head
   B. Reclining with the feet higher than the head
   C. Head down position with feet straight
   D. Semi-recumbent position

4. Following are the indicators of blunt abdominal injury, *except:*
   A. Absence of superficial abdominal reflex
   B. Absence of normal bowel sounds
   C. Falling BP, increasing pulse rate
   D. Referred pain to shoulder tip or back

5. A therapist completes a sensory examination on a patient diagnosed with an incomplete spinal cord injury to assess the C_5 dermatome; the therapist should utilize the:

A. Neck
B. Deltoid area of the lateral arm
C. Thumb and index finger
D. Superior portion of the chest above the axilla

6. A physical therapist instructs a female athlete to complete ten minutes of stretching before beginning her treadmill program. While observing the athlete stretching her hamstrings, he notices repetitive bouncing and a failure to maintain the stretch for more than 5 seconds. Why is this type of stretching considered to be inadequate?

   A. The athlete should maintain each stretch for at least 30 seconds.
   B. The athlete should stretch only after running on the treadmill.
   C. The athlete is activating the stretch reflex.
   D. The athlete should remain activity specific.

7. A physical therapist examines a patient diagnosed with an acute posterior cruciate sprain. The mechanism of injury for the posterior cruciate ligament is:

   A. A forceful landing on the anterior tibia with the knee hyperflexed.
   B. An anteriorly directed force applied to the tibia when the foot is fixed.
   C. A valgus force applied to the knee when the foot is fixed.
   D. Hyperextension, medial rotation of leg with lateral rotation of body.

8. A sports physiotherapist examines joint play movement by placing the joint in its resting position. This position is best described as:

   A. Maximum congruency between the articular surfaces and the joint capsule
   B. Minimum congruency between the articular surfaces and joint capsule
   C. Passive separation of the joint surface is limited.
   D. Parallel to the joint treatment plane

9. The motor examination reveals weakness of calf and hamstrings along with wasting of gluteals, peroneals and

Chapter 2: Emergency Sports Assessment and First Aid

plantar flexors. The corresponding myotome should be recorded as:

A. L2
B. L3
C. S1
D. S2

10. A physiotherapist observes a video on the biomechanics of normal gait. The therapist notes that the subject's knee remain flexed during all of the components of stance phase, *except:*

A. Foot flat
B. Heel strike
C. Midstance
D. Toe off

11. The clinical presentation of transient upper extremity dysesthesia, pain and weakness following an unilateral or contralateral shoulder blow which may be associated with cervical spinal extension, lateral flexion or both resulted in:

A. Burner's syndrome
B. Shoulder hand syndrome
C. Burning hand syndrome
D. Pinched nerve syndrome

12. A 16-year-old high school track participant returns to physical therapy after a physician's appointment. The patient indicates that MRI revealed a tear in medical meniscus of left knee. As you look back on the initial examination, which of the following special tests would you expect to have been positive?

A. Lachman
B. Pivot shift
C. McMurray
D. Apprehension

13. A therapist places a patient's hip in the resting position prior to assessing joint play. Which of the following would be considered as the resting position of the hip?

A. 10° flexion, 15° abduction, slight medial rotation
B. 30° flexion, 30° abduction, slight lateral rotation
C. 30° flexion, 30° adduction, 20° lateral rotation
D. 10° extension, 20° adduction, 20° medial rotation

14. A therapist instructs a patient to close her eyes and hold out her hand. The therapist places a series of different weights in the patient's hand one at a time. The patient is then asked to identify the comparative weight of the objects. This method of sensory testing is used to examine:

A. Barognosis
B. Graphesthesia
C. Recognition of texture
D. Stereognosis

15. The method used by the athletic trainer to remove an inhaled foreign object in the upper airway of an athlete during athletic participation is called?
    A. Upper chest inhibition technique
    B. Delivering a series of rapid thrusts to the upper abdomen
    C. Delivering a series of 4 or 5 short blows to the spine between scapulae
    D. Lower chest inhibition technique

16. A patient is performing exercises on a treadmill, while exercising the patient report his level of perceived exertion as 7 on Borg's ten-point scale. Which word best describe the patient's rate of perceived exertion?
    A. Weak
    B. Moderate
    C. Strong
    D. Very strong

17. A patient positioned in supine on a mat table is instructed to flex her right hip and knee to her chest and hold it. This evaluation technique can be used to assess the length of:
    A. Hamstrings on the left
    B. Hamstrings on the right
    C. Hip flexors on the right
    D. Hip flexors on the left

18. A physical therapist examines a patient's hip range of motion. Which pattern of limitation is typically considered to be a capsular pattern?
    A. Limitation of flexion, abduction and medial rotation
    B. Limitation of flexion, adduction and lateral rotation
    C. Limitation of extension, abduction and lateral rotation
    D. Limitation of extension, adduction and medial rotation

19. The normal flexion range of motion available at atlanto-occipital joint of cervical spine is:
    A. 10°
    B. 15°
    C. 20°
    D. 5°

20. Sacroiliac joint pathology is confirmed by which of the following special tests?
    A. Slump test
    B. Faber's test
    C. Tripod test
    D. Craig's test

21. Following tests are the components of functional strength tests, *except*:

Chapter 2: Emergency Sports Assessment and First Aid

- A. Bench press
- B. Push-ups
- C. Harvard step test
- D. Sit-ups

22. For a head injury patient, the term 'Neural watch' is related to:
    - A. Monitoring of patient's vital sign
    - B. Monitoring of patient's unconscious level
    - C. Verbal reaction to pain
    - D. Monitoring of motor function

23. An anaphylactic shock occurs due to which one of the following?
    - A. Blood loss
    - B. Insufficient pumping of blood by heart
    - C. Allergic reaction
    - D. Loss of body fluid

24. The most appropriate standardized instrument to measure the level of consciousness is:
    - A. Glasgow coma scale
    - B. Rankin scale
    - C. Barthel index
    - D. Sickness impact profile

25. Following are the components of athletic conditioning program, *except:*
    - A. Strength
    - B. Power
    - C. Proprioception
    - D. Nutrition

26. Approximately at 6 hours after head injury, the Glasgow coma scale score of range 9 to 11 indicates which one of the following?
    - A. Normal
    - B. Mild head injury
    - C. Moderate head injury
    - D. Severe head injury

27. A therapist practices assessing joint end feel. The therapist would move accurately classify normal elbow extension end feel as:
    - A. Firm
    - B. Hard
    - C. Soft
    - D. Empty

28. The closed pack position of metacarpophalangeal joint (fingers) is:
    - A. Full extension
    - B. Full flexion
    - C. Full abduction
    - D. Full opposition

29. While examining a patient diagnosed with Achilles tendonitis, a therapist notes that the foot appears to be pronated in standing. Which motion combine to create pronation?
   A. Abduction, dorsiflexion, eversion
   B. Adduction, dorsiflexion, inversion
   C. Adduction, plantar flexion, eversion
   D. Adduction, plantar flexion, inversion
30. The chemical which is most commonly (and currently) being used in cold spray therapy technique during athletic rehabilitation is:
   A. Fluoromethane   B. Ethyl chloride
   C. Xylocaine   D. Hydrocortisone
31. The ratio of chest compression to breaths during two-man cardiopulmonary resuscitation is:
   A. 5:1   B. 10:1
   C. 14:1   D. 14: 2
32. During a soccer game, a player sustains an injury to his right knee joint and cannot continue the game. The physical therapist completes a series of special tests designed to examine the ligamentous integrity of a player's knee. After completing the tests, the therapist is unsure if the laxity is normal or indicative of a ligamentous injury. The most appropriate step to gather more information is to:
   A. Attempt to quantify the millimeters of laxity and compare the values with established norms
   B. Contact the physician and suggest a referral for magnetic resonance imaging
   C. Directly compare the laxity in the involved knee to the laxity in the uninvolved knee
   D. Attempt to identify other special tests that can offer more information on the ligamentous integrity of the knee
33. A physical therapist attempts to place an athlete's hip in the resting position before assessing joint play. Which position would be most consistent with the therapist's objective?
   A. 10° flexion, 15° abduction, slight medial rotation
   B. 30° flexion, 30° adduction, 20° lateral rotation
   C. 30° flexion, 30° abduction, slight lateral rotation
   D. 10° extension, 20° adduction, 20° medial rotation

Chapter 2: Emergency Sports Assessment and First Aid

34. A physical therapist completes a manual muscle test on a hockey player who sustained a laceration in the anterior surface of the forearm. When performing a test on the flexor pollicis brevis, the therapist should direct the force along:
    A. The volar aspect of the proximal phalanx of the thumb
    B. The volar aspect of the distal phalanx of the thumb
    C. The dorsal aspect of the proximal phalanx of the thumb
    D. The dorsal aspect of the distal phalanx of the thumb

35. A physical therapist examines a gymnastic who complains of sacroiliac pain immediately following the event. As part of the on-field examination, the therapist assesses the position of the sacrum by palpating the inferior lateral angles. Which spinal level is most consistent with the inferior lateral angles?
    A. S1 B. S3
    C. S4 D. S5

36. A physical therapist performs a manual muscle test on a collegiate sports person to ascertain whether he has any bilateral upper extremity weakness. The therapist should test the player's scapular adductors by positioning him in:
    A. Prone B. Side lying
    C. Standing D. Supine

37. During the physical examination, a physical therapist, classifies an athlete's end-feel as soft after completing a specific passive movement. Which of the following joint motions would typically produce a soft end-feel?
    A. Hip flexion with the knee extended
    B. Knee flexion
    C. Elbow extension
    D. Forearm supination

38. A 20-year-old female complains of ankle pain while playing volleyball and is suspected of having sprained her ankle. During the examination, she exhibits extreme tenderness to palpation over the sinus tarsi. What ligament is most often associated with tenderness in this case?
    A. Anterior talofibular
    B. Calcaneofibular
    C. Deltoid
    D. Posterior talofibular

39. A physical therapist examines a football player who is suspected of having an acute posterior cruciate ligament sprain. The most common mechanism of injury for the posterior cruciate ligament is:
   A. A forceful landing on the anterior tibia with the knee hyperflexed
   B. An anteriorly directed force applied to the tibia when the foot is fixed
   C. A valgus force applied to the knee when the foot is fixed
   D. Hyperextension and medial rotation of the leg with lateral rotation of the body

40. A football player sustained an injury to his knee joint, and the physical therapist attempts to gain information on the ligamentous integrity of the knee. Which of the following special tests would not provide the therapist with the desired information?
   A. Anterior drawer test
   B. Apprehension test
   C. Lachman test
   D. Pivot shift test

41. A 34-year-old domestic cricket player, while exercising in the gym, suddenly grasps his throat and begins to cough. The physical therapist, recognizing the signs of airway obstruction, should:
   A. Attempt to ventilate
   B. Administer abdominal thrusts
   C. Perform a quick finger sweep of the mouth
   D. Continue to observe the patient, but do not interfere

42. A physical therapist performs rescue breathing on a 22-year weightlifter who collapsed in the physical therapy gym. Which of the following is not accurate when performing rescue breathing on an adult?
   A. Maintain open airway with head tilt/chin lift
   B. Give one breath every five seconds
   C. Pinch nose shut
   D. Continue for 30 seconds; approximately six breaths

43. After observing a 22-year-old collegiate student during an exercise session, a physical therapist concludes that he commonly uses the Valsalva maneuver. Which activity would have the likely probability of producing the Valsalva maneuver?
    A. Lifting a 40 lb package from the floor to a counter at waist level
    B. Walking at 4 mph on a treadmill
    C. Stationary cycling at 80 revolutions per minute
    D. Using an upper extremity ergometer at 40 revolutions per minute

44. A 16-year-old school student participates in an athletic event for the first time. Immediately following the event, a physical therapist determines that the student's respiratory rate is 30 breaths per minute during the examination. What is the first intervention the therapist should perform to help the student slow his respiratory rate?
    A. Pursed-lip breathing
    B. Inspiratory hold
    C. Diaphragmatic breathing
    D. Active cycle of breathing

45. A 20-year-old female basketball player who sustained an ankle injury and is suspected of having lateral ankle instability. She reports that she landed on another player's foot after coming down with a rebound and felt immediate pain. She presents with moderate to severe ecchymosis and swelling along the lateral ankle distal to the lateral malleolus and is tender to palpation in the same region. Which of the following methods would be the MOST relevant ones to assess the ligamentous stability of the ankle?
    A. The therapist applies an anteriorly directed force with the injured player in supine on the proximal tibia with the knee flexed to 30 degrees.
    B. The therapist applies a compressive force to the heel with the injured player in prone and rotates the tibia with the knee flexed to 90 degrees.
    C. The therapist manually dorsiflexes the ankle with the injured player in sitting with the knee in 90 degrees of flexion.

D. The therapist stabilizes the tibia and fibula with the injured player in supine with the foot in 20 degrees of plantar flexion while drawing the talus forward in the ankle mortize.

46. The acronym, 'HOPS' format of evaluating sports injuries stands for:
    A. History of the injury, observation and inspection, palpation, and special testing
    B. History of the injury, observation and identification, palpation, and special testing
    C. History of the injury, observation and identification, palpation, and special treatment
    D. History of the injury, observation and inspection, pain grading, and special testing

47. Which one of the following evaluation formats provides a more detailed and advanced structure for decision making and problem-solving in injury management?
    A. HOPS format
    B. SOAP note format
    C. Visual analogue scale
    D. All of the above

48. A female high school long jumper sustains an ankle injury during practice and immediately reports to the athletic training room. While taking the history, what questions should be asked to identify the cause and extent of this injury?
    A. How did that injury happen?
    B. Briefly narrate the characteristics of the symptoms.
    C. Do you have any related medical history that may have a bearing on the specific injury?
    D. All of the above

49. Immediately after the occurrence of injury, the localized injury site should be inspected. Identify the most appropriate reason for carrying out this inspection:
    A. To rule out any deformity
    B. To rule out swelling
    C. To rule out any discoloration in the skin
    D. All of the above

Chapter 2: Emergency Sports Assessment and First Aid

50. Inspection of the long jumper's injury revealed mild swelling on the anterolateral aspect of the ankle. Based on the information provided concerning the long jumper's condition, the sports physiotherapist palpate to determine the extent and severity of the injury. The bilateral palpation of paired anatomic structures around the ankle joint can detect the following physical findings, *except:*
    A. Swelling
    B. Point tenderness
    C. Muscle strength
    D. Temperature

51. An athlete is suspected of having a head injury and is mobile, the attending sports physiotherapist uses a Pocket Concussion Recognition Tool on the side-line to determine whether any concussion has occurred. The occurrence of which one of the red flags indicates that the player should be removed safely and immediately from the field to seek urgent medical attention.
    A. Repeated vomiting
    B. Seizure or convulsion
    C. Severe and increasing headache
    D. All of the above

52. Skin color can play a significant role during the on-field assessment of endurance athletes. What would be the inference if the skin becomes blue or cyanosis?
    A. Heat stroke
    B. Respiratory distress
    C. Hyperglycemia
    D. Hyperventilation

53. If a long-distance marathon runner experienced a heat stroke leading to breathing difficulty, what emergency intervention is done to give comfort to him?
    A. Slightly elevating the upper part of the body
    B. Placing him in the recovery position
    C. Elevating the lower limbs
    D. Keeping him in the side-lying position

54. During the sports like ice hockey, the athletes wear helmets. If any injury that prone that athlete to an unconscious state without any respiratory distress, what would be the most appropriate response?
    A. The helmet should be removed immediately even though the facemask or visor does not interfere with ventilation.
    B. The helmet should not be removed unless the therapist is absolutely certain that there has not been a neck injury.
    C. The helmet can be removed with the help of another therapist.
    D. None of the above

55. Identify the most appropriate movement sequence to remove an injured but conscious and mobile athlete from the field of play:
    A. Supine lying–Sitting–Kneeling–Supported standing-Unsupported Standing-Walk off the field
    B. Supine lying-Sitting-Kneeling-Unsupported standing-Walk off the field
    C. Supine lying-Kneeling-Sitting-Supported standing-Unsupported standing-Walk off the field
    D. Supine lying-Kneeling-Sitting-Unsupported standing-Walk off the field

56. During the primary assessment, the sports physiotherapist uses several scales to test the severity of an injury or triage the injured athlete. Following scales are employed, *except:*
    A. Galveston Orientation and Amnesia Test
    B. Abbreviated Injury Scale
    C. Circulation, Respiration, Abdomen, Motor, and Speech (CRAMS) Scale
    D. Visual Analogue Scale

57. A 16-point scale used to assess the severity of the injury and provide the survival probabilities of trauma patients is known as:
    A. Trauma index
    B. Trauma scale
    C. CRAMS scale
    D. Injury severity score

Chapter 2: Emergency Sports Assessment and First Aid

58. A 26-year-old male football player having sudden cardiac arrest in the play field. What are the roles of the emergency team?
    A. Immediate care of the athlete
    B. Emergency equipment retrieval
    C. Activation of EMS system
    D. All of the above

59. Breathing emergencies may stem from:
    A. Asthma or allergic reaction
    B. Hyperventilation
    C. Injury to a muscle or bone in the chest
    D. All of the above

60. A 34-year-old motor cyclist undergone severe head injury during the racing. What are the common signals of head and spine injuries?
    A. Blood or other fluids in the ears or nose
    B. Unusual bumps or depressions on the head or over the spine
    C. Both A and B
    D. Has seizures, severe headaches, or slurred speech

61. Which among the following typically produces a more severe injury known as liquefaction necrosis?
    A. Bases
    B. Carbon monoxide
    C. Acids
    D. Toxic fumes

62. When entering the patient's room, you noticed that the patient is lying down on the floor and unconscious. What would the first thing you need to do?
    A. Call for assistance
    B. Check if the patient is breathing
    C. Survey the scene
    D. Perform vital signs assessment

ANSWERS

1. **A.** A positive Thompson's test is indicated by the absence of plantar flexion when the muscle is squeezed and is indicative of a ruptured Achilles tendon (third degree strain).
2. **D.**
3. **B.** The optimal position is reclining with the feet higher than the head. This position will allow available blood to perfuse the brain.
4. **A.**
5. **B.**
6. **C.**
7. **A.** A forceful landing on the tibial tubercle while the knee is at 90 degrees may drive the tibia backwards on the femur rupturing the posterior cruciate ligament.
8. **B.**
9. **C.**
10. **B.**
11. **A.**
12. **C.** McMurray test is used to confirm the meniscal lesion in which the patient is in supine position with the knee completely flexed, the examiner then laterally rotates the tibia and extends the knee to the full range of motion to test the medial meniscus. If there is a loose fragment of the medial meniscus, this action causes a snap or click that is often accompanied by pain.
13. **B.**
14. **A.**
15. **B.** The method so called Heimlich maneuver, which consists of a series of rapid thrusts to the upper abdomen. This can be performed with athlete in either vertical or horizontal position.
16. **D.**
17. **D.** Hip flexors on left side is being assessed by flexing the right hip and knee to the chest and hold it. If there is no flexion contracture, the hip being tested (the straight leg) remains

Chapter 2: Emergency Sports Assessment and First Aid

on the examination table. If the contracture is present, the patient straight leg rises off the table and a muscle stretch end feel will be felt. This evaluation technique is known as Thomas test.

18. A.
19. B.
20. B. Faber's test stands for flexion, abduction, external rotation and the position of hip of the patient to be tested. If the test is positive, it indicates the hip joint may be affected, there may be iliopsoas spasm or the sacroiliac joint may be affected.
21. C.
22. A. Neural watch chart facilitates monitoring of the patient's vital signs. Initially it is performed in every 5 to 15 minutes. Once the patient is stabilized, neural watch recordings may be made every 15 to 30 minutes.
23. C.
24. A. The level of consciousness can be best determined with the use of Glasgow coma scale (GCS). The Glasgow coma scale which is based on eye opening and verbal and motor responses is a practical means of monitoring changes in the level of consciousness through numerical rating. The lowest score is 3 and the highest score is 15.
25. D.
26. C.
27. B. This is a hard unyielding sensation (i.e., painless) felt by the therapist while assessing end elbow extension range of motion of the patient, which occurs due to bone-to-bone approximation.
28. B.
29. A. Pronation of the foot consists of eversion of the heel, abduction of forefoot and dorsiflexion of subtalar and midtarsal joints.
30. A. The cold spray currently being used is fluoromethane, which appears to be safer and more effective than ethyl chloride.
31. A. When performing two-person cardiopulmonary resuscitation, one breath should be administered after every fifth chest compression.

32. **C.** Performing ligamentous testing on an uninvolved joint provides a physical therapist with a valuable baseline that can then be compared to the involved joint.
33. **C.** The hip is a ball and socket joint whose resting position is 30 degrees flexion, 30 degrees abduction, and slight lateral rotation. The close packed position is extension and medial rotation.
34. **A.** The flexor pollicis brevis inserts on the volar aspect of the base of the proximal phalanx of the thumb. The muscle flexes the metacarpophalangeal and carpometacarpal joints of the thumb and assists in opposition.
35. **D.** The inferior lateral angles of the sacrum are formed by the transverse processes of S5.
36. **A.** Scapular adductors including the rhomboids, middle trapezius, and the lower trapezius are tested with the patient in a prone position.
37. **B.** The end-feel associated with knee flexion is typically described as soft due to contact between the posterior calf and thigh or between the heel and buttocks.
38. **A.** The sinus tarsi area is located immediately anterior to the lateral malleolus. The soft tissue depression consists of a tunnel between the calcaneus and talus. The anterior talofibular ligament is often the first ligament affected by an inversion ankle injury.
39. **A.** The posterior cruciate ligament is responsible for preventing posterior displacement of the tibia on the femur. The ligament is most often injured by a direct force on the tibia, which displaces it in a posterior direction in relation to the femur.
40. **B.** Apprehension tests are provocative tests that attempt to simulate the mechanism of injury associated with a selected injury. The primary indication for an apprehension test is to assist with diagnosis. Common apprehension tests include anterior shoulder dislocation and patellar dislocation.
41. **D.** Coughing indicates that the airway is not completely obstructed. As a result, the physical therapist should continue to monitor the patient, however, should not formally intervene. Usually, a patient that is coughing will independently dislodge the object causing the obstruction.

Chapter 2: Emergency Sports Assessment and First Aid

42. D. Rescue breathing is a cardiopulmonary resuscitation technique designed for a patient that exhibits a pulse, but is not breathing. This technique is typically performed on adults for a full cycle of 60 seconds with breaths occurring every five seconds.

43. A. The Valsalva maneuver is an attempt to forcibly exhale with the glottis, nose, and mouth closed. This action produces an increase in intrathoracic and intra-abdominal pressures that lead to decreased venous blood flow to the heart. Patients most commonly utilize the Valsalva maneuver during heavy resistance exercise.

44. A. Pursed-lip breathing may be useful whenever an increase in breathing effort is noted. The intervention naturally slows down respirations and decreases minute ventilation, relieving dyspnea in some patients.

45. D. The presented scenario describes a version of the anterior drawer test of the ankle which is designed to test the integrity of the lateral ankle ligaments, most notably the anterior talofibular ligament.

46. A. The HOPS format uses both subjective information (i.e., history of the injury) and objective information (i.e., observation and inspection, palpation, and special testing) to recognize and identify problems contributing to the condition. The HOPS format focuses on the evaluation component of injury management and excludes the rehabilitation process.

47. B. The SOAP notes format documents patient care and serves as a communication vehicle between the on-site clinicians and other healthcare professionals. The subjective and objective evaluations are identical to those used in the HOPS format; however, two additional components are added to the documentation, viz. assessment and planning.

48. D. A complete history includes information regarding the primary complaint, cause or mechanism of the injury, characteristics of the symptoms, and any related medical history that may have a bearing on the specific condition. This information can provide potential reasons for the symptoms and identify injured structures before initiating the physical examination.

49. **D.** The localized injury site should be inspected for any deformity, swelling (i.e., edema or joint effusion), discoloration (e.g., redness, pallor, or ecchymosis), signs of infection (i.e., redness, swelling, pus, red streaks, or swollen lymph nodes), scars that might indicate previous surgery, and general skin condition (e.g., oily, dry, blotchy with red spots, sores, or hives).

50. **C.** Bilateral palpation of paired anatomic structures can detect eight physical findings: (i) temperature; (ii) deformity; (iii) swelling; (iv) muscle spasm; (v) point tenderness (vi) cutaneous sensation; (vii) crepitus and (viii) pulse. However, muscle strength is measured through manual muscle testing, dynamometry and other functional testing procedures.

51. **D.** According to Pocket Concussion Recognition Tool, if any of the following red flags reported, the player should be moved safely and immediately from the field. If no qualified medical personnel are available, consider transporting him by ambulance for urgent medical attention. The red flags are: (i) repeated vomiting; (ii) seizure or convulsion; (iii) severe and increasing headache; (iv) complains of neck pain; (v) weakness or tingling or burning in arms or legs; (vi) deteriorating conscious state; (vii) unusual behavior change and (viii) double vision.

52. **B.** Cyanosis, or a blue tint to the skin, indicates respiratory distress, as does a gray tint. The most frequent respiratory ailments of athletes are related to a mismatch between airway calibre and increased ventilation caused by exercise. Every endurance athlete has their own limit in endurance training that will produce all the possible respiratory disorders once passed.

53. **A.** Suppose an individual has breathing difficulties or a chest injury or has experienced a heart attack or stroke, it may be desirable to lower blood pressure in the injured parts by slightly elevating the upper part of the body.

54. **B.** Generally, if the patient is unconscious, the helmet should not be removed unless the examiner is certain that there has not been a neck injury. Ideally, the helmet and shoulder pads, if any, should be removed in a controlled setting, such

Chapter 2: Emergency Sports Assessment and First Aid

as the emergency department. Helmets should be removed if the facemask or visor interferes with adequate ventilation.

55. A. If the injury is in the upper limb and the injured part is immobilized, the athlete may first be moved from a supine to a sitting or kneeling position, then from sitting or kneeling to supported standing, to unsupported standing, and finally, the person may walk off the field.
56. D
57. B. Trauma score illustrates the ease of scoring and the survival probabilities expected in trauma patients. This tool provides a dynamic score that monitors changes in the patient's condition and is useful in making triage decisions.
58. D. Direction of EMS to the scene of the emergency. It is the responsibility of emergency responders at the scene to isolate, contain, and neutralize the incident. The ERT will be responsible for managing and directing the activities of the various departments that will be involved in emergency response and recovery.
59. D. A breathing emergency is any respiratory problem that can threaten a person's life. Breathing emergencies happen when air cannot travel freely and easily into the lungs.
60. C. The signs and symptoms of head and spine injuries vary depending on the specific type of injury.
61. A. Bases: Alkaline ingestions cause tissue injury by liquefactive necrosis.
62. C. Survey the scene means to look at something, or to examine something. He sat quietly, surveying the scene around him.

Principles of Athletic Conditioning and Prevention of Sports Injuries

CHAPTER 3

1. At the neuromuscular junction, which substance acts to excite the muscle fibers of the motor unit?
   A. ATP
   B. Serotonin
   C. Creatine phosphate
   D. Acetylcholine

2. Which of the following statements denotes 'ALL or NONE principle'?
   A. A stronger action potential cannot result in a stronger contraction
   B. A stronger action potential always results in a stronger contraction
   C. A weaker action potential always results in a weaker contraction
   D. A stronger action potential always results in a weaker contraction

3. Low actomyosin myofibrillar ATPase activity is the characteristics of which muscle fiber type?
   A. Type I
   B. Type II a
   C. Type II b
   D. Both A and B

4. Which of the following muscle fiber types would be more beneficial for a power lifter?
   A. Type I
   B. Type II a
   C. Type II b
   D. Type III

5. When throwing a basketball, the player's arm is rapidly stretched just prior to throwing the ball. Which of the following structures detects and responds to that stretch by reflexively increasing the muscle activity?
   A. Extrafusal muscle
   B. Pacinian capsule
   C. Golgi tendon organ
   D. Muscle spindle

6. During conventional resistance training, which of the following muscle fiber types will hypertrophy first?
   A. Muscle spindle
   B. Intrafusal muscle
   C. Fast-twitch
   D. Slow-twitch

Chapter 3: Principles of Athletic Conditioning and Prevention...

7. **Following statements are true with respect to adaptations to resistance training, *except:***
   A. Muscle fiber hypertrophy becomes obvious
   B. Strength of the muscle increases
   C. It enhances an athlete's maximum aerobic power
   D. Muscle mass increases

8. **Which muscle fiber type is more prone for atrophy following immobilization?**
   A. Type I fiber
   B. Type II a fiber
   C. Type II ab fiber
   D. Type II b fiber

9. **Following statements are true regarding the fast twitch fibers, *except:***
   A. Fast twitch fibers are used for explosive type activity
   B. Fast twitch fibers have a much higher level of ATP and glycolytic enzyme activity.
   C. Fast twitch fibers are more resistive to fatigue.
   D. Isometric contraction may prevent atrophy of type II fibers during immobilization

10. **The muscle fiber, which is rich in myoglobin, has a high oxidative capacity and a low anaerobic capacity and is recruited for activities demanding endurance is known as:**
    A. Slow-twitch fibers
    B. Fast-twitch fibers
    C. Type II b fiber
    D. Type II a fiber

11. **One liter of oxygen is equal to how many kilocalories?**
    A. 5 Kcal
    B. 10 Kcal
    C. 15 Kcal
    D. 3 Kcal

12. **Following are the components of athletic conditioning program, *except:***
    A. Strength
    B. Proprioception
    C. Power
    D. Nutrition

13. **Following aerobic exercise training, the improvement of the muscles' ability to use energy is a direct result of the following factors, *except:***
    A. Increased levels of oxidative enzymes in the muscles
    B. Increased mitochondrial density
    C. Increased muscle fiber capillary supply
    D. Increasing the speed of exercise

14. Maximum oxygen consumption (VO_2 max) is expressed in terms of the following:
    A. mL/kg per minute
    B. L/g per minute
    C. mL/g per minute
    D. mL/kg per hour
15. "The individual improves in the exercise task used for training and may not in other tasks". This statement follows which training principle?
    A. Overload principle
    B. Specificity principle
    C. Reversibility principle
    D. Overflow principle
16. How much of oxygen is extracted from blood by the myocardial muscle during rest?
    A. 40–50%
    B. 50–60%
    C. 70–75%
    D. 30–40%
17. Following are the effects of deconditioning, *except:*
    A. Decrease in maximum O_2 consumption
    B. Decrease in stroke volume
    C. Decrease in muscular strength
    D. Decrease in respiratory rate
18. Which one of the following energy systems provides energy for short, quick bursts of activity and it is the major source of energy during the first 30 seconds of intense exercise?
    A. The phosphagen system
    B. The anaerobic system
    C. The aerobic system
    D. All of the above
19. Following statements are true regarding the aerobic energy system, *except:*
    A. Glycogen, fats and proteins are fuel sources
    B. No oxygen is required
    C. Predominates over other system after the second minute of exercise
    D. Maximum capacity of system is great (90.0 molATP)
20. The techniques used for improving cardiorespiratory endurance that combines continuous training and circuit training is known as:
    A. Par cours
    B. Fartlek
    C. Interval training
    D. Cariocas training

Chapter 3: Principles of Athletic Conditioning and Prevention... 35

21. Which of the following athletic conditioning components are improved through guided circuit training program?
    A. Strength   B. Cardiovascular
    C. Flexibility   D. All of the above
22. The term 'overtraining' is otherwise called as:
    A. Burnout   B. Overfatigue
    C. Staleness   D. All of the above
23. Following detraining, endurance athletes first notice a decline in maximum:
    A. Strength   B. Oxygen consumption
    C. Power   D. Heart size
24. Maximum anaerobic muscular power is:
    A. Ability of a muscle to exert high force at a high speed
    B. Ability of a muscle to exert high force at a low speed
    C. Ability of a muscle to exert low force at a high speed
    D. Ability of a muscle to exert low force at a low speed
25. High-intensity, low repetition resistance training results in which of the following adaptations?
    A. Increased capillary density
    B. Decreased tidal volume
    C. Improved oxygen extraction
    D. No change in maximum oxygen uptake
26. What will be the target heart rate reserve for a 30-year-old athlete with a resting heart rate of 60 bpm is assigned an exercise intensity of 60–70% of functional capacity?
    A. 138-151 bpm   B. 140-153 bpm
    C. 136-149 bpm   D. 142-155 bpm
27. Which of the following is the method most commonly used to assign and regulate exercise intensity?
    A. Oxygen consumption   B. Heart rate
    C. Rate of perceived exertion   D. Race pace
28. Which of the following types of training is conducted at intensity equal to the lactate threshold?
    A. Pace/temp training   B. Repetition training
    C. Fartlek training   D. Interval training

29. The training program, which is conducted at intensities greater than VO_2 maximum with the work bouts typically lasting between 30 and 90 seconds, is known as:
    A. Fartlek training
    B. Interval training
    C. Repetition training
    D. Intermittent pace training

30. Following are the musculoskeletal system adaptations to aerobic training, *except:*
    A. Increased myoglobin concentration
    B. Increased capillarization in muscle bed
    C. Decreased mitochondrial size and density
    D. All of the above

31. A measure of energy cost of activity at a given exercise velocity is referred to as:
    A. Energy expenditure rate
    B. Fuel utilization rate
    C. Exercise economy
    D. Exercise ergonomics

32. A physical therapist instructs a patient to perform three sets of biceps curls using a piece of light grade elastic tubing. If the therapist's primary objective is to improve the patient's muscle endurance, the MOST appropriate number of repetitions in each set would be:
    A. 5
    B. 10
    C. 30
    D. 90

33. While exercising in a gym, an athletic trainee exhibits many of the signs and symptoms of shock including restlessness, pale skin, and a rapid, weak pulse. The MOST appropriate position for the athletic trainee to promote increased circulation to the vital organs is termed?
    A. Fowler
    B. Semi-Fowler
    C. Modified trendelenburg
    D. Reverse trendelenburg

34. While training an elite athlete, a sports physiotherapist classified throwing motion into six phases considering the purpose and muscle activity. These six phases consist of Wind-up, Early cocking, Late cocking, Acceleration, Deceleration and Follow through. In which one of the following phases, a maximum stress is put on the shoulder?
    A. Phase-II: Early cocking
    B. Phase-III: Late cocking
    C. Phase-IV: Acceleration
    D. Phase-I: Wind-up

Chapter 3: Principles of Athletic Conditioning and Prevention...

35. The system used by the sports physiotherapist to record movement and then to measure positions, angles of joints, speed, and distance of that movement, and also aid them to compare the same actions performed at different times is known:
    A. Human motion analysis
    B. Video analysis software
    C. Biomechanical modeling
    D. Classical mechanics

36. A sports physiotherapist is using the video analysis software during athletic conditioning for the following purposes, *except:*
    A. To capture, edit, and analyze various sport motions
    B. To find the weak parts in the movement which may cause injury, pain, or a drop in the performance
    C. To identify an athlete's biomechanical or movement dysfunction
    D. To provide a clear information on the reasons of injury, muscle weakness, and degree of improvement.

37. Which one of the following are the most common residual disabilities to occur after an acute ankle sprain?
    A. Mechanical instability
    B. Functional instability
    C. Ligament laxity
    D. None of the above

38. The reason for the prophylactic effect of ankle taping is due to which one of the following?
    A. Facilitation of proprioceptive and skin sensory input to the central nervous system.
    B. Sensory cues to plantar surface of the foot are increased
    C. Taping allow more accurate foot placement and reducing the changes of excessive ligamentous strain.
    D. All of the above

39. Ankle support orthotics and braces are commonly used during Sports. Identify the most common reasons for its utility in sports among the following?
    A. Providing mechanical stability
    B. Improve proprioception function
    C. Improve sensorimotor function
    D. All of the above

40. A sports physical therapist plans an appropriate strategy to be employed during the early rehabilitation of an injured soccer player. Which one of the following is the most ones to be advocated to prevent future injuries?
    A. Warm-up with more emphasis on stretching
    B. Strengthening exercises
    C. Proprioceptive exercises
    D. Sports specific skills
41. Which one of the following exercises help to train the lower extremity proprioceptive system through a static activity?
    A. Plyometric exercises
    B. Balance training exercise
    C. Isokinetic exercises
    D. Kinetic chain exercises
42. The type of exercise that includes repetitive, consciously mediated movement sequences performed slowly and deliberately as well as sudden, externally applied perturbations of joint position to initiate reflex "subconscious" muscle contraction is known as?
    A. Isokinetic exercises
    B. Kinetic chain exercises
    C. Proprioceptive exercises
    D. Sport-specific maneuvers
43. Which one of the following exercises incorporate an eccentric preload (a quick eccentric stretch) followed by a forceful concentric contraction and can be performed after near-normal strength in all targeted muscles is achieved?
    A. Isometric exercise B. Isokinetic exercises
    C. Kinetic chain exercises D. Plyometric exercises
44. Following are the examples of Closed-kinetic-chain exercises, *except:*
    A. Leg press B. Vertical jump
    C. Leg curls D. Carioca
45. Which of the following is the player-centered risk factors leading to injuries in Soccer games?
    A. Shoes and shin guards B. Playing surface
    C. Joint instability D. Game rules

Chapter 3: Principles of Athletic Conditioning and Prevention...

46. A sports physiotherapist is planning an exercise program for preventing hamstring injuries in a soccer player. Which of the following exercise is the most optimal choice to prevent hamstring injury?
    A. Nordic exercise
    B. Balance board exercise
    C. Isokinetic exercises
    D. Codman exercise

47. A basketball player is taped for a grade-1 inversion ankle sprain. Which one of the following is the purpose of the utility of elastic tapping in sports?
    A. Provide compression
    B. Provide proprioceptive feedback
    C. Support an injured body part
    D. All of the above

48. Based on an athlete's foot examination, a sports physiotherapist has decided to apply tapping to support the athlete's arch that will enhance him to run or jump effectively. What is the ideal position of the foot while applying taping to support the arch?
    A. Slight dorsiflexion
    B. Slight plantar flexion
    C. Slight inversion
    D. None of the above

49. An athlete is returning to sports after getting rehabilitated for a grade-1 medical meniscus injury of the knee joint. Which one of the following activities are recommended to be carried out before returning to sports?
    A. Sport/activity-specific skill conditioning
    B. Maintain range of motion (ROM) and, joint flexibility
    C. Begin pain-free, isometric strengthening exercises on the affected limb
    D. Instruct the patient on relaxation and coping techniques

50. At the conclusion of the rehabilitation program, the supervising physiotherapist determines whether the individual is ready to return to full activity. Following factors are reviewed to decide the return of the individual to sports?
    A. Muscle flexibility
    B. Proprioception and coordination
    C. Endurance and power
    D. All of the above

51. During aerobic exercise training, the term 'specificity principle' refers to which one of the following?
    A. Increased efficiency of the cardiovascular system and the active muscles
    B. Ability to work for prolonged periods of time and to resist fatigue
    C. Improvement observed in the exercise task used for training and not in other tasks
    D. Improvement observed in the exercise task used for training as well as in other tasks

52. A 20-year-old collegiate football player rehabilitating from a lower extremity injury reports to outpatient physical therapy complaining of soreness in his legs. During the previous session, the student completed lower extremity eccentric strengthening exercises with five-pound weights. The MOST appropriate therapist action is to:
    A. Explain to the player that this is a result of delayed onset muscle soreness and decrease the amount and intensity of the strength training
    B. Explain to the player that this is to be expected and he needs to keep working hard in order to gain additional strength
    C. Increase the intensity of the strength training in order to build up the patient's muscle strength
    D. Stop using weights for strengthening and increase the intensity of closed chain functional exercises

53. A sports physical therapist instructs a volleyball player to perform three sets of biceps curls using a piece of light-grade elastic tubing. If the therapist's primary objective is to improve the player's muscle endurance, the MOST appropriate number of repetitions in each set would be:
    A. 5
    B. 10
    C. 30
    D. 75

54. To improve physical fitness, one of the following basic principles of physical conditioning states that the body or specific muscles must be stressed, and it is called as:
    A. Recuperation principle
    B. Overload principle
    C. Specificity principle
    D. Progression principle

Chapter 3: Principles of Athletic Conditioning and Prevention...

55. Athletes who participate in high-level cardiovascular training should be prepared for their immune system to _____ when they increase their physical training volume from a sedentary level to a moderate level.
    A. Become erratic
    B. Stay the same
    C. Worsen
    D. Improve

56. The "workout hangover," sore and stiff muscles or a feeling of general fatigue in the morning after an exercise training session, is a common symptom of:
    A. Overtraining
    B. Recuperation
    C. Specificity
    D. Progression

57. The purpose of the warm-up is to:
    A. Increase heart rate to get ready for intense activity
    B. Elevate muscle temperature, heart rate, blood pressure, and breathing rate
    C. Elevate muscle temperature and increase blood flow to those muscles engaged in the workout
    D. Elevate blood pressure, heart rate, and breathing rate

58. Heart rate increases in a _____ fashion with energy expenditure.
    A. Fractional
    B. Inverse
    C. Linear
    D. Exponential

59. Although heart rate can also be used to gauge exercise intensity during strength training, the amount of weight and the number of exercise repetitions that can be performed before muscle fatigue occurs is more useful in monitoring _____ during weight lifting.
    A. Progression
    B. Reversibility
    C. Stress
    D. Overload

60. What part of the exercise workout can also reduce the strain on the heart imposed by rapidly engaging in heavy exercise, and reduce the risk of muscle and tendon injuries?
    A. Strength training
    B. Aerobic activity
    C. Warm-up
    D. Cool-down

ANSWERS

1. **D.** Arrival of action potential at the nerve terminal causes release of acetylcholine, which diffuses across the neuromuscular junction causing excitation of the sarcolemma and the fibers contracts.
2. **A.** A stronger action potential cannot result in a stronger contraction. This phenomenon is known as the all or none principle which analogous to firing a gun.
3. **A.** Type I fibers are fatigue resistant, high aerobic power, but they have limited potential for rapid force development as characterized by low actomyosin myofibrillar ATPase activity and low anaerobic power.
4. **C.** Power lifting is the activity requiring near maximal performance, in which most of the motor units are called to play with fast twitch units especially Type II b fibers making more significant contribution to the efforts.
5. **D.** Muscle spindles provide information concerning muscle length and rate of change in length. Spindles indicate the degree to which the muscle must be activated in order to overcome a given resistance. As the load increases, the muscle is stretched to a greater extent, and engagement of muscle spindles results in greater activation of the muscle.
6. **C.** Fast twitch fibers shows greater increases in size than slow-twitch fibers during conventional resistance training.
7. **C.** Resistance training does not enhance an athlete's maximum aerobic power. Moreover, resistance training has no meaningful impact on aerobic power.
8. **A.** Type I fiber is likely to atrophy rapidly following immobilization and is not preserved by isometric contractions.
9. **C.** Slow twitch fibers are more resistive to fatigue, and are the first to be recruited during submaximal exercise.
10. **A.** Slow twitch fibers (Type I) are characterized by a slow contractile response, are rich in myoglobin, have a high oxidative capacity and are recruited during endurance activities. These fibers are used preferentially in low-intensity exercise.
11. **A.** A kilocalorie is the amount of heat necessary to raise 1 kilogram (kg) of water to 1° Celsius and can be expressed in

Chapter 3: Principles of Athletic Conditioning and Prevention... 43

oxygen equivalents .5 kilocalories equals approximately one liter of oxygen consumed.

12. **D.**
13. **D.**
14. **A.** Maximum oxygen consumption is usually expressed relative to body weight, as milliliters of oxygen per kilogram of body weight per minute (mL/kg per minute).
15. **B.** Specificity principle—training for a particular sport or event is dependent on this principle.
16. **C.** The myocardial muscle extracts 70-75% of the oxygen from the blood during rest, its main source of supply during exercise is through on increase in coronary blood flow.
17. **D.** Decrease in respiratory rate.
18. **A.** The phosphagen system provides energy for short, quick bursts of activity. The maximum capacity of system is small (0.7 molATP) and the maximum power of the system is great (3.7 molATP)/min).
19. **B.** Oxygen is required for the aerobic energy system in which ATP is resynthesized in the mitochondria of muscle cell. The ability to metabolize oxygen and other substrates is related to the number and concentration of the mitochondria and cells.
20. **A.** Par cours technique involves jogging a short distance from station to station and performing a designed exercises at each station according to guidelines and direction provided on an instruction board located at each station.
21. **D.** Circuit training program is most definitely an effective technique for improving strength and flexibility. Further, if the pace and work load is maintained at a high level of intensity, the cardiovascular system may benefit from this circuit training program.
22. **D.** Overtraining syndrome is the condition resulting from overtraining. Many alternative terms have been suggested for overtraining including staleness, burnout, chronic overwork, physical overstrain and overfatigue.
23. **B.** Aerobic endurance adaptation are more sensitive to periods on inactivity because of their enzymatic basis. The individual's physiological function reverts to the normal, untrained state following detraining.

24. A.
25. D.
26. A. Working Formula:
Target heart rate = {Heart rate reserve × Exercise intensity} + RHR
Heart rate reserve = Age predicted maximum heart rate- Resting heart rate
Age-predicted maximum heart rate = 220 - age (APMHR)
Working solution:
APMHR= 220 - 30= 190 bpm
HRR= 190 - 60= 130 bpm
THRR (lowest) = (130 × 0.60) + 60= 138 bpm
THRR (highest) = (130 × 0.70) + 60= 151 bpm
27. B.
28. A. Steady pace/temp training is continuous training conducted at an intensity equal to the lactate threshold for durations of approximately 20-30 minutes. The specific purpose is to stress the athlete at a specific intensity and improve energy production for both aerobic and anaerobic metabolism.
29. C.
30. C.
31. C.
32. C. Training programs designed to improve muscle endurance require a significant number of repetitions against a submaximal load. Although no definitive parameters have been established, most sources recommend three to five sets consisting of 15-50 repetitions. Training programs designed to improve muscle strength often are described as two to three sets of 6-12 repetitions.
33. C. Management of shock commonly includes elevating the legs to promote increased circulation to the vital organs. The modified trendelenburg position is characterized by raising the lower extremities without lowering the head and is therefore consistent with the positional management of shock.
34. B. Phase III (late cocking) is the point of maximal external rotation of the shoulder in elite athletes reaching close to 170°. This position of the abducted, externally rotated

Chapter 3: Principles of Athletic Conditioning and Prevention...

shoulder leads to a posterior translation of the humeral head being the point of maximum stress to the anterior capsule.
35. **A.** Human motion analysis (HMA) gives the athlete or the physical therapist clear information on the reasons of injury, muscle weakness, and degree of improvement.
36. **D.** Motion analysis software gives the athlete or the physician clear information on the reasons of injury, muscle weakness, and degree of improvement.
37. **B.** Functional instability of the ankle is one of the most common residual disabilities after an acute ankle sprain and it results from damage to mechanical receptors in the lateral ligaments or muscle/tendon with subsequent partial differentiation of the proprioceptive reflex.
38. **D.** Ankle taping unities the skin of the leg with the plantar surface of the foot that increase the sensory cues to plantar surface, thereby allowing a more accurate foot placement and reducing the changes of excessive ligamentous strain. Taping may help patients with unstable ankles by facilitating proprioceptive and skin sensory input to the central nervous system.
39. **D.** Ankle support orthotics and braces are generally considered effective in providing mechanical stability while restricting joint range of motion. Improvement in proprioception and sensorimotor function has been shown to occur, through stimulation of cutaneous mechanoreceptors near and around the ankle through the application of ankle support and tape.
40. **C.** The concept of doing proprioceptive exercises to regain neuromuscular control initially was introduced in rehabilitation programs. It was considered that because mechanoreceptors are located in ligaments, an injury to a ligament would alter afferent input. Proprioceptive training after an injury would be needed to restore the altered neurologic function.
41. **B.** Balance training is the major category of proprioceptive exercise that trains the proprioceptive system in a mostly static activity. In the lower extremities, these activities include one-legged standing balance exercises, progressive use of wobble board exercises, and tandem exercises in

which a postural challenge (e.g., perturbations) can be applied to the player by the therapist.
42. C.
43. D. Plyometric exercises are increasingly popular neuromuscular control exercise that integrates spinal and brain stem levels and has been an effective addition to upper and lower extremity conditioning and rehabilitation programs. This exercise technique is thought to enhance reflex joint stabilization and may increase muscle stiffness.
44. C. Leg curls is the open kinetic chain exercise where the leg/foot is moving loose in space and not pressing against a surface.
45. C. Player-centered risk factors leading to injuries in Soccer game include joint instability, muscle tightness, insufficient warm-up and stretching, irregular cool down, inadequate rehabilitation, and lack of proprioceptive training.
46. A. The Nordic hamstring exercise is performed standing on the knees on a soft foundation, slowly lowering the body toward the ground using the hamstrings while the feet are held by a partner and it is designed to improve eccentric strength of the hamstring muscles.
47. D. Elastic tape can be used to hold protective pads and dressings in place, provide compression, give proprioceptive feedback, and provide support.
48. B. While taping the arches, the athlete's foot should be in a position of slight plantar flexion.
49. A. Sport/activity-specific skill conditioning will be commenced once the range of motion, muscular strength, and coordination are restored. The athlete should work the affected extremity through functional diagonal and sport-specific patterns before returning to the real sporting event.
50. D. This decision on the individual's return to full activity is based on a review of the individual's ROM and flexibility; muscular strength, endurance, and power; biomechanical skill; proprioception and coordination; and cardiovascular endurance.
51. C. The individual improves in the exercise task used for training and may not improve in other tasks. For example, swimming

Chapter 3: Principles of Athletic Conditioning and Prevention...

may enhance one's performance in swimming events but may not improve one's performance in treadmill running.

52. **A.** Eccentric strength training is linked to a delayed soreness phenomenon where a patient may feel muscle soreness 24 to 48 hours after the actual exercise session. Moderate exercise should continue during the soreness period to assist the patient with adaptation and restoration of muscle function.

53. **C.** Training programs designed to improve muscle endurance require a significant number of repetitions against a submaximal load. Although no definitive parameters have been established, most sources recommend three to five sets consisting of 15–50 repetitions. Training programs designed to improve muscle strength often are described as two to three sets of 6–12 repetitions.

54. **B.** Overload principle basically states that an exercise must become more challenging over the course of a training program in order to continue to produce results.

55. **B.**

56. **A. Overtraining or staleness occurs when an athlete ignores the signs of overreaching and continues to train. Many athletes believe that weakness or poor performance signals the need for even harder training.**

57. **C.** Elevate muscle temperature and increase blood flow to those muscles engaged in the workout.

58. **C.** Heart rate increases in a linear fashion with energy expenditure.

59. **D.** Overload basically states that an exercise must become more challenging over the course of a training program in order to continue to produce results. In the context of strength training, this is done by adding weight to the bar.

60. **C.** Warm-up is a period or act of preparation for a match, performance, or exercise session, involving gentle exercise or practice.

Therapeutic Exercise in Injury Rehabilitation

A. STRETCHING AND WARM-UP

1. A type of stretching typically involves active muscular effort and uses bouncing-type movement in which the end position is not held is known as:
   A. Dynamic stretch
   B. Ballistic stretch
   C. Static stretch
   D. PNF stretch
2. Which of the following stretching techniques decreases muscle spindle stimulation?
   A. Dynamic
   B. Ballistic
   C. Static
   D. Passive
3. Dynamic stretching is most similar to which of the following?
   A. Specific warm up
   B. General warm up
   C. Easy stretch
   D. Static stretch
4. Stimulation of muscle spindles involves a:
   A. Relaxation of GTO'S
   B. Contraction of the stretched muscle
   C. Relaxation of the stretched muscle
   D. Contraction of the reciprocal muscle
5. Following the hold-relax with agonist contraction PNF stretch for the hamstrings, increased flexibility is due to which of the following?
   I. Autogenic inhibition
   II. Reciprocal inhibition
   III. Crossed-extension inhibition
   IV. Stretch inhibition
   A. I and III only
   B. I and II only
   C. I, II and III only
   D. II and IV only
6. An important proprioceptor located within intrafusal muscle fibers that run parallel to extrafusal muscle fibers, monitor changes in muscle length is known as:

Chapter 4: Therapeutic Exercise in Injury Rehabilitation

    A. Muscle spindle   B. Golgi tendon organ
    C. Extrafusal muscle fiber   D. All of the above

7. **Following statements are true about flexibility, *except*:**
   A. Young people are more flexible than older people
   B. Activity level can alter flexibility
   C. Stretching can alter flexibility
   D. Males are more flexible than females

8. **Following are the purposes of giving post-event warm down, *except*:**
   A. For removing lactic acid and other products of metabolism from the muscles.
   B. To reduce stiffness and tightness following the day of event
   C. To allow the athlete to settle down physically and psychologically after the excitement of event
   D. All of the above

9. **Ballistic stretching technique is not advised and is not always a preferred technique in the sports conditioning program because:**
   A. Stretching the reflexively contracted muscle can injure muscle tissue.
   B. Ballistic stretching involves active muscular effort and uses a bouncing-type movement in which end position is not held.
   C. It will not provide actual stretching of muscle, which defeats the purpose of stretching.
   D. All of the above

10. **Which type of flexibility is most essential for the athlete to prevent injury?**
    A. Static flexibility   B. Dynamic flexibility
    C. Both A and B   D. None of the above

11. **What is the minimum time required for the Golgi tendon organs to respond to the increase in muscle tension?**
    A. 30 seconds   B. 4 seconds
    C. 6 seconds   D. 8 seconds

12. **Following are the indications for applying stretching technique, *except*:**

A. ROM is limited because soft tissues have lost their extensibility as the result of adhesions and contractures

B. Restricted motion may lead to structural deformities that are otherwise preventable.

C. May be used as part of a total fitness program designed to prevent musculoskeletal injuries.

D. ROM is limited due to an acute inflammatory or infectious process (heat and swelling) around the soft tissue.

13. Which one of the following therapeutic interventions are applied before and after vigorous exercise to minimize post-exercise muscle soreness?

   A. Stretching
   B. Strengthening exercise
   C. Joint mobilization technique
   D. Endurance training

14. A type of interactive stretching technique that requires feedback from the patient's body to determine the direction, force, and duration of the stretch and facilitate maximum relaxation of tight or restricted tissues is known as:

   A. Muscle energy technique
   B. PNF stretching technique
   C. Myofascial release technique
   D. Neuromuscular facilitation and inhibition techniques

15. The ability of soft tissue to return to its prestretch resting length directly after a short-duration stretch force has been removed is known as:

   A. Extensibility   B. Plasticity
   C. Elasticity   D. Viscosity

16. As a part of a rehabilitation program, a muscle was immobilized in a shortened position for several weeks. The residual effects of prolonged immobilization of the muscle in a shortened position are:

   A. Reduction in the length of the muscle
   B. Reduction in the number of sarcomeres in series within myofibrils
   C. Muscle atrophy and weakness
   D. None of the above

Chapter 4: Therapeutic Exercise in Injury Rehabilitation

17. Which one of the following are the determinants of stretching technique?
    A. Intensity and duration
    B. Frequency and mode
    C. Speed
    D. All of the above
18. A form of flexibility where an active muscle contraction moves a body segment through the available ROM of a joint is known as:
    A. Passive flexibility
    B. Dynamic flexibility
    C. Passive mobility
    D. All of the above
19. The clinical condition where there is an adaptive shortening of the muscle-tendon unit and other soft tissues that either cross or surround a joint, resulting in significant resistance to passive or active stretch and limitation of ROM, which may compromise functional abilities, is known as:
    A. Contracture
    B. Contraction
    C. Muscle tightness
    D. All of the above
20. The basic concept of neuromuscular facilitation and inhibition technique to increase the mobility of soft tissues is:
    A. Relaxing tension in shortened muscles reflexively prior to or during muscle elongation
    B. Sustained or intermittent external, end-range stretch force, applied with overpressure
    C. Elongates a shortened muscle-tendon unit by moving a restricted joint just past the available ROM
    D. Stretch well beyond the normal length of muscle and ROM of a joint and the surrounding soft tissues
21. A type of manipulative procedure that employ voluntary muscle contractions by the patient in a precisely controlled direction and intensity against a counterforce applied by a physiotherapist is known as:
    A. Post-isometric relaxation technique
    B. Muscle energy techniques
    C. Both A and B
    D. None of the above
22. To increase the joint range of motion of an athlete recovering from an injury, a sports physical therapist chooses to apply proprioceptive neuromuscular facilitation using the

hold-relax technique. Which type of contraction is utilized at the endpoint of the available range of motion while applying the hold-relax technique?

A. Isotonic
B. Isometric
C. Isokinetic
D. Eccentric

23. A sports physical therapist attempts to improve an athlete's lower extremity strength. Which proprioceptive neuromuscular facilitation technique would be the most appropriate to achieve the therapist's goals?

A. Contract-relax
B. Rhythmic stabilization
C. Repeated contractions
D. Hold-relax

24. A sports physical therapist instructs a soccer with tight calf muscles to complete a closed kinematic chain standing wall stretch. Prior to beginning the stretch, the therapist positions a folded towel under the medial arch of the soccer's foot. The primary purpose of this action is to limit which one of the following motions?

A. Talocrural dorsiflexion
B. Talocrural plantarflexion
C. Subtalar supination
D. Subtalar pronation

25. The examination of a 19-year-old sprinter reveals a limitation in the straight leg raise of 40 degrees due to inadequate hamstrings length. Which proprioceptive neuromuscular facilitation technique would be the most appropriate to increase his hamstrings length?

A. Contract-relax
B. Rhythmic initiation
C. Rhythmic stabilization
D. Rhythmic rotation

26. A 20-year-old female weightlifter complains of persistent low back pain radiating from the sacrum to the hip joint along the sciatic nerve distribution. On examination, the sports physiotherapist determines that tightness in the right piriformis muscle contributes to the weightlifter's discomfort. In order to stretch the muscle, the weightlifter should be positioned on her left side with the affected hip in:

A. Medial rotation and adduction
B. Lateral rotation and adduction
C. Medial rotation and abduction
D. Lateral rotation and abduction

Chapter 4: Therapeutic Exercise in Injury Rehabilitation

ANSWERS

1. B.
2. C. Static stretching includes the relaxation and concurrent elongation of the stretched muscle, which is performed slowly so that it does not elicit the stretch reflex of the stretched muscles.
3. A. Dynamic stretching is similar to specific warm-up and movements used help to prepare the athlete for competition by allowing him or her to increase sport-specific flexibility.
4. B. Stimulation of muscle spindles involves a contraction of the stretched muscle. If the muscle spindles are not stimulated, the muscle relaxes and allows greater stretch.
5. B. The hold-relax with agonist contraction is the most effective PNF stretching technique due to facilitation via both reciprocal (activation of hip flexors) and antagonist inhibition (activation of hamstrings).
6. A.
7. D. Females are more flexible than males which is mainly due in part to structural and anatomical differences and the type and extent of activities performed.
8. D.
9. D.
10. A. In sports situation, a muscle is forced to stretch beyond its normal active limits which requires enough elasticity to compensate for its additional stretch otherwise the musculotendinous units may be injured.
11. C. The continuous sustained static stretch lasting from 6 to 60 seconds, which is sufficient time for the Golgi tendon organ to begin responding to the increase in tension.
12. D. Application of stretching is contraindicated if there is evidence of an acute inflammatory or infectious process (heat and swelling) or soft tissue healing could be disrupted in the tight tissues and surrounding region.
13. A. Stretching is a commonly proposed therapeutic intervention used to prevent delayed onset muscle soreness (DOMS) and it may be used prior to and after vigorous exercise.
14. C.

15. C.
16. C. The decrease in the overall length of the muscle fibers and their in-series sarcomeres contributes to muscle atrophy and weakness. It has also been suggested that a muscle immobilized in a shortened position, atrophies and weakens occurs at a faster rate than if it is held in a lengthened position over time.
17. D. The determinants of stretching technique include: (i) alignment (positioning a limb or the body), (ii) stabilization (fixation of one site of attachment of the muscle as the stretch force is applied to the other bony attachment), (iii) intensity (magnitude of the stretch force applied), (iv) duration (length of time the stretch force is applied during a stretch cycle), (v) frequency (number of stretching sessions per day or per week), (vi) speed (speed of initial application of the stretch force) and (vii) mode of stretching (form or manner in which the stretch force is applied).
18. B. Dynamic flexibility is the degree to which an active muscle contraction moves a body segment through the available ROM of a joint. It is dependent on the degree to which a muscle contraction can move a joint and the amount of tissue resistance met during the active movement. It is also referred to as active mobility or active ROM.
19. A. The terms contracture and contraction (the process of tension developing in a muscle during shortening or lengthening) are not synonymous and should not be used interchangeably. Contractures are described by identifying the action of the shortened muscle. If a patient has shortened elbow flexors and cannot fully extend the elbow, he/she said to have an elbow flexion contracture.
20. A. Neuromuscular facilitation and inhibition techniques use inhibition or facilitation techniques to assist with muscle elongation, and it is associated with an exercise approach known as proprioceptive neuromuscular facilitation (PNF). These combined inhibition/facilitation/muscle lengthening procedures are often referred to as 'active inhibition', 'active stretching', or 'facilitated stretching'.
21. C. Muscle energy techniques are designed to lengthen muscle and fascia and to mobilize joints. Since the principles

of neuromuscular inhibition are incorporated into this approach, another term used to describe these techniques is post-isometric relaxation.
22. **B.** The hold-relax technique utilizes an isometric contraction at the end of the available range of motion. The athlete is then asked to relax as the physical therapist moves the extremity into the newly gained range.
23. **C.** Repeated contractions is a technique that focuses on movement on one side of the joint. The technique is facilitated by quick stretch and utilizes an isotonic contraction. Providing resistance at the point of weakness can enhance repeated contractions.
24. **D.** Supporting the subtalar joint in a neutral or slightly supinated position limits subtalar pronation and promotes optimal stretching of the calf muscles.
25. **A.** Contract-relax is a proprioceptive neuromuscular facilitation technique utilized to increase range of motion on one side of a joint. This technique utilizes isometric as well as isotonic contractions.
26. **A.** The piriformis muscle assists in abducting and laterally rotating the thigh. As a result, the weightlifter needs to move the involved lower extremity toward hip medial rotation and adduction to stretch the muscle. Tightness or spasm of the piriformis muscle can irritate the sciatic nerve, causing pain in the buttocks and referred pain along the course of the sciatic nerve. This referred pain, called "sciatica", often progresses down the back of the thigh and/or into the low back.

B. RESISTANCE TRAINING

1. The attributes of the sport, which is concerned with the analysis of body and limb movement patterns and muscular involvement is known as:
    A. Movement analysis
    B. Physiological analysis
    C. Injury analysis
    D. Speeds agility analysis
2. When determining a player's resistance training program needs, all of the following factors should be considered, *except*:
    A. Exercise selection
    B. Training load and repetitions
    C. Rest periods
    D. Programs of other similar players
3. An athlete's current condition or level of preparedness to begin a new or revised program is known as:
    A. Training status
    B. Training background
    C. Exercise history
    D. Exercise technique experience
4. The resistance training background of an athlete reveals that the training age of his current program is less than 2 months, his training frequency is less than two per week, his training stress is low and he has minimal exercise technique experience. How you will classify his resistance training status?
    A. Beginner
    B. Intermediate
    C. Advanced
    D. Moderately trained
5. In resistance training program, the term 'Training stress' refers to:
    A. Ability to carry out the given set of exercise
    B. Degree of physical demand imposed on the trainer
    C. Ability to sustain the exercise for longer duration of time
    D. All of the above
6. Following factors may result in impaired muscle performance leading to weakness and muscle atrophy, *except*:
    A. Disuse/inactivity
    B. Injury
    C. Immobilization
    D. Over use

Chapter 4: Therapeutic Exercise in Injury Rehabilitation

7. The most common adaptation to heavy resistance exercise is:
   A. Increase in the maximum force producing capacity of the muscle
   B. Increase in muscle strength
   C. Increase in muscle fiber size
   D. All of the above

8. A sports physiotherapist is designing a conditioning program for enhancing the muscle power of an athlete. Which of the following activities would be more appropriate for enhancing the muscle power?
   A. By reducing the amount of time required to perform greater intensity of exercise.
   B. By increasing the amount of time required to perform lower intensity of exercise.
   C. By increasing the amount of time required to perform greater intensity of exercise.
   D. By reducing the amount of time required to perform lower intensity of exercise.

9. The ability of a muscle to perform low-intensity, repetitive or sustained activities over a prolonged period is known as:
   A. Strength   B. Power
   C. Endurance   D. All of the above

10. The key elements of endurance training program is characterized by:
    A. Low intensity, high repetitions and a prolonged time period
    B. High intensity, low repetitions and a prolonged time period
    C. Low intensity, low repetitions and a prolonged time period
    D. Low intensity, high repetitions and a shorter time period

11. According to the overload principle in a strength-training program, a sports physiotherapist manipulates which of the following variables of exercise to achieve the desired goal?
    A. Increasing the amount of resistance progressively
    B. Increasing the number of repetitions of low load
    C. Increasing the time a muscle contraction is sustained
    D. Decreasing the amount of resistance progressively

12. **Which training principle applies to all body systems and is an extension of Wolff's law?**
    A. Overload principle
    B. SAID principle
    C. Reversibility principle
    D. Overflow principle
13. **Following statements are true regarding the overflow training principle, *except*:**
    A. Carry over of training effects from one variation of exercise to another
    B. Cross training effect can occur from an exercised limb to a non-exercised contralateral limb
    C. Contrary to SAID principle
    D. Detraining after the cessation of resistance exercise
14. **Which type of muscle fiber tends to fatigue slowly?**
    A. Type I fiber
    B. Type II A fiber
    C. Type B fiber
    D. None of the above
15. **Cardiorespiratory fatigue is caused by a combination of the following factors, *except*:**
    A. A decrease in blood sugar (glucose) levels
    B. A decrease in glycogen stores in muscle and liver
    C. A decrease in potassium
    D. A buildup of lactic acid in the muscle
16. **Following statements are true regarding weight training, *except*:**
    A. Increases the size of muscle fiber
    B. Increases strength
    C. Increase in the oxidative potential of muscle
    D. Increases the number of capillaries per muscle fiber
17. **Overload training principle is implemented by increasing following exercise variables, *except*:**
    A. Resistance
    B. Repetitions or sets
    C. Duration of exercise
    D. Speed of movements
18. **The level of strength can be determined by using the following devices, *except*:**
    A. Cable tensiometer
    B. Dynamometer
    C. Nautilus apparatus
    D. Cybex isokinetic dynamometer

Chapter 4: Therapeutic Exercise in Injury Rehabilitation

19. Which device is ideal for developing the power of an athlete?
    A. Orthotron
    B. Nautilus
    C. Cable tensiometer
    D. Universal gym
20. Which is the most important consideration in setting up a weight training circuit?
    A. Number of exercise sets
    B. Exercise order
    C. Resistance of exercise
    D. Number of circuit revolutions
21. In circuit training program, a circuit includes the following sequence of exercises, *except*:
    A. Bench press
    B. Leg press
    C. Sit ups
    D. Uphill running
22. The purpose of advocating velocity spectrum rehabilitation in isokinetic training program is:
    A. To improve strength of the working muscle
    B. To improve muscle performance
    C. To overcome limited physiological overflow of training
    D. To improve function
23. Following statements are true regarding eccentric isokinetic exercise, *except*:
    A. Implemented only after functional ROM has been restored
    B. Performed at slower velocities up to 180° per second for athletes
    C. Introduced only after maximal effort concentric isokinetic exercise can be performed
    D. Appropriate to use in the early phase of rehabilitation program
24. Which exercise equipment is more appropriately used for proprioceptive training of the lower extremity?
    A. BAPS system
    B. Stair master
    C. Pro-fitter
    D. Body blade
25. Which of the following are considered as closed kinetic chain exercises?

I. Squat II. Leg extension
III. Pull up IV. Bench press
A. I and III only B. I, II and III
C. II and IV only D. II, III and IV

26. The axial skeleton consists of the following, *except*:
    A. Vertebral column B. The ribs
    C. Sternum D. Shoulder girdle

27. The most important elements of muscle performance are:
    A. Strength B. Power
    C. Endurance D. All of the above

28. The ability of the neuromuscular system to produce, reduce, or control forces, contemplated or imposed, during functional activities, in a smooth, coordinated manner is known as:
    A. Endurance
    B. Functional muscle strength
    C. Static muscle strength
    D. Activities of daily living

29. Following are the potential benefits of resistance exercise, *except:*
    A. Enhanced muscle performance restoration, improvement or maintenance of muscle strength, power, and endurance
    B. Increased strength of connective tissues: tendons, ligaments, intramuscular connective tissue
    C. Reduced risk of soft tissue injury during physical activity
    D. Increase flexibility and the extensibility of the muscles.

30. According to reversibility principle, the term 'detraining' means:
    A. A reduction in muscle performance, begins within a week or two after the cessation of resistance exercises and continues until training effects are lost.
    B. An increase in muscle performance, begins within a week or two after the beginning resistance exercises and continues until training effects are continued.
    C. A reduction in muscle power, begins within a one or two days after the cessation of resistance exercises and continues until training effects are lost.
    D. All of the above

Chapter 4: Therapeutic Exercise in Injury Rehabilitation

31. A bodybuilder has completed ten sets of bench press with ten repetitions and performed this exercise to the point of exhaustion. After recovery from this strenuous exercise, how much time does it take for force-producing muscle to return to 90% to 95% of the pre-exercise capacity?
    A. 3-4 minutes
    B. 10-15 minutes
    C. 20-30 minutes
    D. 1 hour

32. Considering the age-related changes in muscle and muscle performance through the life span, muscle mass peaks in women during the following ages?
    A. Between 16 and 20 years of age
    B. Between 11 and 14 years of age
    C. Between 21 and 25 years of age
    D. Above 25 years of age

33. Identify the most important skeletal muscle adaptations to resistance exercise.
    A. Increase in tensile strength of tendons, ligaments, and connective tissue in muscle
    B. Increase in ATP and PC storage
    C. Hypertrophy
    D. Increase in motor unit recruitment

34. Which of the following are the important determinants of a resistance exercise program?
    A. Frequency of exercise
    B. Mode of exercise
    C. Exercise order and the duration of exercise
    D. All of the above

35. The amount of resistance (weight) imposed on the contracting muscle during each repetition of an exercise during the resistance training program is known as:
    A. Exercise load
    B. Training load
    C. Both A and B
    D. Neither A nor B

36. A sports physiotherapist is treating an athlete whose injury is in the early stages of soft tissue healing, and the primary goal is to protect the injured tissue. In these circumstances, which one of the following types of exercise intensities is the ideal choice?

A. Low intensity exercise with submaximal loading
B. High intensity exercise with submaximal loading
C. Low intensity exercise with near maximum loading
D. Low intensity exercise with maximum loading

37. During a resistance training program, a high-intensity exercise with a maximum exercise load is applied to accomplish one of the following objectives?
    A. To increase muscle strength, power and muscle size
    B. To improve muscle endurance
    C. To improve muscle flexibility
    D. All of the above

38. The amount of weight that could be lifted and lowered ten times through the full available range of motion is known as:
    A. 1 repetition maximum
    B. 10 repetition maximum
    C. 100 repetition maximum
    D. None of the above

39. A sports physical therapist, while designing an exercise program to improve a shuttle badminton player's muscle endurance, which one of the following exercise strategies is the ideal choice to enhance muscle endurance?
    A. Performing an exercise against a submaximal load for many repetitions
    B. Performing an exercise against a maximal load for low repetitions
    C. Performing an exercise against a submaximal load for low repetitions
    D. Performing an exercise against a near-maximal load for several repetitions until the point of fatigue

40. Besides repetition maximum (RM), identify other suitable alternative methods of determining baseline strength or an initial exercise load.
    A. Cable tensiometry
    B. Isokinetic or handheld dynamometry
    C. A percentage of body weight
    D. All of the above

Chapter 4: Therapeutic Exercise in Injury Rehabilitation

41. A sports physiotherapist plans a leg-press exercise training program for a footballer and how much would be the initial exercise load, beginning with a universal leg press resisted exercise.
    A. 30% of the body weight
    B. 20% of the body weight
    C. 10-20% of body weight
    D. 50% of the body weight

42. When providing an athletic conditioning program, which one of the following statements is true regarding 'exercise order'?
    A. Large muscle groups should be exercised before small muscle groups
    B. Multijoint exercises should be performed before single-joint exercises
    C. Appropriate warm-up, higher intensity exercises should be performed before lower intensity exercises
    D. All of the above

43. During sports conditioning, high-intensity eccentric exercise should be performed less frequently than others because:
    A. these exercises require greater recovery time
    B. to overcome the temporarily fatiguing effects of exercise
    C. to restore from delayed-onset muscle soreness
    D. All of the above

44. Higher incidence of delayed-onset muscle soreness occurs among which one of the following forms of exercise?
    A. High-intensity eccentric exercise
    B. Low-intensity eccentric exercise
    C. High-intensity concentric exercise
    D. Low-intensity concentric exercise

45. During resistance training programs, early strength gains are noticed after 2 to 3 weeks and are primarily due to the following:
    A. Increased vascularization
    B. Hypertrophy
    C. Neural adaptation
    D. All of the above

46. The type of resistance implemented through an isokinetic dynamometer that controls the velocity of active movement during exercise is:
    A. Mechanical resistance
    B. Variable load
    C. Accommodating resistance
    D. Constant load
47. A form of exercise utilized to avoid a portion of the joint's range, which is unstable or to protect healing tissues after injury or surgery is:
    A. Velocity-specific training
    B. Full arc exercise
    C. Short arc exercise
    D. Mode-specific training
48. Identify the most appropriate isometric exercise that decreases muscle spasm and promotes relaxation and circulation after injury to soft tissues during the acute stage of healing:
    A. Stabilization exercise
    B. Muscle setting exercise
    C. Multiple-angle isometrics
    D. Alternating isometrics
49. High-intensity isometric exercises may be contraindicated for patients with a history of cardiac or vascular disorders. The most appropriate precaution to be taken during substantial resistance isometric exercises is:
    A. Avoid breath-holding
    B. Emphasize exhalation during muscle contraction
    C. Encourage rhythmic breathing to be adopted during the exercise
    D. All of the above
50. During sports conditioning, 'Overtraining' leads to a decline in physical performance in healthy individuals participating in high-intensity, high-volume strength and endurance training programs. This overtraining occurs due to:
    A. Inadequate rest intervals between exercise sessions
    B. Too rapid progression of exercises
    C. Inadequate diet and fluid intake
    D. All of the above

Chapter 4: Therapeutic Exercise in Injury Rehabilitation

51. A physical therapist attempts to quantify a patient's endurance level by administering a maximal exercise test. What is the primary limitation of the maximal exercise test?
    A. Maximal exercise testing requires participants to exercise only to the point of volitional fatigue.
    B. Maximal exercise testing does not typically allow a steady state heart rate at each work rate.
    C. Maximal exercise testing is not useful in diagnosing coronary artery disease.
    D. Maximal exercise testing requires progressive stages of increasing work intensities without rest intervals.

52. A physical therapist attempts to obtain information on a patient's endurance level by administering a low-level exercise test on a treadmill. Which of the following measurement methods would provide the therapist with an objective measurement of endurance?
    A. Facial color
    B. Facial expression
    C. Rating on a perceived exertion scale
    D. Respiration rate

ANSWERS

1. **A.** Movement analysis is the component of a need analysis to determine the unique characteristic of the sport. It is mainly related with body and limb movement pattern and muscular involvement in the sport concerned.
2. **D.** Programs of other similar players are not considered while designing a player's resistance training program because resistance training program is individualized according to the need for the player and the nature of sports involved. Strength development should be individualized and determined according to the needs of the athlete.
3. **A.** Training status is an important consideration when designing training program, which includes an evaluation of any current or previous injuries that may affect training.
4. **A.**
5. **B.** Training stress describes the degree of physical demand or stimulus of the resistance training program imposed on the player who is undergoing training.
6. **D.** Factors such as injury, disease, immobilization, disuse or inactivity may result in impaired muscle performance leading to weakness and muscle atrophy.
7. **D.** Following heavy resisted exercise, there will be increase in the maximum force producing capacity of the muscle which results in increase in muscle strength primarily occurs as the result of neural adaptations and an increase in muscle fiber size.
8. **A.** The greater the intensity of exercise and the shorter the time period taken to generate force, the greater the muscle power.
9. **C.** Muscle endurance is the ability of a muscle to contract repeatedly against a load (resistance), generate and sustain tension and resist fatigue over an extended period of time.
10. **A.** Endurance training is characterized by having a muscle contract and lift or lower a light load for many repetitions or sustain a muscle contraction for an extended period of time.
11. **A.** In a strength training program, the amount of resistance applied to the muscle is incrementally and progressively increased.

Chapter 4: Therapeutic Exercise in Injury Rehabilitation

12. **B.** SAID principle applies to all body systems and is an extension of Wolff's law which states that body systems adapt over time to the stresses placed upon them.
13. **D.** Reversibility principle states that adaptive changes, such as increase in muscle strength or endurance in response to a resistance exercise program are transient and reversible unless training induced improvement are regularly used for functional activities in a maintenance program of resistance exercises.
14. **A.** Type I (tonic, slow twitch) muscle fibers generate a low level of muscle tension but can sustain the contraction for a long time, these fibers are geared toward aerobic metabolism and very slow to fatigue.
15. **D.** A buildup of lactic acid in the muscle causes disturbances in contractile mechanism of the muscle resulting in diminished response of muscle to repeated stimulus and is reflected by a progressive decrement in the amplitude of the motor unit potentials leading to local muscle fatigue.
16. **D.** Endurance training results in an increase in the number of capillaries per muscle fiber, but have little or no effect upon the cross-sectional size of the muscle fiber.
17. **D.** Speed of movements has no effect on the strength of muscle.
18. **C.** Nautilus apparatus is used for providing resistance training to strengthen the muscles.
19. **A.** Orthotron is a type of isokinetic device, which conditions the muscle to contract or exert force at an accelerated and fixed speed and has been shown to be useful in the development of power.
20. **B.** Exercise order, which enables one part of the body to recover from exercise while exercising another area and therefore minimizes muscle fatigue.
21. **D.**
22. **C.** Velocity spectrum rehabilitation is advocated in isokinetic training to deal with the problem of limited physiological overflow of training effects from one training speed to another in which exercises are performed across a wide range of velocities.
23. **D.** Eccentric isokinetic exercise is only appropriate in the final phase of rehabilitation program to continue to challenge

individual muscle groups when isolated deficits in strength and power persist.
24. A. Biomechanical ankle platform system (BAPS) is used for proprioceptive training in the upper and lower extremity.
25. A.
26. D. The axial skeleton consists of the skull/cranium, vertebral column, (vertebra C1 through the coccyx), the ribs and the sternum.
27. D. The three elements of muscle performance are strength, power, and endurance, and they can be enhanced by some form of resistance exercise. The extent to which each of these elements is altered by exercise depends on how the principles of resistance training are applied and how factors, such as the intensity, frequency, and duration of exercise are manipulated.
28. B.
29. D. Improved flexibility and the extensibility of the muscles is achieved through the application of stretching technique.
30. A. Detraining occurs within a week or two after the cessation of resistance exercises, and it is imperative that gains in strength and endurance are incorporated into daily activities as early as possible in a rehabilitation program. Following the rehabilitation, it is also advisable that patients should participate in a maintenance program of resistance exercises as an integral component of a lifelong fitness program.
31. A. Following the recovery from acute exercise, the force-producing capacity of muscle returns to 90–95% of the pre-exercise capacity, and it usually takes 3 to 4 minutes, with the most significant proportion of recovery occurring in the first minute.
32. A. Muscle mass peaks in women between 16 and 20 years of age; muscle mass in men peaks between 18 and 25 years of age. Decreases in muscle mass begin to occur as early as 25 years of age.
33. C. Hypertrophy is an increase in the size (bulk) of an individual muscle fiber caused by an increase in myofibrillar volume. After an extended period of moderate- to high-intensity resistance training, usually by 4 to 8 weeks, but possibly as early as 2 to 3 weeks with very high-intensity resistance

Chapter 4: Therapeutic Exercise in Injury Rehabilitation   69

training, hypertrophy becomes an increasingly important adaptation that accounts for strength gains in muscle.

34. **D.** The determinants of a resistance exercise program consist of the following: (i) Alignment of segments of the body during exercise; (ii) stabilization of proximal or distal joints to prevent substitution; (iii) intensity: the exercise load (level of resistance); (iv) volume: the total number of repetitions and sets in an exercise session; (v) exercise order: the sequence in which muscle groups are exercised during an exercise session; (vi) frequency: the number of exercise sessions per day or per week; (vii) rest interval: time allotted for recuperation between sets and sessions of exercise; (viii) duration: total time frame of a resistance training program; (ix) mode of exercise: type of muscle contraction, position of the patient, form (source) of resistance, arc of movement, or the primary energy system utilized; and (x) velocity of exercise.

35. **C.** The amount of resistance imposed on the contracting muscle during each repetition of an exercise is referred to as its exercise load (or training load). To be precise, it is the extent to which the muscle is loaded or how much weight is lifted, lowered, or held.

36. **A.**

37. **A.** If the exercise's goal is to increase muscle strength and power and possibly increase muscle size, a high-intensity exercise with a maximum exercise load has to be applied. Usually, a near-maximum or maximum exercise load is used for training those individuals involved in competitive weight lifting or bodybuilding as well as during conditioning program for individuals with no known pathology.

38. **B.** A repetition maximum (RM) is defined as the greatest amount of weight (load) that a muscle can move through the full, available ROM with control for a specific number of times before fatiguing. 1-RM is used as the baseline measurement of a subject's maximum effort but used a multiple RM, specifically a 10-RM (the amount of weight that could be lifted and lowered ten times through the ROM) during training.

39. **A.** Training to improve muscle (local) endurance involves performing many repetitions of an exercise against a submaximal load. For example, as many as three to five sets of 40 to 50 repetitions against a low amount of weight or a light grade of elastic resistance might be used to improve muscle endurance.
40. **D.** Cable tensiometry and isokinetic or handheld dynamometry are alternatives to a repetition maximum for establishing a baseline measurement of dynamic or static strength. A percentage of body weight has also been proposed to estimate the amount of resistance (load) used in a strength training program.
41. **D.** Bodyweight or partial body weight is considered as a source of resistance if the exercise occurs in an antigravity position. A percentage of body weight has been proposed to estimate how much resistance (load) should be used in a strength training program. For the leg press, 50% of the bodyweight is considered an initial load. These percentages vary for different muscle groups.
42. **D.**
43. **D.**
44. **A.** High-intensity eccentric exercise is associated with greater microtrauma to soft tissues and a higher incidence of delayed-onset muscle soreness than concentric exercise. Therefore, rest intervals between exercise sessions are longer, and exercise frequency is less than with other forms of exercise.
45. **C.** Strength gains observed early in a resistance training program (after 2 to 3 weeks) are primarily neural adaptation. For significant changes to occur in muscle, such as hypertrophy or increased vascularization, at least 6 to 12 weeks of resistance training is required.
46. **C.**
47. **C.** If resistance exercises are performed through only a portion of the available range, it is known as short arc exercise, and they are used to avoid a painful arc of motion or a portion of the range in which the joint is unstable or to protect healing tissues after injury or surgery.

Chapter 4: Therapeutic Exercise in Injury Rehabilitation

48. **B.** Muscle setting exercise involves low-intensity isometric contractions performed against little to no resistance. They are used to decrease muscle pain and spasm and promote relaxation and circulation after injury to soft tissues during the acute stage of healing. Two common examples of muscle setting are the quadriceps and gluteal muscles.
49. **D.** Breath-holding commonly occurs during isometric exercise, mainly when performed against substantial resistance. This is likely to cause a pressor response due to the Valsalva maneuver, causing a rapid increase in blood pressure. Rhythmic breathing emphasizes exhalation during the contraction and should always be performed during isometric exercise to minimize this response.
50. **D.** Overtraining is brought by inadequate rest intervals between exercise sessions, too rapid progression of exercises, and inadequate diet and fluid intake. In healthy individuals, overtraining is a preventable, reversible phenomenon that can be resolved by tapering the training program for some time by periodically decreasing the volume and frequency of exercise (periodization).
51. **A.** Physical therapists gain information on a patient's response to exercise through various subjective and objective measures, however, remain dependent on a patient's willingness to exert a maximal effort in order to collect meaningful data.
52. **D.** Respiratory rate is an objective measure that is used to assess endurance. Respiratory rate typically increases as a patient becomes fatigued.

C. PLYOMETRIC TRAINING

1. In plyometric training, the term 'Amortization' means:
   A. Shortening of agonist muscle fibers
   B. Pause between eccentric and concentric phase
   C. Stretch of the agonist muscle
   D. Stretch shortening cycle time
2. Following are the examples of plyometric warm-up drills, *except*:
   A. Lunging
   B. Zigzag hop
   C. Skipping
   D. Marching
3. Which of the following surfaces is best suited for the performance of plyometric exercises?
   A. Astro Turf field
   B. Suspended wood floor
   C. Asphalt
   D. Trampoline
4. Which of the following areas should be assessed prior to beginning a lower body plyometric training program?
   I. Balance
   II. Strength
   III. Speed
   IV. Lean body mass
   A. I and III only
   B. II and IV only
   C. I, II and III only
   D. All of the above
5. What work-to-rest ratio is more appropriate between sets of plyometric drills?
   A. 1:5
   B. 1:3
   C. 1:4
   D. 1:2
6. Which of the following types of drills is generally considered the most intense?
   A. Bounds
   B. Box jumps
   C. Depth jumps
   D. Jumps in place
7. Which of the following is not a phase of stretch-shortening cycle (SSC)?
   A. Concentric
   B. Isometric
   C. Eccentric
   D. Amortization
8. Which of the following is a primary component of the series elastic component (SEC)?
   A. Muscle fiber
   B. Actin
   C. Ligament
   D. Tendon

Chapter 4: Therapeutic Exercise in Injury Rehabilitation

9. Which of the following structures detects rapid movement and initiates the stretch reflex?
   A. Muscle spindle
   B. Golgi tendon organ
   C. Pacinian corpuscle
   D. Extrafusal muscle fiber

10. Following statements are true about plyometric training, *except*:
    A. Plyometric volume is expressed as the number of repetitions and sets performed during a given training session
    B. Plyometric follows the principles of progressive overload
    C. Mini-trampolines are commonly used for beginning plyometrics
    D. The critical weight for an athlete to avoid high-volume high intensity plyometric exercise is 80 kg so as to overcome the risk of injury

11. Which one of the following statements is true concerning plyometric exercises?
    A. It incorporates an eccentric preload (a quick eccentric stretch) followed by a forceful concentric contraction.
    B. It enhances reflex joint stabilization and may increase muscle stiffness.
    C. It is an effective addition to upper and lower extremity conditioning and rehabilitation programs.
    D. All of the above

12. Plyometric training is used to train the neuromuscular system to react quickly to prepare for sports activities that require rapid starting and stopping movements or quick changes of direction. At which stage of sports injury rehabilitation, this kind of training is employed?
    A. Acute stage of rehabilitation
    B. Subacute stage of rehabilitation
    C. Advanced stage of rehabilitation
    D. All of the above

13. In plyometric training, the rapid eccentric loading phase is termed as:
    A. Stretch cycle
    B. Shortening cycle
    C. Amortization phase
    D. All of the above

14. Which one of the following conditions are contraindicated for the application of plyometric training program?
    A. Presence of inflammation
    B. Pain
    C. Significant joint instability
    D. All of the above
15. Following are the most prominent therapeutic effects of plyometric training program, *except:*
    A. Develop muscle strength and power
    B. Enhance physical performance
    C. Increase arthrokinematics range of motion
    D. Decrease the incidence of lower extremity injury
16. A sports physiotherapy is planning and implementing a plyometric training program for an 18 old gymnastic. Which one of the following parameters are considered while progressing exercise during a plyometric training program?
    A. Exercises should be sequenced from easy to difficult.
    B. Exercises should be progressed in a graduate manner.
    C. Exercises should be individually designed to meet the gymnasts' goal.
    D. All of the above
17. One of the essential criteria to be met by an athlete to begin plyometric training is:
    A. Should have 80-85% level of strength of the involved muscle groups (compared to the contralateral extremity).
    B. Should have a minimum of 50-60% pain-free ROM of the moving joints.
    C. Should have at least 50-60% level of strength of the involved muscle groups (compared to the contralateral extremity).
    D. Should have a minimum of 60-70% pain-free ROM of the moving joints.
18. The intensity of the plyometric exercise can be increased by progressing from simple to complex movements. A sports physiotherapist decided to increase the intensity of the plyometric training by increasing the external resistance. From the following, choose an appropriate method to increase the external resistance.

Chapter 4: Therapeutic Exercise in Injury Rehabilitation

  A. Increase weight belt or vest
  B. Progress from double-leg to single-leg activities
  C. Increase the height of platforms for jumping and hopping activities
  D. All of the above

19. Optimal frequency of plyometric sessions is:
  A. One session per week
  B. Two sessions per week
  C. Three sessions per week
  D. Four sessions per week

20. A sports physiotherapist employs various plyometric exercises for the upper extremities during the final phase of rehabilitation. Which one of the following exercises is not an ideal choice for advanced functional training of upper extremities?
  A. Bilateral chest press and throw in supine position
  B. Bilateral overhead catch and throw in standing position
  C. Hand-to-hand overhead catch and throw
  D. Side-to-side shuffle

21. An injured athlete returning to sporting activities that require strength and power, which one of the following exercises is the ideal choice for the physiotherapist to design a functional training program?
  A. Plyometric drills
  B. Stretch shorting drills
  C. Agility drills
  D. All of the above

22. The type of drills designed to develop coordination (sequencing and timing of movements), balance, and quick neuromuscular responses by practicing activities that include directional changes at varying speeds of movement, irrespective of specific sports' movement patterns is known as:
  A. Agility drills
  B. Sports specific drills
  C. Sports conditioning drills
  D. All of the above

23. An athlete underwent an Achilles tendon repair surgery, and he is in the advanced stage of rehabilitation. Which one of the following statements is true concerning the provision of plyometric exercises to the athlete?
    A. Begin plyometric training in a pool (chest-deep progressing to waist-deep immersion).
    B. Postpone land-based plyometric training and activities that involve high-impact and quick acceleration/deceleration
    C. Wear a tape around the ankle during high-impact, high-velocity activities to minimize the risk of re-rupture of the repaired tendon.
    D. All of the above

24. Among the following plyometric exercises, identify the most suitable one for providing advanced functional training of lower extremities?
    A. Clap push-ups
    B. Dribbling a ball on the floor or against a wall
    C. Bounding and hopping activities
    D. Drop push-ups from a low platform to the floor and back onto the platform

25. A physiotherapist is preparing soccer for sports participation through a plyometric training program. A well-designed plyometric program addresses which one of the following?
    A. Coordination
    B. Efficiency
    C. Speed and power
    D. All of the above

ANSWERS

1. **B.** Amortization or transition phase is the time from the end of the eccentric phase to the initiation of the concentric muscle action, which occurs during phase II of stretch- shortening cycle of plyometric training.
2. **B.** Zigzag hop is a type of lower body plyometric drill, which involves multiple hops and jumps, repeated movements and may be viewed as a combination of jumps in place and standing jumps.
3. **B.** A suspended floor or rubber mat is a good surface for the lower body plyometrics since it possesses adequate shock-absorbing properties so as to prevent injuries.
4. **C.**
5. **A.** The time between sets is determined by proper work-to-rest ratio of 1:5 to 1:10 and is specific to the volume and type of drill being performed in plyometric training.
6. **C.** Depth jumps performed at a height of 48 inches (1.2 m) would provide a significant overload on the muscles. Further, the amount of force to be overcome is so great that the amortization phase is extended and thus the purpose of the exercise is defeated.
7. **B.**
8. **D.** Series elastic component is the workhorse of plyometric exercise which includes some muscular components (i.e., connective tissue), but it is the tendons that constitutes the majority of the series elastic component.
9. **A.** Muscle spindles are proprioceptive organs that are sensitive to the rate and magnitude of a stretch; when a quick stretch is detected, muscular activity reflexively increases.
10. **D.** Athletes who weigh more than 220 lb (100 kg) may be at the increased risk for injury when performing plyometric exercises. Greater weight increases compressive force on joints, thereby predisposing these joints to injury.
11. **D.**
12. **C.** Plyometric training is typically integrated into the advanced phase of rehabilitation of athletes to help them return to high-demand functional activities and sports.

13. **A.** Plyometric training is defined as a system of high-velocity resistance training characterized by a rapid, resisted, eccentric (lengthening) contraction during which the muscle elongates, immediately followed by a rapid reversal of movement with a resisted concentric (shortening) contraction of the same muscle. The rapid eccentric loading phase is the stretch cycle, and the concentric phase is the shortening cycle. The period between the stretch and shortening cycles is known as the amortization phase.
14. **D.**
15. **C.**
16. **D.**
17. **A.** Before initiating plyometric training, an individual should have adequate muscle strength and endurance, and flexibility. Criteria that should be met to begin plyometric training usually include 80–85% level of strength of the involved muscle groups (compared to the contralateral extremity) and 90–95% pain-free ROM in the moving joints. Sufficient strength and stability of proximal regions of the body (trunk and limb) for balance and postural control are necessary prerequisites.
18. **D.** Methods for increasing external resistance include a weight belt or vest, heavier weighted balls, or heavier grade elastic resistance; progressing from double-leg to single-leg activities; and increasing the height of platforms for jumping and hopping activities.
19. **B.** The optimal frequency of plyometric sessions is two sessions per week, which allows a 48- to 72-hour recovery period between sessions. Maximum training benefits typically occur within an 8- to 10-week duration.
20. **D.** Side-to-side shuffle targets the lower extremity, and it requires postural stability and balance because of the quick changes of direction involved. Here, the patient takes several quick side steps to the right and then back to the left and repeat. This exercise requires rapid contractions of the hip abductors and adductors against body weight during each change of direction.
21. **D.** If the athlete is returning to activities that require strength and power, incorporate plyometric drills. Plyometric

Chapter 4: Therapeutic Exercise in Injury Rehabilitation

training, also referred to as stretch-shortening drills or agility drills, is designed to improve power and develop quick neuromuscular responses. This form of training is appropriate during the advanced rehabilitation phase for selected patients intending to return to high-demand work- or sport-related activities.

22. **A.** Agility drills are designed to develop coordination (sequencing and timing of movements), balance, and quick neuromuscular responses. Drills involve practicing movements that include directional changes at varying speeds of movement. Activities include maneuvering around or stepping over obstacles in the environment first while walking and then while running, pivoting, cutting, or hopping.

23. **D.**

24. **C.** Hopping is also known as four-quadrant jumps performed using two lines on the floor intersecting at right angles as a guide where the athlete jumps forward, backward, side-to-side, and diagonally from one quadrant to another, using quick directional changes. Bounding is a series of forward jumps across a floor. Both are used for functional training of lower extremities.

25. **D.** Plyometric exercises take an important part in rehabilitation programs for the athletes to prepare them for the demands of their sport and safe return to sport activities. A well-designed plyometric program offers coordination, efficiency, speed, and power in preparation for sport participation.

CHAPTER 5
Basic Concepts in Injury Rehabilitation

1. Rehabilitation programs are influenced by the following factors, *except*:
   A. The severity of injury
   B. The stage of tissue healing
   C. Strength of injured muscle of the limb
   D. Joint swelling
2. Which of the following components are to be measured during and at the end of the rehabilitation program?
   A. Strength of each muscle group
   B. Power of each muscle group
   C. Functional use of the injured limb in the required sport
   D. All of the above
3. Which of the following should be emphasized during the early stage of injury rehabilitation (joint is under immobilization)?
   A. Cardiovascular fitness
   B. Isometric contractions
   C. Muscle stimulation
   D. All of the above
4. Which of the following exercises are to be prescribed towards the final stage of injury rehabilitation when the athlete demonstrates pain free range of motion and has 90% of power strength and endurance of opposite leg and feels stable both clinically and subjectively?
   A. Circuit training program
   B. Sport specific skills
   C. DAPRE techniques
   D. Extrinsic exercises
5. Following statements are true regarding isotonic exercises, *except*:
   A. Joint is moved through a range of motion against the resistance of a fixed weight
   B. Delorme PRE program is a form of isotonic exercise
   C. Isotonic exercise consists of concentric and eccentric work
   D. Intensity or resistance is constant throughout the range of motion

Chapter 5: Basic Concepts in Injury Rehabilitation

6. An isotonic resistance training consists of three sets of 10 repetitions, which are performed at 100%, 75% and 50% of the ten-repetition maximum is known as:
   A. Oxford technique
   B. Delorme technique
   C. DAPRE technique
   D. All of the above

7. An accommodating variable resistance exercise in which the speed of motion is set and the resistance accommodates to match the force applied is known as:
   A. Isotonic exercise
   B. Isokinetic exercise
   C. Isometric exercise
   D. Isoinertial contractions

8. The purpose of providing controlled motion of the injured structure during remodeling phase is:
   A. Structural adaptation of injured tissue
   B. Functional adaptation of the injured tissue
   C. To make adhesions flexible
   D. All of the above

9. According to severity of symptoms, the phase II of inflammatory response to micro trauma is:
   A. Pain all the time with significant functional disability
   B. Pain during and after activity with significant functional disability
   C. Pain during and after activity with no significant functional disability
   D. Pain after activity only

10. Which is the weakest part of growth plate in which separation usually occurs in the event of an injury?
    A. Resting layer
    B. Zone of proliferating cells
    C. Zone of hypertrophied cells
    D. Zone of provisional calcification

11. A sports physiotherapist designs an exercise program for an athlete recovering from a lower extremity injury. A single

most important factor in an exercise program designed to increase muscle strength is:
A. The recovery time between exercise sets
B. The number of repetitions per set
C. The duration of exercise session
D. The intensity of exercise

12. All are the phases of healing following injury, *except*:
A. Inflammation
B. Remodeling
C. Reconditioning
D. Repair

13. A sports physical therapist examines an athlete who has been diagnosed with an anterior talofibular ligament sprain. The athlete exhibits signs of inflammation in the ankle region, including heat, swelling, redness, and pain. This phase of inflammation and repair is BEST termed:
A. Inflammatory phase
B. Proliferative phase
C. Maturation phase
D. Chronic phase

14. A natural sequence of events will follow to repair the damaged tissue, restore homeostasis and normal function in a soft tissue injury. Identify the proper series of this event to occur following a soft tissue injure from the following options?
A. Inflammation-Bleeding-Proliferation-Remodeling
B. Bleeding-Inflammation-Proliferation-Remodeling
C. Bleeding-Proliferation-Inflammation-Remodeling
D. Bleeding-Inflammation-Remodeling-Proliferation

15. What would be the most appropriate body tissue response following a primary injury that occurs due to sporting events?
A. Cell membranes get disrupted due to the mechanical force resulting from an injury
B. There is a loss in homeostasis and subsequent cell death
C. There may be involvement of ligament, tendon, muscle, nerve, and connective tissues
D. All of the above

16. The acronym 'PRICE' stands for:
A. Protection, rest, ice, compression, elevation
B. Protection, rest, immersion, compression, elevation

Chapter 5: Basic Concepts in Injury Rehabilitation

    C. Protection, rest, ice, concussion, elevation
    D. Protection, rest, insertion, compression, elongation

17. Following are primary goals of physiotherapy during the early phases (i.e., phase 1 and 2) of tissue healing and repair, *except*?
   A. To reduce pain
   B. To limit and reduce inflammatory exudates
   C. To increase the muscle strength and control
   D. To promote new tissue growth and fiber realignment

18. A sports physiotherapist is applying strapping to an athlete diagnosed with an anterior talofibular ligament of the ankle. What would be the most appropriate ankle joint position to use strapping during the early stages to protect the talofibular ligament from stresses?
   A. Apply strapping to control inversion and plantar flexion
   B. Apply strapping to control eversion and dorsiflexion
   C. Apply strapping to control dorsiflexion
   D. None of the above

19. The primary reason for applying ice in immediate early injury management is:
   A. To cool the affected tissues
   B. To minimize secondary tissue damage
   C. To reduce the metabolic demands of the neighboring cells
   D. All of the above

20. When deciding on the dosage of cryotherapy application, the physical therapist considers the following parameters, *except*?
   A. The size of the injury
   B. The depth of the tissues injured
   C. Subcutaneous fat depth
   D. Mechanism of injury

21. Following are primary goals of physiotherapy during the remodeling stage (phase 4) of tissue healing, *except:*
   A. Promoting collagen growth and tissue realignment
   B. Increasing muscle strength/control
   C. To reduce metabolic demands of tissue
   D. Maximizing function

22. The most common electrotherapy modalities that appear to have a direct action on the tissue repair process is:
    A. Ultrasound
    B. Laser
    C. Pulsed shortwave diathermy
    D. All of the above

23. A sports physical therapist treats a patient rehabilitating from an Achilles tendon repair using cryotherapy. Among the following options, which cryotherapy agent would provide the most significant magnitude of tissue cooling?
    A. Frozen gel packs
    B. Fluori-Methane spray
    C. Ice massage
    D. Cold water bath

24. A physical therapist elects to treat an athlete with a first-degree ankle sprain using a contrast bath. Among the following temperature ranges, which temperatures would be the most appropriate when preparing the cool and warm water?
    A. 9° C and 34° C
    B. 14° C and 38° C
    C. 19° C and 45° C
    D. 23° C and 48° C

25. A physical therapist administers a contrast bath to a long-distance runner rehabilitating for his lateral ankle sprain. The therapist begins the first cycle by immersing the injured ankle in warm water for three minutes and then immediately moves the ankle into cold water. How long should the therapist leave the ankle in the cold water?
    A. 30 seconds
    B. 1 minute
    C. 3 minutes
    D. 5 minutes

26. A physical therapist determines to provide aquatic therapy for a 33-year football player. Which condition would not be considered a contraindication to aquatic therapy?
    A. Infectious disease
    B. Urinary tract infection
    C. Raynaud's disease
    D. Fever

Chapter 5: Basic Concepts in Injury Rehabilitation

27. A physical therapist planning to administer phonophoresis on a 19-year-old tennis player diagnosed with impingement syndrome palpates the insertion of the supraspinatus. Which one of the following bony landmarks best indicates this site?
    A. Lesser tubercle of the humerus
    B. Greater tubercle of the humerus
    C. Supraspinatus fossa of the scapula
    D. Deltoid tuberosity of the humerus

28. A physical therapist reads in an existing medical record that a gulf player who underwent elbow surgery will be seen in physical therapy two times a week for an additional three weeks. In using a S.O.A.P. note format, this information would appear in which section?
    A. Subjective section
    B. Objective section
    C. Assessment section
    D. Plan section

29. Which one of the following interventions is the most appropriate one to promote the healing of injured tissues during the chronic/return to functional stage of the tissue repair process?
    A. Monitor response of tissue to exercise progression
    B. Decrease intensity of the exercise if pain or inflammation increases
    C. Protect healing tissue with assistive devices, splints, tape, or wrap
    D. Teach safe body mechanics

30. Considering the severity of tissue injury, which one of the following statements is the most appropriate indicator of grade 2 injury?
    A. Near-complete or complete tear or avulsion of the tissue with severe pain.
    B. Moderate pain requires stopping the activity, and when the tissue is palpated, it dramatically increases the pain.
    C. Mild pain at the time of injury that occur within the first 24 hours
    D. All of the above

31. The clinical condition resulting from the tendon's degeneration due to repetitive microtrauma is known as:
    A. Tenovaginitis
    B. Tendinosis
    C. Tendinitis
    D. Tendinopathy

32. Identify the common adverse effects of giving a complete or continuous immobilization of tissue during the acute stage of tissue healing after an injury?
    A. Adherence of the developing fibrils to surrounding tissue
    B. Weakening of connective tissue
    C. Changes in articular cartilage
    D. All of the above

33. Physical therapists employ the following therapeutic interventions to maintain the integrity and function of associated areas nearer to the injured site during the acute stage of tissue healing, *except:*
    A. Active-assistive exercises
    B. Free exercises
    C. Stretching and resistance exercises
    D. Modified aerobic exercises

34. A sports physiotherapist is designing a care plan for a hockey player diagnosed with an acute grade 2 medial meniscus injury of the right knee joint. Identify the most appropriate choice of intervention to develop the neuromuscular control, muscle endurance, and strength in involved and related muscles of the knee joint during the second week of post-injury rehabilitation?
    A. Submaximal isometric exercises within patient's tolerance
    B. Initiate active range of motion exercises
    C. Protected weight bearing, and stabilization exercises
    D. All of the above

35. From the following options, the most appropriate intervention to overcome exercise-induced muscle soreness that either does not decrease after 4 hours or not resolved after 24 hours is:

A. Design an appropriate warm-up program
B. Increase the frequency of exercise
C. Either modify or reduce the intensity of the exercise
D. None of the above

36. Following are the most appropriate therapeutic interventions used during the early subacute stage of tissue healing after an initial muscle injury, *except:*
   A. Protected weight-bearing exercises
   B. Muscular endurance exercises.
   C. Eccentric and progressive resisted exercises
   D. Multiple-angle, submaximal isometric exercises

37. Among the following, which is the most appropriate therapeutic technique applied to gain mobility of scar tissue?
   A. Stretching
   B. Cross friction massage
   C. Finger kneading
   D. Gliding techniques

38. Types of injuries that are resulting from repetitive tasks, forceful exertions, vibrations, mechanical compression, or sustained postures involving both musculoskeletal and nervous systems are known as:
   A. Cumulative trauma disorders
   B. Repetitive strain injuries
   C. Overuse syndrome
   D. All of the above

39. A volleyball player returning to sports requires greater-than-normal demand activities and progressed further to do intense exercises. Choose the appropriate training that helps the player to return to sports participation?
   A. Plyometrics
   B. Agility training
   C. Skill development training
   D. All of the above

40. A sports physical therapist orders a wheelchair with a reclining back for a patient in a rehabilitation hospital.

Which type of leg rests would be the most appropriate for the wheelchair?

A. Swing-away
B. Detachable
C. Elevating
D. Fixed

41. A sports physical therapist prepares to select an assistive device for a patient rehabilitating from a lower extremity injury. Which of the following would be of least importance when choosing an assistive device?

A. The patient's level of understanding
B. The patient's height and weight
C. The patient's upper and lower extremity strength
D. The patient's level of coordination

42. An athlete rehabilitating from a total hip replacement receives home physical therapy services. The patient is currently full weight-bearing and can ascend and descend stairs independently. The athlete expresses that her goal following rehabilitation is to walk one mile each day. The most appropriate plan to accomplish the patient's goal is to:

A. Continue home physical therapy services until the athlete's goal is attained
B. Refer the athlete to an outpatient orthopedic physical therapy clinic
C. Design a home exercise program that emphasizes progressive ambulation
D. Admit the athlete to a rehabilitation hospital

43. A sports physical therapist designs an exercise program for a patient rehabilitating from a lower extremity injury. A single most important factor in an exercise program designed to increase muscular strength is:

A. The recovery time between exercise sets
B. The number of repetitions per set
C. The duration of the exercise session
D. The intensity of the exercise

44. A physical therapist employed in a rehabilitation hospital treats a patient status post-traumatic brain injury. During the treatment session, the therapist notices that the patient's toes are discolored below a bivalved lower extremity cast. The cast was applied approximately five hours ago in an attempt to reduce a plantarflexion contracture. The most appropriate therapist action is to:
    A. Document the observation in the medical record and continue to monitor the patient's circulation
    B. Contact the staff nurse and request that the cast is removed
    C. Refer the patient to an orthotist
    D. Remove the cast

45. A physical therapist examines a 30-year-old male rehabilitating from a meniscus repair. The physician orders indicate the patient is nonweight bearing on the involved lower extremity. The most appropriate gait pattern for the patient is:
    A. Two-point
    B. Three-point
    C. Four-point
    D. Swing-to

ANSWERS

1. **C.** Rehabilitation should not be focused on strength of injured muscle group, instead all muscles of the limb need to be exercised concentrating on those that are weaker. However, the limitations imposed by the injury or surgery should be observed.
2. **D.** Before releasing the athlete for full activity, the components, such as strength, power, endurance and functional utility of the injured limb should equal measurements obtained from the opposite injured side.
3. **D.** During the early stage of injury rehabilitation, when a joint is immobilized, the emphasis should be on cardiovascular fitness and isometric contractions. Exercising the opposite limb may evoke a crossover reaction and maintain the muscles of the opposite limb. Muscle stimulation is also frequently used at this stage.
4. **B.** Sport specific skills with progressively complex drills are incorporated during the final stage of rehabilitation. The exercises are designed to improve proprioception and co-ordination and it should be adapted to the specific needs of the athlete's particular position in a sport.
5. **D.** The amount of weight is fixed, and usually determined by the 'Sticking point' or weakest part of the range of motion of the lift. This means that, except for this point, the muscles moving the weight are working at below-maximum intensity and it is not constant.
6. **A.** Oxford technique is just opposite to delorme technique in which the weight is taken off rather than added on. This method is probably less effective and is seldom used in sports medicine.
7. **B.** Isokinetic exercise is made popular by cyber and the orthotron machines and the possible speed setting range from 0° per second to 300° per second. Strength is usually developed between 60° per second and 120° per second and power at 180° per second.
8. **D.** Controlled motion of injured tissue will influence their structure when they are healed. If the limb is completely immobilized during the recovery process, the tissue may heal

Chapter 5: Basic Concepts in Injury Rehabilitation

fully but poorly adapted functionally with little chance for change. Further controlled motion will make the adhesions to be flexible and thus allow tissue to move easily on each other.

9. **C.**
10. **C.** Zone of hypertrophied cells are the weakest part of the growth plate and are the area through which separation usually occurs in the event of an injury.
11. **D.**
12. **C.**
13. **A.** The inflammatory phase, generally lasting six days, represents body tissue's initial reaction to an injury—cellular injury results in changes in metabolism and the introduction of materials that initiate the inflammatory response. Signs of inflammation include redness, tenderness to touch, and increased temperature.
14. **B.** This healing and tissue repair process starts with a short period of tissue bleeding due to the disruption of small blood vessels and capillaries. Immediately following this bleeding period, a complex cascade of biochemical events proceeds, triggering an inflammatory reaction. The inflammatory process initiates the proliferation of new tissue cells, which eventually remodel to restore normal tissue function.
15. **D.** The primary injury is the damage to cells caused by the direct injury mechanism, be that a crush, contusion, or strain force. The cells damaged by this mechanical force may have their cell membranes disrupted, causing a loss in homeostasis and subsequent cell death. Many tissue types may also be involved, including ligament, tendon, muscle, nerve, and connective tissues.
16. **A.** PRICE is a mnemonic for the principal interventions commonly used in the immediate early stages following tissue injury. It stands for protection, rest, ice, compression, elevation.
17. **C.** One of the goals of physiotherapy during the tissue proliferation stage (phase 3) is to increase muscle strength and control.
18. **A.** If anyone injured their anterior talofibular ligament in their ankle, it will be necessary during the early stages to protect

this structure from stresses into inversion and plantarflexion while allowing eversion and dorsiflexion movements.

19. D. The application of cryotherapy enables more cells to survive the ischemic phase, thus minimizing secondary tissue damage. To maximize the therapeutic effects of cryotherapy, an optimal tissue temperature reduction of 10–15° is required, and it can reduce the number of cells damaged overall; the healing and repair process will be quicker, hence speeding up return to function.

20. D.

21. C.

22. D. Ultrasound, pulsed shortwave diathermy (PSWD), and laser therapy can influence the normal physiological processes of tissue repair, particularly the early inflammatory stage. This machine-generated energy is absorbed by the tissue (to varying degrees depending on the type), resulting in a change in one or more physiological events. It results from the energy being absorbed by the tissues resulting in a physiological shift, which is referred to as the therapeutic effect.

23. C. Ice massage is a form of cryotherapy most commonly used over small areas, such as a muscle belly or tendon. Usually, ice massages are often administered using ice cups. Due to the direct contact of the ice and the target area, 5–10 minutes is the typical treatment time.

24. B. The cooler water temperature should range from 12–20°C, while the warmer water temperature should range from 27–40°C.

25. B. The ratio of heat to cold when using a contrast bath is most commonly expressed as 3:1 or 4:1.

26. C. Raynaud's disease is a peripheral vascular disorder characterized by abnormal vasoconstriction of the extremities upon exposure to cold or emotional distress. Although Raynaud's disease can be considered a contraindication for selected forms of cryotherapy, it is not contraindicated for aquatic therapy.

27. B. The supraspinatus originates on the supraspinous fossa of the scapula and inserts on the greater tubercle of the humerus and it is innervated by suprascapular nerve.

Chapter 5: Basic Concepts in Injury Rehabilitation

28. **D.** The plan section of a S.O.A.P. note typically includes the frequency and expected duration of physical therapy services.
29. **D.** Educating the injured sportsperson about safe body mechanics is carried out during the chronic stage/return to function phase of tissue healing.
30. **B.** The grade 2 (second degree) tissue injury is characterized by moderate pain that requires stopping the activity. Stress and palpation of the tissue significantly increase the pain. When the injury is to ligaments, some of the fibers are torn, resulting in increased joint mobility.
31. **B.**
32. **D.** Complete or continuous immobilization should be avoided during the acute stage of tissue healing whenever possible as it can lead to adherence of the developing fibrils to surrounding tissue, weakening of connective tissue, and changes in articular cartilage.
33. **C.** Stretching and resistance exercises should not be performed at the site of the inflamed or swollen tissue during the acute stage of tissue healing. The intensity (dosage) of movement should be gentle enough, so the fibrils are not detached from the site of healing. Too much activity, too soon, is painful and reinjures the tissue
34. **D.** During the subacute phase of tissue healing, it is advisable to progress multiple-angle isometric exercises within the patient's tolerance; begin cautiously with mild resistance; initiate an active range of motion (AROM), protected weight-bearing, and stabilization exercises. As the range of motion (ROM), joint play, and healing improve, progress isotonic exercises with increased repetitions. Emphasize control of exercise patterns and proper mechanics. Progress resistance later in this subacute stage.
35. **C.** Exercise progressions may cause some temporary soreness that can last 4 hours. However, if exercise or activity pain comes on earlier or is increased over the previous session leading to increased stiffness and decreased ROM over several exercise sessions, those activities, exercise, or stretching maneuvers that are too stressful should be modified or reduced in intensity.

36. **C.** Eccentric and heavy-resistance exercises (such as PRE) may cause added trauma to muscle and are not used in the early subacute stage after muscle injury since the weak tensile quality of the healing tissue could be jeopardized.
37. **B.** Cross-fiber massage is used at the site of muscle scar tissue or tendon adhesions to gain scar tissue mobility. The intensity and duration of the technique are progressively increased as the tissue responds.
38. **D.** A repetitive strain injury (RSI) is an injury to part of the musculoskeletal or nervous system caused by repetitive use, vibrations, compression or long periods in a fixed position. Other common names include repetitive stress disorders, cumulative trauma disorders (CTDs), and overuse syndrome.
39. **D.** While returning to the chronic stage (i.e., functional stage) of tissue healing, emphasis is given to designing exercise drills that simulate the sports activities using a controlled environment with specific, progressive resistance and plyometric drills. As the player demonstrates capabilities, increase the repetitions and speed of the movement. Progression is made by changing the environment and introducing surprise and uncontrolled events into the activity.
40. **C.** Elevating leg rests promote patient comfort and stability when the wheelchair is in a reclined position.
41. **B.** Assistive devices can easily be adjusted to accommodate individuals of various height and weight.
42. **C.** The patient's goal of walking one mile each day does not warrant continued physical therapy services. Physical therapists should avoid overutilization of physical therapy services, however, should assist patients to achieve individual goals through activities, such as a home exercise program.
43. **D.** Gains in strength are greatest when a muscle is exercised against resistance at maximal intensity.
44. **D.** Discoloration of the patient's toes may be an indication that the cast is too tight and may be impeding the patient's circulation. Since the cast is bivalved, the cast can be easily removed by the physical therapist.

45. **B.** A three-point gait pattern can be used when a patient is able to bear weight on one lower extremity, but is nonweight bearing on the other. The gait pattern requires good upper extremity strength and the use of crutches or a walker. A swing-to gait pattern infers bilateral lower extremity weakness requiring the extremities to be advanced simultaneously.

Shoulder and Arm Injuries

1. What type of falling technique has to be adapted by the player in order to prevent shoulder injuries?
   A. Fall on outstretched arm
   B. Fall on the point of the shoulder
   C. Roll on the shoulder
   D. All of the above

2. Which type of tackling technique is more prone to cause shoulder dislocation?
   A. Arm is abducted and externally rotated
   B. Arm is adducted and internally rotated
   C. Arm is adducted and externally rotated
   D. Arm is abducted and internally rotated

3. What are the points to consider in order to prevent shoulder injuries?
   A. Falling techniques
   B. Shoulder pad placement
   C. Tackling technique
   D. All of the above

4. Which group of athletes is more prone for sternoclavicular joint sprain?
   A. Cricketers
   B. Wrestlers
   C. Tennis players
   D. Swimmers

5. What does it mean by shoulder pointer injury?
   A. Fracture of the shaft of the clavicle
   B. Osteolysis of the distal clavicle
   C. Acromioclavicular joint sprains
   D. Contusion to the outer end of the clavicle

6. What does it meant by shoulder separations?
   A. Acromioclavicular joint separations
   B. Sternoclavicular joint separations
   C. Glenohumeral dislocation
   D. Scapulothoracic joint separations

Chapter 6: Shoulder and Arm Injuries

7. **What is the commonest mechanism of injury for acromioclavicular joint sprains?**
   A. Falls on the point of the shoulder
   B. Roll over the shoulder
   C. Both A and B
   D. None of the above

8. **Which external device is used to immobilize the acromioclavicular joint?**
   A. Donut pad
   B. Figure of eight sling
   C. Kenny Howard sling
   D. U slab

9. **What are the complications of acromioclavicular joint sprain?**
   A. Spur formation
   B. Soft-tissue calcification
   C. Osteolysis of distal clavicle
   D. All of the above

10. **Which type of dislocation is common in glenohumeral joint?**
    A. Anterior dislocation
    B. Posterior dislocation
    C. Medial dislocation
    D. Lateral dislocation

11. **What is the mechanism of injury for anterior dislocation of shoulder?**
    A. Internal rotation, abduction
    B. External rotation, abduction
    C. Internal rotation, adduction
    D. External rotation, adduction

12. **How can we identify the anterior dislocation of shoulder by physical examination?**
    A. Arm is held with slight external rotation and abduction
    B. Arm is held in adduction and internal rotation
    C. Limited external rotation
    D. All of the above

13. **How can we identify posterior dislocation of shoulder by physical examination?**
    A. Arm is held with slight external rotation and abduction
    B. Limited internal rotation of the arm
    C. Arm is held in adduction and internal rotation
    D. All of the above

14. What defect is known as Bankart lesion in shoulder joint?
    A. Defect of posterolateral glenoid labrum
    B. Defect of anterior glenohumeral ligaments and glenoid labrum
    C. Defect of inferior glenoid labrum
    D. Defect of posteroinferior glenoid labrum
15. Which view of radiograph is good to identify the Hill-Sachs lesion?
    A. AP view in internal rotation
    B. AP view in external rotation
    C. West point modification of the axillary view
    D. Stryker notch view
16. Which is the common direction of getting sternoclavicular dislocation?
    A. Superior
    B. Posterior
    C. Anterior
    D. Inferior
17. Which is the commonest site of fracture of clavicle?
    A. Middle third
    B. Medial third
    C. Lateral third
    D. All of the above
18. What is the mechanism of injury in anterior sternoclavicular dislocation?
    A. Blow on the posterolateral aspect of the clavicle
    B. Blow on the anterolateral aspect of the clavicle
    C. Blow on the anterior aspect of the clavicle
    D. Blow on the posterior aspect of the clavicle
19. Which directional movement of acromion leads to acromioclavicular joint separation in a fall on to the lateral aspect of the shoulder?
    A. Downward, laterally and posteriorly relative to the clavicle
    B. Upward, laterally and posteriorly relative to the clavicle
    C. Upward, medially and anteriorly relative to the clavicle
    D. Downward, medially and anteriorly relative to the clavicle
20. Which are the methods of reduction of glenohumeral joint dislocation?

A. Modified hippocratic method
B. Hippocratic method
C. Kocher's maneuver
D. All of the above

21. **Where is the tender spot in the recurrent anterior subluxation of the shoulder?**
    A. Insertion/origin of transverse humeral ligament
    B. Insertion/origin of the inferior glenohumeral ligament
    C. Over the deltoid muscle
    D. Over the teres minor muscle insertion

22. **Which is the suitable mechanism in order to create a posterior dislocation of the glenohumeral joint?**
    A. Force drives the humeral head backward while the arm is in extension and internal rotation
    B. Force drives the humeral head backward while the arm is in extension and external rotation
    C. Force drives the humeral head backward while the arm is in flexion and internal rotation
    D. Force drives the humeral head backward while the arm is in abduction and external rotation

23. **Which are the reduction methods for posterior dislocation of the glenohumeral joint?**
    A. Longitudinal forward traction with the elbow bend
    B. Downward pressure on the humeral head
    C. Adduction of the arm, then external rotation followed by internal rotation
    D. All of the above

24. **Which tendon gets trapped in the impingement of the rotator cuff?**
    A. Supraspinatus   B. Infraspinatus
    C. Teres minor   D. Latissimus dorsi

25. **Which group of swimmers will get the vascular impairment of supraspinatus tendon?**
    A. Butterfly stroke   B. Back stroke
    C. Diving   D. Breast stroke

26. Snapping feeling of the shoulder will happen in which range for impingement syndrome?
    A. Abduction between 0°-30°
    B. Abduction between 70°-120°
    C. Abduction between 0°-60°
    D. Abduction between 120°-180°
27. In rotator cuff tear, which are the muscles possibly getting involved?
    A. Supraspinatus tendon
    B. Infraspinatus
    C. Tendon of the long head of biceps
    D. All of the above
28. Which is the common direction of getting subluxation of biceps tendon?
    A. Laterally
    B. Medially
    C. Anteriorly
    D. Superiorly
29. What are the causes of getting thoracic outlet syndrome?
    A. Compression of the neurovascular bundle between the inferior and middle scalene muscles
    B. Costoclavicular syndrome
    C. Compression under the pectoralis minor muscles
    D. All of the above
30. The athlete sitting with shoulder pulled backward and downward. The arm is in 30 degree of abduction and extension. Name the special test for thoracic outlet syndrome:
    A. Military brace test
    B. Allen's test
    C. Adson's test
    D. Hyper flexion-abduction test
31. Pendulum exercise in clockwise and counter clockwise, forward punch-pull back and shoulder shrugs are collectively known as:
    A. Codman's exercises
    B. Kerlan's shoulder exercises
    C. Elastic tubing exercises
    D. Hand exercises

Chapter 6: Shoulder and Arm Injuries

32. What is the meaning of "catch up" in abnormal scapular biomechanics?
    A. More distal links have to work at a higher level of activity to compensate for the loss of the proximally generated force.
    B. More proximal links have to work at a higher level of activity to compensate for the loss of the proximally generated force
    C. More proximal links have to work at a higher level of activity to compensate for the loss of the distally generated force.
    D. More distal links have to work at a higher level of activity to compensate for the loss of the distally generated force.
33. What is snapping scapula?
    A. Trapezius muscle weakness
    B. Serratus anterior weakness
    C. Scapulothoracic bursitis
    D. Nodule forms in the supraspinatus tendon
34. Who is credited with the first anatomic description of the rotator cuff tear?
    A. JG Smith   B. Wilk
    C. Andrews   D. Codman
35. Who has done the first surgical repair of the rotator cuff?
    A. Smith   B. Henry Pott
    C. Codman   D. Campbell
36. What are the causes of getting rotator cuff injuries?
    A. Outlet impingement
    B. Impingement secondary to Glenohumeral instability
    C. Abutment of the cuff tendon in the glenoid rim
    D. All of the above
37. In which position of arm, the supraspinatus tendon seems more hypovascular?
    A. Adduction   B. Abduction
    C. Flexion   D. Extension
38. What is sourcil sign?
    A. Anterior marginal tear of rotator cuff
    B. Inferior marginal tear of rotator cuff
    C. Sclerosis on the under surface of the acromion
    D. Sclerolysis of the under surface of the acromion

39. Who described the use of radio-opaque contrast for the detection of rotator cuff tears?
    A. Mc Miller   B. Willk
    C. Andrews   D. Lindblom
40. Who described anterior acrominoplasty?
    A. Neer   B. Paulow
    C. Bankart   D. Hill-Sach
41. Who reported posterior inferior glenoid lesion in the throwing athlete?
    A. Bankart   B. Bennett
    C. Hill-Sach   D. Paulow
42. Which are the structures that get involved in posterior inferior glenoid labrum lesion?
    A. Exostosis at the insertion of the long head of the triceps
    B. Laberal lesions of posterior inferior aspect
    C. Both exostosis at the insertion of the long head of the triceps and laberal lesions
    D. Laberal lesions and teres minor tear
43. Which is the best view of X-ray to identify the posterior inferior glenoid lesion?
    A. Bennett view   B. Anteroposterior view
    C. Axillary view   D. Posteroanterior view
44. Maximal external rotation of shoulder reaches in which phase of the pitching motion?
    A. Winding-up   B. Stride
    C. Arm-cocking   D. Follow-through
45. Range of motion of joints in the arm during arm cocking in pitchers are:
    A. Elbow flexion of 60°, arm external rotation of 90° and arm abduction of 30°
    B. Elbow flexion of 95°, arm external rotation of 170° and arm abduction of 94°
    C. Elbow flexion of 60°, arm external rotation of 170° and arm abduction of 94°
    D. Elbow flexion of 135°, arm external rotation of 90° and arm abduction of 30°

Chapter 6: Shoulder and Arm Injuries

46. Which muscle will work more in arm cocking phase?
    A. Serratus anterior   B. Infraspinatus
    C. Teres minor   D. Subscapularis
47. Repetitive injury of translation plus rotation to the anterosuperior labrum is referred as:
    A. Shoulder grinding factor   B. Codman paradox
    C. Painful arc   D. Shoulder steering
48. Which is the site of lateral laxity in divers shoulder?
    A. Anterolateral   B. Posterolateral
    C. Anterosuperior   D. Inferior
49. Which site of the labrum shows laxity in throwers?
    A. Posterosuperior labrum
    B. Posteroinferior labrum
    C. Anterosuperior glenoid labrum
    D. Anteroinferior glenoid labrum
50. Which are the muscles that will involve in rotator cuff tear of throwing shoulder?
    A. Supraspinatus   B. Infraspinatus
    C. Both A and B   D. Teres major
51. An extracapsular ossification of the posteroinferior glenoid in the older long time throwers is known as:
    A. Bennett's disease   B. Throwers exostosis
    C. Both A and B   D. Adhesive capsulitis
52. In footballers which site of the glenoid labrum is frequently injured?
    A. Posterior glenoid labrum   B. Anterior glenoid labrum
    C. Inferior glenoid labrum   D. Superior glenoid labrum
53. Superior labrum anterior to posterior (SLAP) injuries are common for which group of sports people?
    A. Footballers   B. Overhead athletes
    C. Skiers   D. Rowing
54. What is the mechanism of injury of anterior labrum?
    A. Shoulder abduction, flexion and external rotation
    B. Shoulder abduction, flexion and internal rotation
    C. Shoulder abduction, extension and internal rotation
    D. Shoulder abduction, extension and external rotation

55. In modified blocking techniques the elbow should be in:
    A. Full extension   B. Slight flexion
    C. Full flexion   D. All of the above
56. Which are the forces that lead to a superior labral lesion?
    A. Traction and compression
    B. Shear
    C. Rotational forces
    D. All of the above
57. Which nerve gets injured in anterior dislocation of shoulder?
    A. Median nerve   B. Ulnar nerve
    C. Both A and B   D. Axillary nerve
58. Which sports activity leads to injury of spinal accessory nerve commonly?
    A. Wrestling   B. Cricket
    C. Football   D. Skiers
59. Which nerve will get injured during the late cocking phase of the throwing motion?
    A. Spinal accessory   B. Long thoracic nerve
    C. Suprascapular nerve   D. Axillary nerve
60. During the deceleration phase of throwing, which joint gets more force?
    A. Glenohumeral joint   B. Radiohumeral joint
    C. Wrist   D. Ulnohumeral joint
61. What are the movements taking place in swimmer's shoulder:
    A. Abduction/forward flexion/internal rotation
    B. Abduction/forward flexion/external rotation
    C. Abduction/extension/internal rotation
    D. Abduction/extension/external rotation
62. In which position of shoulder, the vascular filling of the supraspinatus tendon is prevented?
    A. Shoulder abduction
    B. Shoulder adduction
    C. Shoulder external rotation
    D. Shoulder internal rotation
63. What is the most common type of anterior dislocation of the shoulder?

A. Subglenoid dislocation   B. Subclavicular dislocation
C. Intrathoracic dislocation   D. Subcoracoid dislocation

64. A 25-year-old male athlete is diagnosed with a first-degree acromioclavicular sprain. The injury occurred two days ago after being checked in to the boards while playing hockey. Which of the following would you not expect to be true during the initial examination?
    A. Increased elevation of the clavicular end of the acromion
    B. Inability to bring the arm completely across the chest
    C. Inability to fully abduct the arm throughout the full range of motion
    D. Point tenderness on palpation of the injury site

65. A patient diagnosed with right shoulder adhesive capsulitis is limited to 25 degrees of lateral rotation. Which mobilization technique would be indicated with this limitation?
    A. Lateral distraction and anterior glide
    B. Medial distraction and posterior glide
    C. Lateral distraction and posterior glide
    D. Medial distraction and inferior glide

66. Which progressive resistive exercise would function to strengthen the infraspinatus and teres minor?
    A. Extension of the shoulder with dumb bell weights
    B. Flexion of the shoulder with dumb bell weights
    C. Lateral rotation of the shoulder with elastic tubing
    D. Medial rotation of the shoulder with elastic tubing

67. A volleyball player is referred to physical therapy after sustaining a grade I acromioclavicular joint sprain. Common therapeutic management for this injury includes all of the following, *except*:
    A. Ice massage
    B. Progressive active range of motion
    C. Trapezius and deltoid strengthening
    D. Temporary immobilization

68. Posterior dislocation of the shoulder is considered acute if diagnosed with one of the following periods from injury?
    A. Within 8 weeks   B. Within 6 weeks
    C. Within 6 months   D. Within 12 weeks

69. Which one of the following injury mechanisms leads to acute posterior shoulder dislocation in athletes?
   A. Any dislocating force applied to the anterior aspect of the shoulder with the arm in the flexed, adducted, and internally rotated position
   B. Any dislocating force applied to the posterior aspect of the shoulder with the arm in the flexed, adducted, and internally rotated position
   C. Any dislocating force applied to the posterior aspect of the shoulder with the arm in the flexed, abducted, and externally rotated position
   D. Any dislocating force applied to the anterior aspect of the shoulder with the arm in the flexed, adducted, and externally rotated position.

70. The impaction fracture of anteromedial aspect of the humeral head following posterior SLAP is:
   A. Reverse Hill–Sachs lesion
   B. Reverse Bankart lesion
   C. Hill–Sachs lesion
   D. Kim lesion

71. The most commonly applied physical tests to detect posteroinferior instability of the glenohumeral joint is known as:
   A. Kim test
   B. Jerk test
   C. McMurray test
   D. Crank test

72. The most common site for the occurrence of fracture clavicle is:
   A. Medial end of the clavicle
   B. At the junction of middle and inner third of clavicle
   C. At the junction of middle and outer third of clavicle
   D. Lateral end of the clavicle

73. The type of direct event causing injury to acromioclavicular joint during sports is:
   A. Tackling
   B. Pulling
   C. A fall on the outstretched hand
   D. Loading the upper shoulder while someone lies on the sides

Chapter 6: Shoulder and Arm Injuries

74. According to Sage-Salvatore acromioclavicular (ACL) and coracoclavicular (CCL) ligaments injury classification, type II injury refers to:
    A. Both ACL and CCL ruptured, clavicle is displaced upwards
    B. Rupture of ACL, sprain of CCL
    C. Inferior dislocation with clavicle towards base of the neck
    D. Minor sprain to acromioclavicular ligaments
75. The etiology of glenoid labral injuries stems from which one of the following actions during volleyball sport?
    A. Repetitive overhead actions creating excessive inferior humeral traction forces
    B. During the cocking phase of throwing and pitching
    C. Both A and B
    D. None of the above
76. The most accurate description for the type IV 'superior labrum anterior to posterior' ('SLAP') lesion is:
    A. The labral attachment to the glenoid rim is firmly intact but evidence of degeneration is present.
    B. The superior biceps–labral complex attachment is subsequently detached from the glenoid rim.
    C. The superior labrum sustains a bucket-handle lesion extending into the biceps tendon with potential displacement into the joint.
    D. The superior labral meniscoid rim sustains a bucket handle lesion with potential displacement into the joint with intact biceps tendon and labral attachment.
77. A sports physiotherapist is devising an exercise program for an athlete diagnosed with anterior shoulder instability. Which of the following exercises must be either avoided or modified during the program?
    A. Shrugging
    B. Elbow-curl
    C. Push-up
    D. Weight bearing exercises
78. While treating patients with traumatic shoulder instability, the primary objective of early-stage physical therapy management is:
    A. Restore full joint mobility and increase glenohumeral joint strength and dynamic stability

B. Reduce joint pain and inflammation and promote healing through proper immobilization

C. Full restoration of strength, dynamic stability and proprioception

D. Maintain muscular endurance, strength, dynamic stability and functional range of motion

79. Which one of the following special tests is primarily developed to assess acromioclavicular joint pathology?
    A. O'Brien's test
    B. Neer's tests
    C. Spurling's test
    D. Hawkins-Kennedy

80. Which one of the following special tests are applied to determine a compromise in the rotator cuff function with a specific focus on supraspinatus muscle?
    A. Cross adduction test
    B. Resisted external rotation tests
    C. Empty can test
    D. Speed test

81. A physical therapist performs a manual muscle test on a patient with bilateral upper extremity weakness. The therapist should test the patient's scapular adductors with the patient positioned in:
    A. Prone   B. Side lying
    C. Standing   D. Supine

82. An athlete diagnosed with right bicipital tendinitis performs upper extremity resistance exercises using a piece of elastic tubing. What muscle is emphasized when laterally rotating the involved extremity against resistance?
    A. Pectoralis major   B. Teres major
    C. Subscapularis   D. Teres minor

83. During the palpation examination of an injured throwball player's shoulder joint, which of the following signs would indicate a suspected pathology needing further investigation?
    A. Muscle spasm   B. Tenderness
    C. Edema   D. All of the above

Chapter 6: Shoulder and Arm Injuries

84. While observing a patient from the lateral view through a theoretical 'plumb-line', the common observation of a forward head posture is:
    A. Chin pokes forward, upper cervical spine extension and the lower cervical spine flexion
    B. Chin pokes forward, upper cervical spine flexion and the lower cervical spine extension
    C. Chin pokes forward, lower cervical spine flexion and the upper cervical spine extension
    D. Chin pokes forward, lower cervical spine extension and the upper cervical spine flexion

85. A sports physiotherapist examines the functionality of individual muscles and the associated myofascial through muscle length tests. Which one of the following statements is true to attain accuracy in testing?
    A. Appropriately fixing the muscle insertion while allowing the proximal bone to move distally to decrease the muscle length
    B. Appropriately fixing the muscle origin while allowing the insertion bone to move distally to increase the muscle length
    C. Tightening the muscles at the insertion bone level
    D. Fixing the muscle both at the origin and insertion bone level while allowing insertion bone to move distally to increase the muscle length to increase the muscle length

86. A positive 'piano key sign test' of an injured athlete shoulder is the indicative of which one of the following pathologies?
    A. Sternoclavicular joint sprain
    B. Glenohumeral joint instability
    C. Acromioclavicular joint instability
    D. Rotator-cuff lesions

87. A physical therapist is examining a basketball player who complains of pain in his shoulder, and the application of the 'painful arc test' elicits pain during the outer range of abduction (i.e., around 170-180°). Which one of the following conditions that you suspect which warrant further investigation?
    A. Subacromial impingement
    B. Acromioclavicular joint pathology

C. Sternoclavicular joint pathology
D. Subacromial bursa pathology

88. A baseball pitcher is complaining of limitation in internally rotating his shoulder, and the examination reveals a tightness in the posteroinferior capsule of shoulder and an alteration in the position of the total arc of humeral rotation at 90° abduction of the shoulder. Which one of the following pathologies do you suspect?
    A. Glenohumeral internal rotation deficit
    B. Glenohumeral extension deficit
    C. Glenohumeral external rotation deficit
    D. Glenohumeral flexion deficit

89. During the acute management of sports-related musculoskeletal injuries, the acronym 'POLICE' stands for:
    A. Protection, observation, loading, ice compression, and elevation
    B. Protection, observation, leveraging, ice compression and elevation
    C. Protection, optimal loading, ice compression, and elevation
    D. Protection, optimal leveraging, ice compression, and elevation

90. A sport physiotherapist is planning a four-stage return-to-sport rehabilitation protocol to progress an athlete from the stage of acute symptom management to return to sporting activities. Which one of the following is the most ideal treatment technique to employ in the fourth stage of the rehabilitation?
    A. Restoration of movement through passive exercises
    B. Normalization of shoulder arthrokinematics
    C. Strengthening exercises
    D. Incorporating sports specific skills

91. A high school student is referred to with an acute anterior shoulder subluxation. Which one of the following is the classical conservative treatment suggestive of managing this patient during the acute stage?
    A. 3-6 weeks of immobilization with the arm rests on the body in internal rotation

Chapter 6: Shoulder and Arm Injuries

    B. 3-6 weeks of immobilization with the arm rests on the body in external rotation

    C. 3-6 weeks of immobilization with the arm rests on the body in neutral rotation

    D. Suggesting absolute bedrest without a brace

92. A 42-year-old javelin thrower with a 40-degree limitation in right shoulder flexion and a 35-degree limitation in lateral rotation is unable to perform a number of activities of daily living. Which activity would be the most difficult for the patient using the right upper extremity?

    A. Tucking in shirt   B. Combing hair
    C. Eating   D. Washing the left shoulder

93. A physical therapist treats a patient diagnosed with adhesive capsulitis with continuous ultrasound and mobilization. The patient has a significant range of motion deficits and has been unable to return to work as a physical education instructor. Which objective finding provides the best support from the current treatment regimen?

    A. A decrease in the patient's pain level using a visual analog scale

    B. Improved patient compliance with an established home exercise program

    C. A 10 degree increase in passive glenohumeral abduction range of motion

    D. A subjective report of warmth in the shoulder during and after ultrasound treatment

94. A patient positioned standing with their arm positioned at their side with 90 degrees of elbow flexion completes shoulder medial and lateral rotation exercises using a piece of elastic tubing. Which plane of the body is utilized with this activity?

    A. Coronal   B. Frontal
    C. Sagittal   D. Transverse

95. A physical therapist treats a 45-year-old female diagnosed with adhesive capsulitis. The therapist administers small amplitude, rhythmic oscillations at the limit of the available range of motion. This description best describes:

    A. Grade I oscillations   B. Grade II oscillations
    C. Grade III oscillations   D. Grade IV oscillations

ANSWERS

1. **C.**
2. **A.**
3. **D.** The athlete should learn not to fall over outstretched arm or the point of the shoulder, but rather to roll over so as to avoid the shock of impact. Shoulder dislocations are more frequently encountered through poor tackling technique; particularly the arm is abducted and externally rotated while trying to stop the ball carrier. The points which have to be considered in order to prevent the shoulder injuries are falling technique, shoulder pad placement, tackling technique, muscle development, warm-up techniques, throwing techniques, etc.
4. **B.** The most common injury to the sternoclavicular joint is sprain, which occurs particularly in such activities as football and wrestling.
5. **D.**
6. **A.**
7. **A.** The mechanism of injury includes the athlete falls on the point of the shoulder, falls on the outstretched, etc.
8. **C.** One of the best methods of immobilization of acromioclavicular joint is Kenny Howard sling.
9. **D.** The complication of Acromioclavicular joint injury includes pain, disability, decrease ROM, degeneration changes, soft tissue calcification, osteolysis, cosmetic deformity.
10. **A.**
11. **B.**
12. **A.** In anterior dislocation, arm is held with slight external rotation and abduction and the patient has difficulty with internal rotation of the arm.
13. **C.** In posterior dislocation, arm is held with adduction and internal rotation and patient has difficulty with external rotation.
14. **B.** Bankart's lesion is an injury involving the anterior glenohumeral ligaments and glenoid labrum, which become separated from the articular surface of the anterior glenoid neck during a traumatic anterior dislocation.

15. **D.** The west point modification of the axillary view can be obtained to look specifically for bony Bankart lesions, whereas the Stryker notch view can be obtained to look for humeral head or Hill-Sachs defects.
16. **C.** Overall anterior sternoclavicular dislocations occur three times more often than posterior dislocation.
17. **A.** Most clavicular fractures occur in the diaphysis or middle third whereas medial third fractures are exceedingly rare.
18. **B.** The medial clavicle will displace anteriorly with a blow to the anterolateral aspect of the shoulder, where as a posterior sternoclavicular dislocations occurs often a blow on the posterolateral shoulder.
19. **D.** Codman pointed out, the causes, the acromion to be driven downward, medially, and anteriorly relative to the clavicle.
20. **D.**
21. **B.** Tenderness may be found at the insertion of the inferior glenohumeral ligament anteriorly and origin of the ligament posteriorly.
22. **C.** The force drives the humeral head backward while the arm is in flexion (usually below 90°-0°) and internal rotation. The head slips out posteriorly and comes to rest under the acromion process.
23. **D.**
24. **A.** The lesion consists of the rotator cuff tendons (especially the supraspinatus tendon) and the tendon of the long head of the biceps being squeezed against the anterior edge of the acromion and the coracoacromial ligament.
25. **A.** In sports, such as swimming, particularly in the butterfly, where the swimmer is required to rotate the arm on the shoulder many hundreds, if not thousands of times a day, there may be interference with the blood supply to the supraspinatus tendon, leads to tendonitis.
26. **B.** Snapping feeling or sensation may occur when the arm is brought from an external to an internally rotated position or when the arm is abducted between 70° and 120°.
27. **D.** A rotator cuff tear results from an acute shoulder injury. It most frequently involves the supraspinatus tendon, but it may also includes the infraspinatus and the tendon of the long head of the biceps.

28. **B.** In its cause over the humeral head, the biceps tendon is angulated approximately 30° medially, so that tightening of the biceps together with external rotation of the arm tends to cause the tendon to bowstring toward the medial side. Most subluxation is though it to occur in the medial direction, but some cases of lateral subluxation has been noted.
29. **D.**
30. **A.**
31. **B.**
32. **A.** The kinetic chain is the most efficient system for developing appropriate energy and force to be delivered to the hand. The scapula and shoulder are pivoted links in the chain, funneling the force from the large segments, the legs and the trunk, to the smaller rapidly moving small segments of the arm. If the scapula does become deficient in motion or position, transmission of the large generated forces from the lower extremity to the upper extremity is impaired. This creates a deficiency in resultant maximum force that can be delivered to the hand or creates a situation of 'catch up' in which the more distal links have to work at a higher level of activity to compensate for the loss of the proximally generated force.
33. **C.** Scapulothoracic bursitis (snapping scapula) is demonstrated by painful crepitus or snapping over the superomedial or inferomedial borders. This usually occurs with arm abduction or scapular retraction.
34. **A.** JG Smith an English anatomist, is credited with the first anatomic discretion of a rotator cuff tear published in his report in the London Medical Gazette in 1834.
35. **C.** Codman is credited with performing the first surgical repair of the rotator cuff. He published the results of tendon repair in two patients in 1911.
36. **D.** Numerous etiologies have been proposed for rotator cuff injuries including outlet impingement, impingement secondary to glenohumeral instability, abutment of the cuff tendon in the glenoid rim, tensile load or shear injury to the tendon fibers and avascular zones within the tendon.
37. **B.** Rathbun and Macnab demonstrated a hypovascular zone in the loading edge of the supraspinatus tendon when the

Chapter 6: Shoulder and Arm Injuries

arm was abducted when compared with the adducted arm. This area corresponds to the critical zone where rotator cuff degeneration is most frequently seen.

38. **C.** In large and massive rotator cuff tears, sclerosis may be present on the under surface of the acromion called the sourcil sign.
39. **D.** Lindblom described the use of radio-opaque contrast for the detection of rotator cuff tears in 1939.
40. **A.** Classic treatment for the management of the impingement syndrome has been the anterior acrominoplasty as described by Neer in 1972.
41. **B.** In 1947, Bennett reported a posterior inferior glenoid lesion in the throwing athlete with posterior shoulder pain.
42. **C.** It is the lesion of labrum in association with exostosis at the insertion of the long head of the triceps.
43. **A.** The lesions of posterior inferior calcifications best visualized with a Bennett view of the shoulder. This view is taken in the anteroposterior plane with the arm abducted and externally rotated and the X-ray beam angle 5° cephalad.
44. **C.** In arm cocking, the shoulder abducted 90° and the elbow flexed 90°, maximal external rotation of the humerus reaches limits between 150 and 180°.
45. **B.** Average positions include elbow flexion of 95°, arm external rotation of 170° and arm abduction of 94° through motion analysis.
46. **A.** Electromyography of the early arm-cocking phase reveals that the trapezius and serratus anterior positions the glenoid through scapular protraction and upward rotation at 60% of maximal voluntary isometric contraction (MVIC).
47. **A.** Any force that shifts the humeral head to glenoid rim during internal rotation causes the humeral head to be reseated off-center thus impinging the labrum and eventually leading to labral tearing. This repetitive injury of translation plus rotation to the anterosuperior labrum is referred to as the "shoulder-grinding factor".
48. **D.** In diver's shoulder-shoulder is held in a position of maximal straight overhead forward flexion plus internal rotation. At dive entry, superior loading forces are great and subtle inferior capsular laxity develops.

49. A. Arthroscopic finding in throwers is partial tearing of the posterior supraspinatus and the anterior infraspinatus in conjunction with fraying of the posterosuperior glenoid labrum.
50. C. Rotator cuff tears in the throwing shoulder are usually partial, spanning from the mid supraspinatus to mid infraspinatus.
51. B. Throwers exostosis is an extracapsular ossification of the posteroinferior glenoid rarely seen except in older long time throwers. This condition was originally considered to be a traction osteophyte of the long head of the triceps.
52. A. Interior linemen in football appear to be the group at greatest risk for sustaining these injuries to the posterior glenoid labrum. Blocking technique that place the arm in a position of forward flexion and internal rotation with the elbows locked in extension appear to be responsible for most of these injuries.
53. B. SLAP injuries to the superior glenoid labrum are seen in both overhead throwing athletes and those involved in contact sports.
54. D. Movements that produce the combination of shoulder abduction, extension and external rotation generate forces that stress the anterior labrum and capsule and this is the typical position seen in traumatic anterior shoulder dislocation.
55. B. Modified blocking techniques that place the elbow in slight flexion may help prevent these injuries. By unlocking the elbow, the triceps and pectoralis musculature may absorb some of the load applied to the arm and reduce the sheer stress being transferred to the posterior labrum.
56. A. Most injuries to the superior glenoid labrum are produced by one of two mechanisms; traction and compression. Traction mechanism may occur suddenly and violently, such as during water skiing or as a result of repetitive overhead throwing motions. The compression mechanism that may be more common in contact sports typically results from a fall on the outstretched arm with the arm in a position of slight abduction and forward flexion.
57. D.

Chapter 6: Shoulder and Arm Injuries

58. **A.** Sports related spinal accessory nerve injuries have reportedly occurred in wrestling and hockey.
59. **C.** The mechanism of injury is due to the traction produced on the nerve during the late cocking phase of the throwing motion. This motion causes nerve entrapment at the spinoglenoid notch that result in isolated infraspinatus palsy.
60. **A.**
61. **B.**
62. **B.**
63. **D.**
64. **A.**
65. **A.**
66. **C.**
67. **D.** A grade I acromioclavicular sprain often results in point tenderness and mild discomfort during selected portions of shoulder range of motion. There is no deformity present with only mild stretching of the supporting ligaments. As a result, immobilization would not typically be warranted.
68. **B.** Posterior dislocation is considered acute if it has been diagnosed within six weeks from injury, whereas, after six months, it is considered chronic.
69. **A.** An acute posterior dislocation is the result of a force being applied to the anterior aspect of the shoulder with the arm to the side or through the long axis of flexed, adducted, and internally rotated arm. In both situations the dislocating force is directed posteriorly.
70. **A.** Reverse Hill–Sachs lesion, also called a McLaughlin lesion, is defined as an impaction fracture of anteromedial aspect of the humeral head following posterior dislocation of the humerus.
71. **A.** Kim test is a test to confirm the posterior instability/torn posterior or posteroinferior labrum. The therapist grasps the elbow with one hand and the scapular with the other and elevates the patient's arm to 90° of adduction and internal rotation with the patient seated. The arm is moved horizontally across the body. A sudden clunk indicates a positive result as the humeral head slides off the back of the

glenoid. When the arm is returned to the original position, a second jerk may be produced by the humeral head returning to the glenoid.

72. **C.** About 80% of the fracture clavicle occurs at the junction of middle and outer third.
73. **C.** An indirect force due to fall on the outstretched hands is the most common mechanism causing injury to acromioclavicular joint during sports.
74. **B.**
75. **C.** The etiology of labral injuries commonly stems from repetitive overhead actions creating excessive inferior humeral traction forces, particularly in volleyball serving or spiking, and in the cocking phase of throwing and pitching.
76. **C.**
77. **C.**
78. **B.** The early-stage management goals for traumatic shoulder instability aimed at reducing joint pain and inflammation and promote healing while protecting the damaged tissues and initiating the restoration of joint mobility and dynamic stability. These goals are achieved by initial immobilization using a simple sling, accompanied by isometric contractions of the dynamic stabilizers.
79. **A.** O'Brien's active compression test was primarily developed for the assessment of acromioclavicular joint pathology following a patient's demonstration of what reproduced their shoulder pain.
80. **C.** Empty can test: The arm is placed in 30° of flexion and abduction in the plane of the scapula with the elbow fully extended and thumb pointing down (empty can test) toward the floor. The patient is asked to raise the arm against resistance applied by the examiner over the forearm. If the arm flops down with pain, it is indicative of a rotator cuff tear.
81. **A.** Scapular adductors including the rhomboids, middle trapezius, and the lower trapezius are tested with the patient in a prone position.
82. **D.** The teres minor is a lateral rotator of the shoulder while the pectoralis major, teres major, and subscapularis are medial rotators of the shoulder.

Chapter 6: Shoulder and Arm Injuries

83. **D.** Palpating in an anteroposterior direction, the sports therapist should assess for and record any muscular spasm, tenderness, deformity, edema, or joint effusion around the musculoskeletal structures, which may indicate the pathological source.
84. **A.** A common observation is that of a forward head posture, where the chin pokes forward, the upper cervical spine extends and the lower cervical spine flexes. Postural deviations observed in forward head posture involve a downwardly rotated, anteriorly tilted and protracted scapula, leading to a reduction of the subacromial space during arm elevation.
85. **B.** Accuracy in muscle testing requires fixation of the origin while the insertion bone is moved distally to increase the muscle length.
86. **C.** A positive piano key sign 'test' is indicated by depression and elevation of the clavicle in response to the inferiorly directed pressure and its subsequent release, which may indicate acromioclavicular joint instability and/or coracoclavicular ligament sprain or separation.
87. **B.** During the application of 'painful arc test', if pain is experienced more in the outer range of abduction (around 170-180°), this may indicate pathology of the acromioclavicular joint, warranting further investigation.
88. **A.** 'GIRD' (glenohumeral internal rotation deficit) is commonly occurring in tennis players and baseball pitchers who experience a notable loss in degrees of glenohumeral internal rotation of the throwing shoulder compared with the non-throwing shoulder and it is caused by posteroinferior capsular tightness.
89. **C.** 'POLICE' is an acronym that stands for protection, optimal loading, ice compression, and elevation. It promotes and guides safe and effective loading in acute soft tissue injury management.
90. **D.** The return to sports phases generally focuses on incorporating sport-specific drills. Sport specific training is simply fitness and performance training designed specifically for athletic performance enhancement.

91. **A.** The typical conservative treatment for managing acute anterior shoulder subluxation includes 3-6 weeks of immobilization in which the arm rests on the body in internal rotation.
92. **B.** A patient requires 30-70 degrees of horizontal adduction, 105-120 degrees of abduction, and 90 degrees of lateral rotation to independently comb their hair.
93. **C.** Continuous ultrasound can be used to increase periarticular extensibility in a patient diagnosed with adhesive capsulitis. A 10 degree increase in passive glenohumeral abduction range of motion following ultrasound application and mobilization demonstrates that the patient is making objective progress.
94. **D.** The transverse plane is horizontal and divides the body into upper and lower portions. Medial and lateral rotation occur in the transverse plane around a vertical axis.
95. **D.** Grade IV oscillations are used primarily as stretching maneuvers.

CHAPTER 7

Elbow Injuries

1. What type of loading in the elbow leads to lateral tennis elbow?
    A. Eccentric
    B. Concentric
    C. Isometric
    D. All of the above
2. In which muscle may locate pain in lateral tennis elbow?
    A. Extensor carpi radialis longus
    B. Extensor carpi radialis brevis
    C. Supinator
    D. Palmaris longus
3. In posterior tennis elbow which muscle gets affected?
    A. Flexor carpi radialis origin
    B. Pronator teres origin
    C. Triceps insertion
    D. Anconeus insertion
4. Why throwing athletes develop medial epicondylitis?
    A. Distraction
    B. Compression
    C. Varus stress
    D. Valgus stress
5. In golfers, which type of tendinosis can we expect?
    A. Medial tendinosis of the dominant elbow and lateral tendinosis of the nondominant elbow
    B. Lateral tendinosis of the dominant elbow and medial tendinosis of the nondominant elbow
    C. Medial tendinosis of both elbows
    D. Lateral tendinosis of both elbows
6. Which intrinsic risk factor leads to over use injury?
    A. Training errors
    B. Inflexibility and instability
    C. Poor technique
    D. Bad equipment
7. The condition where it is predisposed to the development of overuse injuries with complaints of multiple sites of tendon degeneration and pain, often without an impressive history of overuse is known as?
    A. Miliary syndrome
    B. Metastatic syndrome
    C. Mesenchymal syndrome
    D. None of the above

8. What can we suspect if point of maximum tenderness is distal to the level of radial head?
   A. Involvement of ECRB along with EDC
   B. Lateral epicondylitis
   C. Anterior interosseous nerve entrapment
   D. Posterior interosseous nerve entrapment
9. The point of maximum tenderness for the radial tunnel syndrome is at?
   A. Proximal edge of the supinator
   B. Underneath the mobile wad of Henry
   C. Approximately 4 to 5 cm distal to the lateral epicondyle
   D. All of the above
10. Medial tennis elbow usually represents which muscle involvement?
    A. Pronator teres
    B. Flexor carpi radialis
    C. Both A and B
    D. Flexor sublimus
11. Which one is the differential diagnosis for medial elbow pain?
    A. MCL injury
    B. Ulnar neuropathy
    C. Snapping medial triceps tendon
    D. All of the above
12. The anterior band of MCL is best palpated in which position of elbow?
    A. 30°-60° flexion
    B. 135° flexion
    C. 60°-90° flexion
    D. 10°-20° flexion
13. What is the cause of getting posterior tennis elbow?
    A. Chronic hyperextension overload
    B. Chronic valgus laxity
    C. Chronic flexion overload
    D. Chronic varus laxity
14. Positive provocative supinator testing suggests?
    A. Lateral tennis elbow
    B. Medial tennis elbow
    C. Radial tunnel syndrome
    D. Both A and C

15. Which activity should be avoided during treatment in patients with medial tennis elbow?
    A. Grasping or lifting with both supination and pronation of forearm
    B. Grasping or lifting with forearm pronated
    C. Grasping or lifting with forearm supinated
    D. All of the above
16. What is the use of providing larger racquet grip for tennis player?
    A. Greater the palmar flexion of the wrist and the less tension on the origin of forearm extensor muscle
    B. Lesser the dorsiflexion of the wrist and the less tension on the origin of forearm extensor muscle
    C. Greater the dorsiflexion of the wrist and the less tension on the origin of forearm extensor muscle
    D. None of the above
17. How will you measure the working length of the hand in tennis player?
    A. Proximal palmar crease to the tip of the middle digit's radial border
    B. Distal palmar crease to the tip of the middle digit's radial border
    C. Distal palmar crease to the tip of the ring digit's radial border
    D. Proximal palmar crease to the tip of the ring digit's radial border
18. In off-center impaction of tennis which muscle group is more prone for injury?
    A. Extensors of forearm
    B. Flexors of forearm
    C. Shoulder flexors
    D. Shoulder abductors
19. Which of the following technical factors has to be advised for a tennis player in order to avoid tennis elbow?
    A. Mid-sized graphite composite light weight racket
    B. Looser strings
    C. Strings of smaller gauge
    D. All of the above

20. What is the influence of counterforce bracing in order to prevent stress on tendons and muscle?
    A. Prevent full muscular expansion there by not allowing a maximal contraction
    B. Decreases intrinsic muscular forces to the muscles injured tendinous origin
    C. Helps to decrease elbow angular acceleration
    D. All of the above
21. In which phase of throwing motion, there are tremendous forces generated in the elbow?
    A. Deceleration phase   B. Acceleration phase
    C. Cocking   D. Wind-up
22. These are the phases of throwing motion, *except*:
    A. Wind-up   B. Cocking
    C. Acceleration   D. Mid-swing
23. What is the clinical phrase coined to explain the injuries including medial tension injuries, lateral compression injuries and posterior elbow impaction injuries in throwing motion?
    A. Varus extension overload
    B. Valgus extension overload
    C. Varus flexion overload
    D. Valgus flexion overload
24. Medial tension injuries of elbow occur in which group of people?
    A. Gymnastics   B. Baseball pitchers
    C. Skiers   D. Football players
25. Which ligament is the main stabilizer in order to prevent medial tension injuries?
    A. Transverse band of the ulnar collateral ligament
    B. Posterior band of the ulnar collateral ligament
    C. Anterior band of the ulnar collateral ligament
    D. Fibers of lateral collateral ligament
26. Which phase of throwing motion is more prone for posterior impaction injuries?
    A. Wind-up   B. Cocking up
    C. Acceleration phase   D. Deceleration phase

27. Which type of dislocation is common in elbow joint?
    A. Posterolateral dislocation   B. Posteromedial
    C. Direct lateral   D. Anterior dislocation
28. The term valgus extension overload refers to:
    A. Lateral tension injuries
    B. Anterior impingement injuries
    C. Posterior impingement injuries
    D. Medial impingement injuries
29. What is the pathoanatomy of valgus extension overload?
    A. Osteophyte formation   B. Loose bodies
    C. Articular cartilage defect   D. All of the above
30. In ulnar collateral ligament injury the most painful phase of throwing is:
    A. Wind-up   B. Cocking up
    C. Acceleration   D. Deceleration
31. If the radiographic findings include medial epicondylar enlargement, fragmentation, breaking and separation of the medial epicondyle in response to excessive throwing, the condition is known as:
    A. Little league elbow   B. Medial traction apophysitis
    C. Both A and B   D. Avulsion fracture
32. Who described the osteochondritis of the capitulum first?
    A. Woodward   B. Bianco
    C. Panner   D. Palmer
33. Which type of contracture is common in elbow?
    A. Extension   B. Flexion
    C. Valgus   D. Varus
34. Nonseptic olecranon bursitis is seen commonly in which type of sports people?
    A. Basketball player   B. Skiers
    C. Tennis players   D. Football linemen
35. Name the tunnel formed by fibrous tissue where the ulnar nerve passes through the intermuscular septum and it enters the posterior compartment:
    A. Ligament of Ansari   B. Lacertus fibrous
    C. Arcade of Struthers   D. All of the above

36. What are the causes of getting ulnar neuropathy?
    A. Subluxation of the nerve   B. Ganglion
    C. Rheumatoid arthritis   D. Osteoarthritis
    E. All of the above
37. Which type of athletes is more prone for ulnar nerve injury?
    A. Throwing athletes   B. Football players
    C. Cross-country skiing   D. Badminton players
38. Pronator syndrome occurs in which type of sports people?
    A. Weight lifters   B. Gymnastics
    C. Racquet sports   D. All of the above
39. In pronator syndrome, where does the median nerve gets compressed?
    A. Between the ligament of Struthers and fibrous band of flexor digitorum superficialis
    B. At the level of lacertus fibrous
    C. Intramuscular course through the pronator teres
    D. All of the above
40. Which one among these is a pure motor neuropathy?
    A. Anterior interosseous syndrome
    B. Pronator syndrome
    C. Both A and B
    D. Radial tunnel syndrome
41. Name the anastomosis in which the ulnar nerve combines with the anterior interosseous nerve?
    A. Blalock   B. Tausing
    C. Martin Grueber   D. Morris
42. In which position the pronator quadratus can be tested in order to identify its isolated function?
    A. Elbow fully flexed   B. Elbow fully extended
    C. Elbow at 90° flexion   D. All of the above
43. Sites of compression of posterior interosseous nerve include:
    A. Vascular leash of Henry
    B. Extensor carpi radialis brevis
    C. Archade of Froshe
    D. All of the above

44. What structures at the elbow are most susceptible to injury in the throwing athlete?
    A. Lateral collateral ligament
    B. Extensor carpi radialis longus and brevis
    C. Anterior oblique medial collateral ligament
    D. Pronator teres
45. An osteochondral focal lesion that commonly involves the capitulum humeri with the highest incidence between 10 to 15 years is termed as:
    A. Osteoarthritis   B. Septic arthritis
    C. Osteochondral fractures   D. Osteochondritis dissecans
46. Name the injury that causes Panner's elbow in 5–10 years aged children playing sports such as baseball and throwing.
    A. Lateral compression   B. Medial compression
    C. Anterior compression   D. Posterior compression
47. Which of the following sports activities often lead to the Humeral-olecranon conflict?
    A. Volleyball   B. Baseball
    C. Javelin throw   D. All of the above
48. Anterior coronoid humeral conflict is most frequently seen in sportspersons such as:
    A. Rugby players   B. Weight lifters
    C. Football players   D. Both A and B
49. In weight lifters, name the condition that occurs due to the repeated flexion and traction mechanism leading to the osteophyte and loose bodies formation on the coronoid process and humeral coronoid fossa.
    A. Humeral-olecranon conflict
    B. Anterior coronoid humeral conflict
    C. Radial head fracture
    D. Coronoid process fracture
50. Throwers having a hypertrophied forearm flexor mass (attached to the medial epicondyle) compress _____ nerve during muscle contraction.
    A. Radial nerve   B. Median nerve
    C. Ulnar nerve   D. Posterior interosseous nerve

51. **Name the test used to evaluate the posterolateral rotatory instability (PLRI) of the elbow joint.**
    A. Lateral pivot-shift test
    B. Cozen test
    C. Mill's test
    D. Golfer's elbow test

52. **Name the apprehension sign observed in cases with posterolateral rotary instability of the elbow joint.**
    A. Posterior impingement sign
    B. Chair sign
    C. Push-up sign
    D. Both B and C

53. **What are the provocative maneuvers used to examine the valgus stability of the elbow joint?**
    A. Static valgus stress test
    B. Moving valgus stress test
    C. Milk test
    D. All of the above

54. **Which kind of sports persons experience olecranon stress fractures resulting from repetitive microtrauma caused by olecranon impingement or excessive triceps tensile stress?**
    A. Football players
    B. Throwing athletes
    C. Runners
    D. Hockey players

55. **Which of the following factors causes lateral epicondylitis among tennis players?**
    A. Too small grip
    B. String tension
    C. Poor racquet dampening
    D. All of the above

56. **A "late" mechanically poor backhand in tennis players leads to:**
    A. Lateral epicondylitis
    B. Medial epicondylitis
    C. Cubital tunnel syndrome
    D. None of the above

57. **What advice can be given for the tennis players experiencing tennis elbow?**
    A. Reduce string tension
    B. Use large grip size
    C. Use a better dampening racquet
    D. All of the above

Chapter 7: Elbow Injuries

58. Identify the brace used in the treatment of tennis elbow:
    A. Lateral counterforce brace (tennis elbow strap)
    B. Wrist splint
    C. Both A and B
    D. Elbow extension splint
59. Choose the special tests used to assess the tennis elbow:
    A. Mill's test   B. Cozen's test
    C. Both A and B   D. Wartenberg's sign
60. Name the type of stretching used for treating the elbow flexion contracture in throwing athletes.
    A. High-intensity, short-duration stretching
    B. Low-load long-duration stretching
    C. Ballistic stretching
    D. None of the above
61. High-intensity, short-duration stretching is contraindicated in treating the limited elbow range of motion as it may lead to:
    A. Elbow laxity   B. Ulnar nerve injury
    C. Myositis ossificans D. None of the above
62. Name the other terms for medial epicondylitis.
    A. Flexor-pronator tendinitis
    B. Golfer's elbow
    C. Pitcher's elbow
    D. All of the above
63. Name the muscles that need to be strengthened to prevent the tennis elbow.
    A. Extensor carpi radialis longus
    B. Extensor carpi radialis brevis
    C. Supinator
    D. All of the above
64. What are the manual therapy techniques used in the management of tennis elbow?
    A. Mulligan's mobilization with movement (lateral glide)
    B. Mills manipulation
    C. Both A and B
    D. Eccentric exercises for wrist flexors

65. Name the muscles that need to be strengthened to minimize the valgus stress on the elbow during the throwing motion.
    A. Biceps
    B. Wrist flexors
    C. Pronators
    D. All of the above
66. Name the clinical condition in which "Pouring coffee from a pot with an extended elbow" is a typical pain-provoking daily life activity.
    A. Medial epicondylitis
    B. Students' elbow
    C. Tennis elbow
    D. Little league elbow
67. Name the clinical condition which characterizes pain during resisted flexion and pronation of the wrist with elbow extension.
    A. Lateral epicondylitis
    B. Golfer's elbow
    C. Nursemaid's elbow
    D. Baker's elbow
68. What are the physiotherapy treatment methods that used to reduce the force elicited from the common extensor origin?
    A. Taping
    B. Orthosis
    C. Both A and B
    D. Ultrasound therapy
69. Mention the muscle which can be tested by applying resistance to the third metacarpal bone with elbow fully flexed position.
    A. Extensor carpi radialis brevis
    B. Extensor carpi radialis longus
    C. Extensor carpi ulnaris
    D. Extensor pollicis longus
70. Name the muscle which can be tested by applying resistance to the second metacarpal bone with 30° elbow flexed position?
    A. Extensor carpi radialis brevis
    B. Extensor carpi radialis longus
    C. Extensor carpi ulnaris
    D. Extensor pollicis longus
71. Which muscle needs to be strengthened in patients diagnosed to have ulnar collateral ligament injury of the elbow?

A. Extensor carpi radialis longus
B. Flexor carpi ulnaris
C. Flexor digitorum superficialis
D. Both B and C

72. Name the deep heat physiotherapeutic modality used in the management of lateral epicondylitis.
    A. Ultrasound therapy
    B. Cryotherapy
    C. Hot packs
    D. Infrared radiation

73. Which of the following muscles provide the dynamic stability against valgus stress of the elbow?
    A. Flexor digitorum superficialis
    B. Flexor carpi ulnaris
    C. Palmaris longus
    D. All of the above

74. The inflammation of the subcutaneous bursa overlying the olecranon process between the skin and the triceps tendon is termed as:
    A. Olecranon bursitis
    B. Student's elbow
    C. Both A and B
    D. Tennis elbow

75. The "return-to-sport" stage of management of tennis elbow (extensor tendinopathy) typically includes:
    A. Plyometrics
    B. Agility
    C. Sports skills practice
    D. All of the above

76. Name the sports movement pattern commonly associated with flexor tendinopathy related to the common flexor origin at the medial epicondyle.
    A. Backhand stroke
    B. Forceful kick
    C. Baseball pitch
    D. None of the above

77. A 21-year-old cricket player rehabilitating from a radial head fracture is examined in physical therapy. During the examination, the physical therapist notes that the player appears to have an elbow flexion contracture. Which of the following would not serve as an appropriate active exercise technique to increase range of motion?
    A. Contract-relax
    B. Hold-relax
    C. Maintained pressure
    D. Rhythmic stabilization

78. Formula one care racer suffers a chemical burn on the cubital area of the elbow. Which position would be the most appropriate for splinting of the involved upper extremity?
    A. Elbow flexion and forearm pronation
    B. Elbow flexion and forearm supination
    C. Elbow extension and forearm pronation
    D. Elbow extension and forearm supination
79. On examination, the therapist identifies excessive medial displacement of the elbow during ligamentous testing. Which ligament is typically involved with medial instability of the elbow?
    A. Annular
    B. Radial collateral
    C. Ulnar collateral
    D. Volar radioulnar
80. A physical therapist examines a gulf player referred to physical therapy with olecranon bursitis. During the initial examination, the therapist identifies diffuse swelling in the elbow joint. Which of the following joints would be affected with swelling in the elbow complex?
    A. Ulnohumeral joint
    B. Ulnohumeral and radiohumeral joints
    C. Radiohumeral and proximal radioulnar joints
    D. Ulnohumeral, radiohumeral, and proximal radioulnar joints
81. A sports physical therapist performs goniometric measurements for elbow flexion with a tennis player in supine. In order to isolate elbow flexion, the therapist should stabilize the:
    A. Distal end of the humerus
    B. Proximal end of the humerus
    C. Distal end of the ulna
    D. Proximal end of the radius
82. A 23-year-old male athlete is seen in physical therapy with a complaint of pain and soreness in his elbow. When applying ultrasound for vigorous heating to the extensor carpi radialis brevis, the therapist should direct the ultrasound energy to the:

A. Anterior aspect of the elbow
B. Medial aspect of the elbow
C. Lateral aspect of the elbow
D. Posterior aspect of the elbow

83. A 21-year-old male was playing rugby when he sustained an injury to his right elbow during a fall. The patient states that his arm was outstretched to break the fall when another player fell into his elbow. He presents with marked edema along the medial aspect of the elbow and a 15-degree carrying angle. Which of the following structures would MOST likely be involved?
    A. Annular ligament
    B. Ulnar collateral ligament
    C. Radial collateral ligament
    D. Biceps brachii

84. A physical therapist completes a dorsal glide of the humeroradial articulation with a patient in supine. When performing this mobilization technique, the therapist should stabilize the:
    A. Distal humerus from the lateral side of the patient's arm
    B. Distal humerus from the medial side of the patient's arm
    C. Proximal humerus from the lateral side of the patient's arm
    D. Proximal humerus from the medial side of the patient's arm

85. A physical therapist records the end-feel associated with forearm supination as firm in the medical record. Which of the following is not consistent with an end-feel categorized as 'firm'?
    A. Muscular stretch
    B. Capsular stretch
    C. Soft tissue approximation
    D. Ligamentous stretch

ANSWERS

1. **A.** Eccentric loading of the lateral elbow tendons include racquet sports, throwing sports and swimming in addition to occupational activities that require stressful forearm use such as carpentry, plumbing, and textile production leads to lateral tennis elbow.
2. **B.**
3. **C.** Medial tennis elbow typically presents with pain over the flexor pronator mass and posterior tennis elbow with pain over the triceps insertion.
4. **D.** Throwing athletes tend to develop medial tendinosis (epicondylitis) because of the valgus stress experienced.
5. **A.**
6. **B.** Intrinsic risk factors relate to biomechanical abnormalities that are specific to the individual patient. These include deconditioning, weakness, inflexibility and instability and overall less durable collagen framework. Extrinsic risk factors are related to the stress applied to the arm and include training errors, poor technique, bad equipment or a poor work environment.
7. **C.** There may be a subset of people particularly predisposed to the development of overuse injuries. This patient complains of multiple sites of tendon degeneration and pain, often without an impressive history of overuse. The term mesenchymal syndrome is used to describe them. Routine laboratory and rheumatologic screening tests are characteristically normal.
8. **D.** If point of maximum tenderness is distal to the level of radial head, posterior interosseous nerve entrapment (radial tunnel syndrome) should be suspected.
9. **D.** The point of maximum tenderness for the radial tunnel syndrome is at the proximal edge of the supinator, underneath the mobile wad of Henry, approximately 4–5 cm distal to the lateral epicondyle.
10. **C.** Medial tennis elbow usually represents tendinosis of the pronator teres and flexor carpi radialis.
11. **D.** The differential diagnosis of medial elbow pain includes injury to the medial collateral ligament, ulnar neuropathy,

cubital tunnel syndrome and a snapping medial triceps tendon.
12. **A.** The anterior band of the MCL (it is the most significant structural component) is best palpable with the elbow gently flexed 30° to 60°.
13. **A.** Chronic hyperextension overload leads to posterior tennis elbow, such as throwing athletes.
14. **D.** Provocative supinator testing elicits symptoms of radial tunnel syndrome. Pain on supination may also be present in lateral tennis elbow but without tenderness over the nerve.
15. **B.** Grasping or lifting with the forearm pronated (palms down) should be avoided and the patient should be shown how to lift with the forearm supinated.
16. **C.** The larger the grip that is used, the greater the dorsiflexion of the wrist and the less tension on the origin of the forearm extensor muscle.
17. **D.** The circumstances of the racquet handle should correspond to the working length of the hand. This is the distance from the proximal palmar crease to the tip of the ring digit, measured along the ring digits radial border.
18. **A.** Off-center impaction has been shown to cause increased electromyography activity in the forearm extensors and may contribute to the formation of tennis elbow.
19. **D.** A clinical observation is that, a midsized graphite composite light-weight racquet offers the best protection. Looser stringing increases the dwell time of the ball on the racquet, thus decreasing the shock that must be absorbed by the arm. Strings of smaller gauge have more "give" than thicker ones, so a player with tennis elbow may be advised not to use a string any thicker than 1.3 mm.
20. **D.** The major mechanism of braces action is to prevent full muscular expansion, there by not allowing a maximum contraction. This decreases intrinsic muscular forces to the muscles injured tendinous origin. Counterforce bracing has been shown to decrease elbow angular acceleration and decrease electromyographic activity of the forearm muscles in players of all skill levels for both one handed back hand, without a concomitant decrease in strength output.

21. **B.** During the acceleration phase of the throwing motion, tremendous forces are generated in the elbow. The elbow is placed in an extreme valgus position which generates tremendous tensile force across the medial elbow and compensatory forces laterally.
22. **D.** The throwing motion is divided into five basic phases: wind-up, cocking, acceleration, deceleration and follow through.
23. **B.** Valgus extension overload is the clinical phrase coined to explain the injuries that occur during the throwing motion. These injuries include medial tension injuries, lateral compression injuries and posterior elbow impaction injuries.
24. **B.** Medial tension injuries are the result of the valgus stress across the medial elbow during the throwing motion. These occur mainly during the arm cocking and acceleration phase, but there is also some valgus stress during the deceleration phase. It occurs in Baseball pitchers.
25. **C.** The main stabilizer of valgus stress is the anterior band of the ulnar collateral ligament.
26. **D.** Posterior impaction injuries occur primarily during the deceleration phase of throwing, at which time the elbow experiences both extension and valgus forces that result in the olecranon impacting against the posteromedial humerus.
27. **A.** The mechanism of an elbow dislocation is usually a fall on the outstretched arm, with a hyperextension load to the elbow with either a valgus or varus force, resulting in the more common posterolateral dislocation.
28. **C.** Valgus extension overload is a term that refers posterior impingement overload.
29. **D.** The extension force results in osteophyte formation at the tip of olecranon with fibrous tissue deposition in the olecranon fossa. Loose bodies may form and with continued abutment of the olecranon tip against the humeral fossa with a valgus load, posteromedial osteophyte forms on the olecranon, with an articular cartilage defect on the humerus as a result of continued impingement.
30. **B.** The athlete complains of medial elbow pain often this will only be symptomatic with this force of throwing and is most

painful during the cocking portion of the throw where the maximum stress is placed across the ligament.
31. **A.** Little league elbow was described in term of radiographic findings, including medial epicondylar enlargement, fragmentation, breaking and separation of the medial epicondyle in response to excessive throwing. It is also referred to as medial epicondylitis or a medial traction apophysitis.
32. **C.** Panner first described osteochondritis of the capitulum in 1929.
33. **B.**
34. **D.** Nonseptic bursitis is thought to be the result of repetitive microtrauma. It is often seen in football linemen and hockey players.
35. **C.** In the distal arm, the ulnar nerve passes through the intermuscular septum where it enters the posterior compartment. The fibrous tissue forming the tunnel through the septum is called the Arcade of Struthers.
36. **E.** Causes of the ulnar neuropathy include subluxation of the nerve, a ganglion, ancones epitrochlearis muscle, rheumatoid arthritis or osteoarthritis.
37. **A.** Athletic injuries to the ulnar nerve are most common in throwing athletes.
38. **D.** Pronator syndrome may occur in grasping sports due to repetitive stress such as weight lifting, gymnastics or racquet sports.
39. **D.** The compression of the median nerve occurs between the ligament of Struthers and the fibrous band where the nerve runs deep to the flexor digitorum superficialis. The nerve may also be compressed at the level of lacertus fibrous or the intramuscular course through the pronator teres.
40. **A.** Anterior interosseous syndrome is a pure motor neuropathy of the muscles supplied by the anterior interosseous nerve.
41. **C.** If a Martin Grueber anastomosis is present in which the ulnar nerve combines with the anterior interosseous nerve, then the ulnar intrinsic and the flexor digitorum profundus to the other fingers may be involved.

42. **A.** Pronator quadratus strength can be tested by fully flexing the elbow and comparing pronation strength to the uninvolved side. Elbow flexion removes the pronator teres and fully isolates the pronator quadratus.
43. **D.** Sites of compression of radial tunnel syndrome include fibrous bands at the radiocapitular joint, the vascular leash of Henry, extensor carpi radialis brevis, the arcade of Frohse and the distal supinator.
44. **C.**
45. **D.** Osteochondritis dissecans is represented by an osteochondral focal lesion that generally involves the capitulum humeri and with the greatest incidence between 10 and 15 years.
46. **A.** Panner's disease is due to the lesion from lateral elbow compression, characteristic of children practicing sports like baseball and throwing.
47. **D.** Humeral-olecranon conflict is most frequently seen in throwing sports, such as volleyball, handball, baseball, javelin, etc.
48. **D.** Anterior coronoid humeral conflict is most frequently seen in the population of rugby players, fighters, weight lifters (lifting sports).
49. **B.** In anterior coronoid humeral conflict, the repeated flexion and traction mechanism typical of lifting in the long-term could lead to the osteophyte and loose bodies formation on the coronoid process and at the level of the humeral coronoid fossa.
50. **C.** Throwers often having a hypertrophied forearm flexor mass (attached to the medial epicondyle) that compresses the ulnar nerve during muscle contraction.
51. **A.** The posterolateral rotatory instability test of the elbow is also known as the lateral pivot-shift test. It is described as the most sensitive examination technique for diagnosing posterolateral rotatory instability.
52. **D.** Two active apprehension signs of posterolateral rotatory instability of the elbow joint are chair sign and push-up sign.
53. **D.** Provocative maneuvers to assess the valgus stability are static valgus stress test, moving valgus stress test, and milk test.

54. **B.** Olecranon stress fractures in throwing athletes may occur due to repetitive microtrauma caused by olecranon impingement or excessive triceps tensile stress.
55. **D.** The contributing factors of lateral epicondylitis include incorrect grip size, string tension, poor racquet "dampening," and underlying weak muscles of the shoulder, elbow, and arm. Tennis grips that are too small often exacerbate or cause tennis elbow.
56. **A.** The most common cause of tennis elbow/lateral epicondylitis in tennis players is a "late," mechanically poor backhand that places excess force across the extensor wad; that is, the elbow "leads" the arm.
57. **D.** Tennis players may reduce racquet string tension, change the size of the grip (usually to a larger grip), and change to a better dampening racquet.
58. **C.** Lateral counterforce brace for elbow (lateral epicondylitis). Place the brace two fingerbreadths distal to the lateral epicondyle (snug). Some authors recommend 6–8 weeks' use of a wrist splint positioned in 45° of dorsiflexion.
59. **C.** Cozen's test and Mill's test are the special tests used to diagnose lateral epicondylitis.
60. **B.** Low-load, long-duration stretching is advocated for restoration for elbow extension among throwing athletes with elbow flexion contracture.
61. **C.** High-intensity, short-duration stretching is contraindicated in treating the limited elbow range of motion as it may produce myositis ossificans.
62. **D.** The other terms of medial epicondylitis are golfer's elbow, flexor-pronator tendinitis, and pitcher's elbow.
63. **D.** Proper conditioning and the specific regime of strengthening exercises to the extensor carpi radials longus and brevis as well as supinator forms the basis of preventive program of tennis elbow.
64. **C.** Management of tennis elbow includes Mulligan's lateral glide treatment and Mills manipulation maneuver to reduce pain and improve function.
65. **D.** The biceps, wrist flexors, and pronators greatly reduce valgus stresses on the elbow during the throwing motion.

66. **C.** Pouring coffee from a pot with an extended elbow is a typical pain-provoking daily life activity in tennis elbow.
67. **B.** The condition which characterizes pain during resisted flexion and pronation of the wrist with elbow extension is Golfer's elbow.
68. **C.** The forces elicited from the common extensor origin can be transferred or reduced using taping, epicondylitis bandage, or orthosis stabilizing the wrist.
69. **A.** The extensor carpi radialis brevis is tested with the elbow fully flexed, and resistance applied to the third metacarpal bone.
70. **B.** For lateral epicondylitis, testing of the extensor carpi radialis longus is performed with the elbow flexed 30° and resistance applied to the second metacarpal bone.
71. **D.** Because the flexor carpi ulnaris and flexor digitorum superficialis overlay the UCL, strengthening exercises for these muscles can assist the UCL in resisting valgus stresses at the elbow.
72. **A.** For the treatment of lateral epicondylitis, ultrasonography with hydrocortisone cream of 0.05% concentration as a coupling agent, has been reported as a useful modality.
73. **D.** Flexor digitorum superficialis, palmaris longus and flexor carpi ulnaris, originating at the medial epicondyle provide dynamic stability against valgus stress of the elbow.
74. **C.** The inflammation of the subcutaneous bursa overlying the olecranon process between the skin and the triceps tendon is termed as olecranon bursitis or student's elbow.
75. **D.** In the management of extensor tendinopathy, the return-to-sport stage typically includes progression to full function involving plyometrics, agility and sports skills practice.
76. **C.** Whether acute or chronic, flexor tendinopathy is commonly associated with such sports movement patterns as the golf-swing follow-through, the baseball pitch and the javelin throw.
77. **C.** Maintained pressure is an effective technique that can be used to increase the range of motion by facilitating local muscle relaxation; however, it is a passive technique.

Chapter 7: Elbow Injuries 141

78. **D.** Splinting in the position of elbow extension and slight forearm supination will effectively limit contractures and maximize functional use of the upper extremity.
79. **C.** The medial collateral ligament, also termed the ulnar collateral ligament, is a fan-shaped ligament that restricts the ulna's medial angulation on the humerus. The ligament extends from the medial epicondyle to the medial margin of the ulna's trochlear notch and is assessed for potential instability by applying a valgus force to the distal forearm.
80. **D.** The elbow complex consists of the ulnohumeral, radiohumeral, and proximal radioulnar joint. Each of the joints is affected by swelling in the elbow complex.
81. **A.** The distal end of the humerus should be stabilized when measuring elbow flexion. Failure to adequately stabilize the humerus permits shoulder flexion.
82. **C.** The extensor carpi radialis brevis originates from the common extensor tendon from the lateral epicondyle of the humerus. As a result, the most appropriate area to direct ultrasound energy is the lateral aspect of the elbow.
83. **B.** When a patient is in the anatomic position the normal carrying angle for a male is between 5 and 10 degrees. The angle is created by the long axis of the humerus and the long axis of the ulna. Any angle in excess of 10 degrees is considered cubitus valgus. The ulnar collateral ligament is the primary restraint to excessive cubitus valgus force.
84. **B.** The humeroradial articulation is formed by the convex capitulum articulating with the concave radial head. A dorsal glide is used to increase elbow extension. The lateral orientation of the radius would necessitate the therapist stabilizing the patient's distal humerus from the medial side of the patient's arm.
85. **C.** Soft tissue approximation is associated with a soft end feel. An example of a soft end feel is created by contact between the soft tissue of the posterior leg and the posterior thigh during knee flexion.

Wrist and Hand Injuries

1. Garden spade deformity is seen following:
   A. Colle's fracture
   B. Smith's fracture
   C. Barton's fracture
   D. Bennett fracture
2. Negative ulnar variance means:
   A. Ulna shorter than radius
   B. Ulna longer than radius
   C. Radius and ulna equal in length
   D. Absence of ulna
3. Intersection syndrome is related to excessive friction between which contacting soft tissues?
   A. Abductor pollicis longus, extensor pollicis brevis and extensor carpi radialis longus, extensor carpi radialis brevis
   B. Extensor pollicis longus, extensor pollicis brevis and extensor carpi radialis longus, extensor carpi radialis brevis
   C. Extensor pollicis longus, abductor pollicis longus and extensor carpi radialis longus extensor carpi radialis brevis
   D. Extensor pollicis brevis, adductor pollicis and extensor carpi radialis longus, extensor carpi radialis brevis
4. Which tendon is commonly ruptured in squash players?
   A. Extensor carpi radialis
   B. Extensor carpi ulnaris
   C. Extensor indices
   D. Extensor pollicis longus
5. Fracture of radial styloid process is called as:
   A. Chopart's fracture
   B. Chance fracture
   C. Cotton's fracture
   D. Chauffeur's fracture
6. Injury to which of the following nerve leads to "Handle-Bar Palsy"?
   A. Radial
   B. Median
   C. Ulnar
   D. Musculocutaneous

Chapter 8: Wrist and Hand Injuries

7. "Terry Thomas Sign" results due to widening of space between which carpal bones?
   - A. Trapezium and trapezoid
   - B. Trapezium and scaphoid
   - C. Lunate and capitate
   - D. Scaphoid and lunate
8. Avascular necrosis of scaphoid bone is known as:
   - A. Hauser's disease
   - B. Preiser's disease
   - C. Kienbock's disease
   - D. Pellegrini Stieda disease
9. Injury to which of the following arteries is leads to "Catcher's Hand"?
   - A. Radial
   - B. Ulnar
   - C. Brachial
   - D. Axillary
10. Which joint disruption leads to Type II perilunate instability?
    - A. Scapholunate
    - B. Lunotriquetral
    - C. Capitolunate
    - D. Lunotrapezoid
11. Scapholunate angle more than 65° indicates the presence of which structure instability?
    - A. Dorsal intercalated segmental instability
    - B. Volar intercalated segmental instability
    - C. Perilunate instability
    - D. Triangular fibrocartilage complex instability
12. Gymnasts show a high incidence for:
    - A. Dorsal wrist pain
    - B. Ulnar impaction syndrome
    - C. Scaphoid fracture
    - D. Distal radial epiphysis stress fracture
13. According to Weber's longitudinal column theory of wrist, the "Control Column" is formed by:
    - A. Distal radius, proximal scaphoid, trapezoid, base of 2nd and 3rd metacarpal
    - B. Lunate, capitate, hamate, base of 3rd and 4th metacarpal
    - C. Distal ulna, triangular fibrocartilage complex, base of 4th and 5th metacarpal
    - D. Scaphoid, trapezium, trapezoid and base of 1st metacarpal
14. In the wrist joint, "Space of Poirier" is known as area of:
    - A. Potential weakness
    - B. Maximal stability
    - C. No muscle attachment
    - D. None of the above

15. Madelung deformity affects which joint?
    A. Wrist joint   B. Shoulder joint
    C. Ankle joint   D. Hip joint
16. Carpometacarpal bossing is a painless firm mass over dorsal aspect of hand at the base of:
    A. Middle finger   B. Ring finger
    C. Little finger   D. Index finger
17. Ballottement provocation test is performed to confirm the instability of:
    A. Scapholunate ligament
    B. Arcuate ligament
    C. Lunotriquetral ligament
    D. Triangular fibrocartilage complex
18. Murphy's sign indicates:
    A. Lunate dislocation   B. Scaphoid dislocation
    C. Capitate dislocation D. All of the above
19. In the oval ring theory, conceptualizing the carpus as a dynamic ring was proposed by:
    A. Navarro et al.   B. Taleisnik et al.
    C. Weber et al.   D. Lichtman et al.
20. Compound palmar ganglion is most often caused due to:
    A. Osteoarthritis   B. Syphilis
    C. Tuberculosis   D. Trauma
21. Traumatic subluxation of extensor carpi ulnaris is caused due to forceful movements consisting of:
    A. Pronation, radial deviation, extension
    B. Supination, ulnar deviation, flexion
    C. Pronation, ulnar deviation, extension
    D. Supination, radial deviation, extension
22. All are the features of scaphoid cast, *except*:
    A. The cast extends up to the metacarpal heads
    B. The hand is kept in the tumbler position
    C. It is an above elbow cast
    D. In case of thumb, the cast extends up to the interphalangeal joint

23. Which ligament avulsion injury leads to hook of hamate fracture?
    A. Pisohamate ligament
    B. Ulnar collateral ligament
    C. Transverse carpal ligament
    D. Radial collateral ligament
24. Type II traumatic fibrocartilage complex injury is:
    A. Tear in central cartilagenous disc
    B. Avulsion of triangular fibrocartilage from ulnar styloid process
    C. Tear of palmar third of triangular fibrocartilage and ulnocarpal ligament involvement
    D. Avulsion of triangular fibrocartilage complex from radial attachment and fracture of distal radius
25. Piano keys test indicates:
    A. Instability of distal radioulnar joint
    B. Instability of 2nd and 3rd carpometacarpal joints
    C. Stability of capitate bone
    D. Degenerative joint disease of metacarpophalangeal joint
26. Shuck test is used to detect:
    A. Radiocarpal instability
    B. Kienbock's disease
    C. Scaphoid instability
    D. All of the above
27. What is the normal capitolunate angle?
    A. 30°–60°
    B. 0°–30°
    C. 0°–15°
    D. 0°–60°
28. Avulsion fracture of pisiform bone results from rupture of which structure?
    A. Flexor carpi ulnaris
    B. Pisohamate ligament
    C. Pisotriquetral ligament
    D. All of the above
29. The term "Catch-up Clunk" is referred to which pathological condition?
    A. Lunotriquetral ligament injuries
    B. Ulnar midcarpal instability
    C. Torn triangular fibrocartilage complex
    D. Scapholunate injuries

30. To assess the integrity of the collateral ligaments, the athletic trainer should apply which type of force to the joints?
    A. Lateral
    B. Medial
    C. Anterior
    D. Posterior
31. Disruption of terminal extensor mechanism at the distal interphalangeal joint leads to:
    A. Mallet finger
    B. Drop finger
    C. Baseball finger
    D. All of the above
32. Which tendon is ruptured in "Jersey Finger"?
    A. Flexor digitorum superficialis
    B. Flexor digitorum profundus
    C. Flexor pollicis longus
    D. Extensor indicis
33. What is the other name of Button-hole deformity?
    A. Ape thumb deformity
    B. Swan neck deformity
    C. Boutonniere deformity
    D. None of the above
34. Which ligament is injured in Skier's thumb?
    A. Ulnar collateral ligament
    B. Radial collateral ligament
    C. Transverse ligament
    D. Oblique retinacular ligament
35. According to American Society for Surgery of the hand, the normal limit of two point discrimination in finger-tip is:
    A. 3-4 mm
    B. 6 mm
    C. 6-10 mm
    D. 11-15 mm
36. In which type of sports activity, hypertrophy of metacarpophalangeal joint takes place?
    A. Boxing
    B. Tennis
    C. Squash
    D. Karate
37. According to Leddy and Packer, what is the explanation for Type III classification of flexor digitorum profundus tendon rupture.
    A. Profundus avulsed with a small bone fragment
    B. Large bony fragment caught at A4 pulley of tendon sheath
    C. Comminuted fracture of distal phalanx
    D. Both vincula has disrupted

38. Which structure at the proximal interphalangeal joint is injured leading to pseudoboutonniere deformity?
    A. Volar plate
    B. Collateral ligament
    C. Extensor mechanism
    D. Oblique retinacular fibers
39. Boxer's fracture is:
    A. 5th metacarpal base fracture
    B. 5th metacarpal shaft fracture
    C. 5th metacarpal neck fracture
    D. 5th metacarpal head fracture
40. Bennett's fracture dislocation is difficult to manage conservatively because of the pull of which muscle?
    A. Palmaris longus
    B. Palmaris brevis
    C. Extensor pollicis longus
    D. Flexor pollicis longus
41. The special test performed for hypothenar hammer syndrome is:
    A. Watson's test
    B. De Quervain's test
    C. Stress test
    D. Allen test
42. Injury to which of the following nerve leads to Bowler's thumb?
    A. Palmar cutaneous branch of median nerve of thumb
    B. Ulnar digital sensory nerve to thumb
    C. Palmar digital sensory branch of radial nerve to thumb
    D. Radial digital sensory nerve to thumb
43. In proximal interphalangeal volar plate injuries, mention the mechanism of injury involved:
    A. Hyperflexion
    B. Hyperextension
    C. Jamming force
    D. Hyperabduction
44. Stener lesion encountered in complete rupture of ulnar collateral ligament of thumb, which aponeurosis is found between the two ends of torn ligament?
    A. Adductor aponeurosis
    B. Abductor aponeurosis
    C. Palmar aponeurosis
    D. Flexor aponeurosis
45. Tenderness at anatomical snuffbox is characteristic of:
    A. De Quervain's disease
    B. Scaphoid fracture
    C. Radial styloid fracture
    D. All of the above

46. Acute infection of the fingertip pulp space of the hand is called as:
    A. Paronychia
    B. Ganglion
    C. Stye
    D. Whitlow
47. Interphalangeal joint should always be immobilized in which position?
    A. Extension
    B. Flexion
    C. Neutral position
    D. Either flexion or extension does not matter
48. Which of the following fractures is known as Rolando's fracture?
    A. Fracture base of 5th metacarpal
    B. Intra-articular fracture of base of 1st metacarpal
    C. Fracture neck of 2nd metacarpal
    D. Fracture neck of ulnar styloid process
49. Mallet thumb results from avulsion of which tendon?
    A. Abductor pollicis longus
    B. Flexor pollicis longus
    C. Extensor pollicis longus
    D. Adductor pollicis
50. Which alignment of the hand and wrist is most difficult to evaluate and maintain?
    A. Flexion
    B. Extension
    C. Rotation
    D. Opposition
51. Improperly treated proximal interphalangeal joint injuries to fingers can lead to:
    A. Coach's finger
    B. Trainer's finger
    C. Athlete's finger
    D. Player's finger
52. An injury to the middle finger may also affect which of the following metacarpals?
    A. 2nd metacarpal
    B. 3rd metacarpal
    C. 4th metacarpal
    D. 5th metacarpal
53. It is easier to mobilize a finger joint that has been fixed in— for several weeks than a joint that has been fixed in:
    A. Flexion, extension
    B. Extension, flexion
    C. Abduction, adduction
    D. Adduction, abduction

54. Nine hole peg test is used to assess:
    A. Fine coordination
    B. Gross manual dexterity
    C. Finger dexterity
    D. Gross coordination
55. When the hand is at rest, what is the normal alignment of the fingers?
    A. Slightly flexed
    B. Maximally flexed
    C. Slightly extended
    D. Maximally extended
56. Boyes test is positive in case of which pathology?
    A. Torn central slip of extensor hood
    B. Ruptured flexor digitorum profundus
    C. Paratenonitis between flexor pollicis longus and flexor indices
    D. None of the above
57. Extrinsic minus thumb is due to the weakness of:
    A. Extensor pollicis longus
    B. Extensor pollicis brevis
    C. Abductor pollicis
    D. Adductor pollicis
58. Period of immobilization (splinting) for collateral ligament injuries of the finger metacarpophalangeal joints is:
    A. 6 weeks
    B. 5 weeks
    C. 1 week
    D. 3 weeks
59. In grade III dorsal dislocation of metacarpophalangeal joint of thumb there is:
    A. Avulsion of volar plate proximally
    B. Volar lip of the proximal phalanx rests on the dorsum of the metacarpal head with entrapment of volar plate
    C. Base of the proximal phalanx will eventually rest on the dorsum of the metacarpal head
    D. The collateral ligaments remain intact and the metacarpal head does not sublux through the volar capsular defect
60. When can an athlete with a grade III ulnar collateral ligament rupture safely return to sports if protected with a splint or playing cast?
    A. At 2 weeks
    B. At 6 weeks
    C. When strength is 90% of normal
    D. When pain and swelling subsides

61. The stability of ulnar collateral ligament of thumb is checked by asking the patient to perform:
    A. Thumb-Index pinch
    B. Key pinch
    C. Precision grip
    D. Power grip
62. A therapist can palpate the bony structures of the wrist and hand, which of the following structure would not be identified in the distal row of carpals?
    A. Capitate
    B. Triquetrum
    C. Hamate
    D. Trapezoid
63. Name the athletic activity which leads to the triangular fibrocartilage injury.
    A. Racquet sports
    B. Basketball
    C. Judo
    D. All of the above
64. Name the mechanism of injury which leads to the traumatic athletic injuries of the triangular fibrocartilage complex (TFCC)?
    A. Fall on the outstretched hand
    B. Hyperpronation injury to the forearm
    C. A and B
    D. Hyperflexion injury to the elbow
65. The positive fovea sign indicates the presence of:
    A. Triangular fibrocartilage complex (TFCC) injury
    B. Radial collateral ligament injury
    C. Carpal fracture
    D. Extensor carpi ulnaris injury
66. The ulnocarpal stress test is a provocative test for:
    A. Carpal tunnel syndrome
    B. Ulnocarpal abutment syndrome
    C. Scaphoid fracture
    D. None of the above
67. What is the test used to isolate distal radioulnar joint pathology?
    A. Mill's test
    B. Purdue pegboard test
    C. Piano key test
    D. Boyes test

Chapter 8: Wrist and Hand Injuries

68. Which of the following ones does not fall under the groups of carpal instabilities?
    A. Dorsal intercalated segment instability (DISI)
    B. Humeroradial joint subluxation
    C. Palmar intercalated segment instability (PISI)
    D. Ulnar translocation
69. Name the carpal instability in which the lunate is abnormally extended relative to the radius?
    A. Dorsal intercalated segment instability (DISI)
    B. Palmar intercalated segment instability (PISI)
    C. A and B
    D. Dorsal translocation
70. The test which used to detect the abnormal motion between the lunate and scaphoid is:
    A. Boyes test   B. Bunnel-Littler test
    C. Scaphoid ballottement test D. Phalen's test
71. Special test for scapholunate instability is:
    A. Linschied test   B. Bunnel-Littler test
    C. Watson test   D. Phalen's test
72. Which ligament injury leads to the progressive flexion of the scaphoid and migration of the scaphoid away from the lunate and results in dorsal intercalated segment instability (DISI) pattern of carpal collapse?
    A. Lunotriquetral interosseous ligament (LTIL)
    B. Ulnotriquetral (UT) ligament
    C. Ulnolunate (UL) ligament
    D. Dorsal part of scapholunate interosseous ligament (SLIL)
73. _____ injury commonly occur in ball-catching sports such as football, basketball, baseball, and softball.
    A. Mallet finger   B. Jersey finger
    C. Ganglion cysts   D. Metacarpal fracture
74. A mallet finger deformity is readily observed as the athlete is:
    A. Unable to actively flex the wrist
    B. Unable to actively extend the wrist
    C. Unable to actively flex the distal phalanx
    D. Unable to actively extend the distal phalanx

75. Mallet finger injury is treated with the splinting of the DIP joint in slight hyperextension for the duration of:
    A. 1-2 weeks B. 3-4 weeks
    C. 6-8 weeks D. 12-14 weeks
76. Which finger is commonly involved in the Jersey finger injury?
    A. Mallet finger B. Ring finger
    C. Little finger D. Middle finger
77. Which muscle is isolated by blocking PIP joint motion while actively flexing the DIP joint of a finger?
    A. Flexor digitorum profundus
    B. Flexor pollicis longus
    C. Flexor carpi ulnaris
    D. Flexor digitorum superficialis
78. The postoperative rehabilitation protocol of the Jersey finger includes:
    A. Dorsal block splint B. Tendon gliding exercises
    C. Sports-specific activities D. All of the above
79. Name the condition which involves irritation of the extensor pollicis brevis and abductor pollicis longus tendon of the wrist among the players of racquet sports, gymnasts, and golfers.
    A. Mallet finger B. Jersey finger
    C. De Quervain tenosynovitis D. Boutonneire injuries
80. Special test for De Quervain tenosynovitis is:
    A. Finkelstein test B. Boyes test
    C. Bunnel-Litter test D. Formet's sign
81. Which of the following type of fist is the tendon gliding exercise?
    A. Full fist B. Intrinsic-plus position
    C. Intrinsic-minus position D. All of the above
82. Lack of active flexion of the distal interphalangeal (DIP) joint of the finger indicates the diagnosis of:
    A. Flexor pollicis longus avulsion
    B. Flexor digitorum superficialis avulsion
    C. Extensor pollicis longus avulsion
    D. Flexor digitorum profundus avulsion

83. **In gamekeeper's thumb, the integrity of the ulnar collateral ligament is assessed by:**
    A. Valgus stress testing with the MCP joint of the thumb in 30 degrees of flexion
    B. Valgus stress testing with the MCP joint of the thumb in 60 degrees of flexion
    C. Valgus stress testing with the MCP joint of the thumb in 90 degrees of flexion
    D. Valgus stress testing with the MCP joint of the thumb in 30 degrees of extension

84. **_____ is a compression neuropathy of the ulnar digital nerve of the thumb.**
    A. Skier's thumb   B. Bowler's thumb
    C. Gamekeeper's thumb   D. Mallet finger

85. **Exercises prescribed by 3 months after repair of TFCC tear include:**
    A. Weighted wrist curls
    B. Four-way diagonal upper extremity patterns using dumbbells
    C. Wall-falling
    D. All of the above

86. **Name the exercises which means of static muscle contractions to generate active tension of the finger flexors and impose controlled stress on the repaired tendon.**
    A. Thrower's ten exercises   B. Tendon gliding exercises
    C. Place-and-hold exercises   D. None of the above

87. **Name the exercise that is prescribed for the flexor tendon repaired digit with the patient wearing either a dorsal blocking splint or a tendodesis splint.**
    A. Progressive resisted exercises
    B. Place-and-hold exercises
    C. Finger extension exercises
    D. Stretching exercises

88. **Name the position to be avoided at 6–8 weeks since that position places extreme tension on the repaired flexor tendon.**
    A. Finger extension combined with wrist extension
    B. Finger flexion combined with wrist flexion

C. Finger flexion combined with wrist extension
D. None of the above

89. Exercises to reduce extensor lag of the fingers include:
    A. Isolated MCP extension
    B. Isolated PIP and DIP extension
    C. Terminal-range IP extension
    D. All of the above

90. Sign of a ruptured flexor digitorum profundus tendon in the ring finger of a football player is:
    A. Finkelstein test   B. Tinel's sign
    C. Boyes test   D. Sweater finger sign

91. A flexed or dropped posture of the DIP joint and an inability to actively extend the DIP joint is the hallmark finding of a:
    A. Jersey finger   B. Mallet finger
    C. Boutonniere deformity   D. None of the above

92. Which type of strapping keeps the thumb position in neutral and apply an anchor around proximal wrist?
    A. Boxer's wrap
    B. Wrist and hand strapping
    C. Thumb hyperextension strapping
    D. Thumb spica

93. Which condition shows a painful snapping phenomenon that occurs as the finger flexor tendons suddenly pull through a tight A1 pulley portion of the flexor sheath?
    A. Flexor tendonitis   B. Extensor tendonitis
    C. Trigger finger   D. Jersey finger

94. What is the hallmark finding of the mallet finger?
    A. Flexed or dropped posture of the DIP joint
    B. Inability to actively extend the DIP joint
    C. Inability to straighten the DIP joint
    D. All of the above

95. Which of the following condition shows repetitive pressure on the thumbhole of the bowling ball results in the formation of perineural fibrosis?
    A. Skier's thumb   B. Digital nerve injury
    C. Boxer's thumb   D. Ganglion cyst

Chapter 8: Wrist and Hand Injuries

96. Which movement is limited in basilar joint arthritis of the thumb?
    A. Palmar abduction and opposition of thumb
    B. Palmar adduction and opposition of thumb
    C. Flexion of thumb
    D. Extension of thumb
97. Which one of the following stress tests is more suitable for radial collateral ligament?
    A. Wrist adduction   B. Wrist abduction
    C. Axial compression   D. Piano key
98. Which one of the following tests is not suitable for lunotriquetral shear test?
    A. Ballottement   B. Axial grind
    C. Reagan's   D. Shuck
99. What is the optimal position to splint the hand after injury or surgery to prevent ligament shortening and possible fixed deformity?
    A. Wrist flexion, MCP extension, IP extension, and thumb adduction.
    B. Wrist radial deviation, MCP extension, IP extension, and thumb adduction
    C. Wrist extension, MCP flexion, IP extension, and thumb abduction
    D. Wrist ulnar deviation, MCP flexion, IP extension, and thumb abduction
100. When the tendons receive their blood supply through synovial folds known as:
    A. Vincula   B. Mesotendon
    C. Paratenon   D. Tendon sheath
101. Cheiralgia paresthetica is otherwise called as:
    A. Allen test   B. Scaphoid shift test
    C. De Quervain's disease D. Wartenberg's disease
102. Identify the deformity in the finger where there is proximal interphalangeal joint flexion and distal interphalangeal joint and MCP joint hyperextension?
    A. Boutonnière   B. Swan neck
    C. Mallet finger   D. Jersey finger

103. Name the fluid-filled lump that grows out of a joint or tendon sheath similar to a balloon on a stalk.
    A. Flexor tendon laceration
    B. Ganglion cyst
    C. Bursa
    D. Synovium
104. Which action involves clamping an object with partially flexed fingers against the palm of the hand?
    A. Prehension
    B. Holding
    C. Power grip
    D. Pinching
105. Which exercise are beneficial for grip strengthening and wrist stabilization?
    A. Wrist exerciser
    B. Dumbbells
    C. Exercise ball
    D. Putty
106. What type of exercises encourages wrist motion and general upper-body strengthening during wall push-ups?
    A. Active assisted
    B. Resisted
    C. Closed-kinetic-chain
    D. Open-kinetic-chain
107. In ape hand deformity, wasting of the thenar eminence of the hand occurs as a result of:
    A. Axillary nerve palsy
    B. Median nerve palsy
    C. Ulnar nerve palsy
    D. Radial nerve palsy
108. Which deformity is caused by adhesions or shortening of the extensor communis tendon proximal to the metacarpophalangeal joint?
    A. Extensor plus
    B. Flexor plus
    C. Abduction plus
    D. Adduction plus
109. Which tool can be used to measure the hand grip?
    A. Pinch meter
    B. Pinch gripper
    C. Jamar dynamometer
    D. Hand exerciser

110. Which one of the following tests is not functional assessment of the hand?
    A. Jebson–Taylor
    B. Purdue pegboard
    C. Crawford small parts dexterity
    D. DASH

111. Which nerve compression shows paresthesia on the half of the ring finger and the entire little finger?
    A. Median
    B. Ulnar
    C. Radial
    D. Posterior interosseous

112. Which technique can be used to check the joint play movements of the individual carpal bones?
    A. Kaltenborn technique
    B. Maitland technique
    C. Mulligan technique
    D. McKenzie technique

113. Which one of the following is not the wrist arcuate line?
    A. Along the distal margin of the scaphoid, lunate and triquetrum
    B. Along the proximal margins of the scaphoid, lunate, and triquetrum
    C. Along the distal aspects of these bones
    D. Along the proximal margins of the capitate and hamate

114. When the digits shift to the ulnar side of hands at MCPs (common with RA), the deformity is called:
    A. Ulnar nerve palsy
    B. Radial nerve palsy
    C. Ulnar drift
    D. Carpal tunnel syndrome

115. What is the most common type of fracture occurring from a fall on an outstretched with dislocation of radial head?
    A. Colle's fracture
    B. Elbow dislocation
    C. Low end of humerus fracture
    D. Supracondylar fracture

116. An isolated contraction of the extensor digitorum produces:
    A. Ape thumb
    B. Clawing of the finger
    C. Ulnar drift
    D. Swan neck deformity

117. While applying a lateral glide, the patient actively flexes or extends the wrist and then applies a passive stretch force with his other hand at the end of the range. Which of the following technique increase wrist flexion or extension?
   A. Maitland mobilization
   B. Kaltenborn technique
   C. Peripheral joint mobilization
   D. Mobilization with movement

118. Which surgical procedure corrects wrist deformity and gives the patient stability and relief from pain with only some compromise of function despite the loss of joint motion?
   A. Arthrodesis
   B. Total wrist arthroplasty
   C. Resection arthroplasty
   D. Soft tissue arthroplasty

Chapter 8: Wrist and Hand Injuries

ANSWERS

1. **B.** Garden spade deformity is seen following fracture of distal radius, in which the distal fragment displaces volarly and proximally.
2. **A.** Negative ulnar variance means, the ulna is, on average 9 mm shorter than radius.
3. **A.** The abductor pollicis longus and extensor pollicis brevis muscles cross the extensor carpi radialis longus and extensor carpi radialis brevis tendons several centimeters proximal to extensor retinaculum. Excessive friction between contacting soft tissues is described in weightlifters, skiers and racquetball players.
4. **D.** Overuse often leads to extensor pollicis longus tenosynovitis and rupture, where pain is localized over Lister's tubercle.
5. **D.**
6. **C.** Cyclist may develop handle bar palsy by chronic pressure on the ulnar nerve as it traverses Guyon's canal.
7. **D.** Terry Thomas sign is a widening of the space between the scaphoid and the lunate produced by disruption of the intercarpal scapholunate ligament.
8. **B.** Depending on the sports, the wrist is subject to significant loading, which can create stress fractures, thereby damaging the blood supply and reducing the inflow to few vessels. Scaphoid, lunate, capitate is particularly susceptible to avascular necrosis. Avascular necrosis of scaphoid bone is known as Preiser's disease.
9. **B.** Repetitive trauma to the ulnar artery along its course through Guyon's canal to its digital branches can cause both thrombosis and aneurysm called catcher's hand seen in cyclists and handball players.
10. **C.**
11. **A.** In dorsal intercalated segmental instability, the concavity of the lunate will be tilted dorsally, marring the normal linear relationship between the distal radius, lunate, capitate and 3rd metacarpal.
12. **B.** Ulnar impaction syndrome may result from an epiphyseal injury caused by excessive compression force on the maturing distal radius leading to positive ulnar variance.

13. **A.** Control column is directed ulnarly and forces generated by the hand are ultimately directed radially, i.e., choice (A) which is the force column of the wrist.
14. **A.** Space of Poirier is found between volar ligaments, which are arranged in a double V, with capitate at the apex of the broad V and lunate at the apex of the smaller V. The lunocapitate ligament defect leads to carpal subluxation.
15. **A.**
16. **D.** Carpometacarpal bossing corresponds to osteophyte formation around the joint as a consequence of tendon insertion pull or arthritis. More firm and immobile. It occurs over dorsal aspect of hand at the base of the index finger.
17. **C.** The examiner grasps the triquetrum between the thumb and second finger of one hand and the lunate with the thumb and second finger of other hand. The examiner then moves the lunate up and down noting any laxity, crepitus or pain that indicates a positive test for lunotriquetral instability.
18. **A.** In murphy's sign when the athlete makes a fist, knuckle formed by metacarpal heads levels with the adjoining knuckles which indicates lunate dislocation.
19. **D.**
20. **C.** Tuberculosis is the most common cause of the condition known as compound palmar ganglion and one of its striking clinical features happens to be cross infection.
21. **B.** Forceful supination, ulnar deviation and flexion as in tennis player's forehand stroke can lead to a tear of extensor carpi ulnaris sheath at distal ulna, resulting in subluxation of extensor carpi ulnaris ulnarly and volarly with ulnar deviation of wrist in supination.
22. **C.** A scaphoid cast is a below elbow cast extending to the metacarpals and in case of thumb extending up to the interphalangeal joint. The wrist is held in dorsiflexion and slight radial deviation.
23. **C.**
24. **B.** Many racquet, rowing and batting sports require strong wrist action for effective performance. Wrist hyperrotation or even a fall may overload the triangular fibrocartilage complex and produce intrasubstance tears or perforations of the load bearing cushion or disc leading to instability.

Chapter 8: Wrist and Hand Injuries

25. **A.** Patient sits with both arms pronated. Examiner's index finger can push down on the distal ulna as one would push on a piano key. A positive test is indicated by a difference in mobility and production of pain indicating instability of distal radioulnar joint.
26. **D.** Shuck test: The examiner holds the patient's wrist flexed and asks the patient to actively extend the finger against resistance. This test is used to detect the radiocarpal stability, Kienbock's disease, and scaphoid instability.
27. **C.**
28. **D.** All these structures are attached to the pisiform bone and are responsible for its avulsion fracture when stretched.
29. **B.** In ulnar midcarpal instability, patient complains of ulnar sided pain and a clunk that occurs with ulnar deviation and pronation. This term represents abnormally flexed proximal carpal row "catching-up" as it reduces into the extended position late in ulnar deviation.
30. **A.**
31. **D.** Ruptures of terminal extensor tendon is common in sports requiring catching or hitting a ball with one's hand. The end of the finger is struck by the ball, which forces the distal interphalangeal joint into acute flexion. The flexed deformity of distal segment is frequently referred to as "mallet or baseball finger", although "drop finger" is more accurate and descriptive term.
32. **B.** Flexor digitorum profundus tendon attaches to the volar base of the distal phalanx and functions to flex the distal interphalangeal joint. Mechanism of injury is generally a forced extension of a distal interphalangeal joint that is actively flexing, such as in football when a tackler has a hold of an opponent's jersey and the opponent breaks away, forcing the gripping flexed finger into extension.
33. **C.** Disruption of the extensor mechanism at the dorsum of the proximal interphalangeal joint level leads to a boutonniere or button-hole deformity in which there is loss of active extension at proximal interphalangeal joint and secondary hyperextension at distal interphalangeal joint.
34. **A.** In skier's who fall with their thumb in a extended position, the ski pole, which is caught between the thumb and index

finger, can force the metacarpophalangeal joint into such a hyperextended position, rupturing the ulnar collateral ligament.
35. B.
36. D. History of repeated striking of the fist against a post as part of practice routine, the karate players present with a mass that moves with the extensor apparatus. The mass represents hypertrophy of extensor mechanism and is called as hypertrophic infiltration tendonitis.
37. B.
38. A. McCues and colleagues have pointed out that some volar plate injuries at the proximal interphalangeal joint that is seen late present with flexion deformities at the proximal interphalangeal joint and an extension at the distal interphalangeal joint that resembles boutonniere deformity.
39. C. Fracture occurs from direct impact as when a closed fist strikes a blunt object such as a wall. This causes fracture of metacarpal neck just proximal to the metacarpal head.
40. D.
41. D. Ischemia of the hand and fingers secondary to repetitive blunt trauma is called hypothenar hammer syndrome. Constant trauma to the hypothenar area may cause spasm of the ulnar artery, thrombosis and aneurysm of hand. The special test for the hypothenar hammer syndrome is Allen test.
42. B. Bowler's thumb involves the ulnar digital sensory nerve to thumb and may be so painful as to incapacitate the bowler. Contributing factors may be heavy or oversized ball, improper bore spread, poor bowling technique leading to neuroma formation.
43. B. Injury to the volar plate at the proximal interphalangeal joint is a common entity associated with a jammed finger. The mechanism involving hyperextension injury to the proximal interphalangeal joint rupturing the volar plate.
44. A. In Stener lesion, there is interposition of adductor aponeurosis of the torn ulnar collateral ligament with complete disruption, which presents healing in the case. Early operative intervention is recommended.
45. D.

Chapter 8: Wrist and Hand Injuries

46. **D.** Whitlow: Accumulation of pus or fluid in the confined tissue spaces of the fingertip produces marked pressure that can shut off the blood supply and cause early necrosis of bone. Also known as "felon".
47. **A.** Interphalangeal joints should always be immobilized in extension, for this is the position in which ligaments are at their longest and do not stiffen following splinting.
48. **B.** Rolando's fracture is actually a fracture dislocation of the base of first metacarpal.
49. **C.** Tendon injuries to thumb are commonly to extensor mechanism. A mallet thumb secondary to avulsion of extensor pollicis longus and boutonniere deformity occurs after central slip injury takes place.
50. **C.**
51. **A.** The proximal interphalangeal joint is especially vulnerable to injury in athletic competition. They are treated on the sideline by the coach, trainer or the player himself. They return to competition with unprotected use of finger, long before healing takes place. The result is, in 2–3 weeks' time, a painful, stiff and deformed finger develops termed as coacher's finger.
52. **B.** The third metacarpal is in direct relationship with the third (middle) finger.
53. **B.** The soft tissues are in lengthened position in extension, which enhances early return to movement than the position of flexion where soft tissues undergo shortening.
54. **C.** In nine-hole peg test the patient places nine 3.2 cm peg in a 12.7 by 12.7 cm board and then removes them. The score is the time taken to do this task. It is used to assess the finger dexterity.
55. **A.**
56. **A.** The Boyes test is used to assess the torn central slip of extensor hood. The examiner holds the finger to be examined in slight extension at the proximal interphalangeal joint. Patient is asked to flex distal interphalangeal joint. Inability to flex the distal interphalangeal joint is considered as positive test.
57. **B.** The extensor pollicis brevis tendon is stretched and cannot extend the metacarpophalangeal joint leading to extrinsic minus thumb.

58. **D.** Splinting the metacarpophalangeal joint in flexion for 3 weeks has been the recommended treatment in case of metacarpophalangeal collateral ligament injuries followed by buddy taping.
59. **B.**
60. **D.**
61. **A.**
62. **B.**
63. **D.** Injury to the triangular fibrocartilage can occur as a result of athletic activity ranging from racquet sports to basketball to contact sports like judo.
64. **C.** Traumatic athletic injuries of the TFCC result from a fall on the outstretched hand or hyperrotation injury to the forearm.
65. **A.** When the pressure is applied on the foveal region of the ulnar side of the wrist between flexor carpi ulnaris and extensor carpi ulnaris, it replicates the patient's pain. This represents either a foveal disruption of TFCC and/or ulnotriquetral ligament injury.
66. **B.** The ulnocarpal stress test (nakamura test) is a provocative test for ulnocarpal abutment syndrome (degenerative injury to the TFCC).
67. **C.** The piano key test is an excellent test to isolate distal radioulnar joint pathology.
68. **B.** The carpal instabilities can be classified into four groups: dorsal intercalated segment instability (DISI), palmar intercalated segment instability (PISI), ulnar translocation, and dorsal translocation.
69. **A.** In DISI, the lunate is abnormally extended relative to the radius.
70. **C.** Scapholunate ballottement test is an attempt to detect abnormal motion between the lunate and scaphoid.
71. **C.** The Watson test is used to test the scapholunate instability.
72. **D.** The primary stabilizer of the scaphoid is the dorsal part of the scapholunate interosseous ligament (SLIL). Injury of this ligament leads to progressive flexion of the scaphoid and migration of the scaphoid away from the lunate. It results in DISI pattern of carpal collapse.

73. **A.** Mallet finger injury often occurs in ball-catching sports, such as football, basketball, baseball, and softball.
74. **D.** A mallet finger deformity is readily observed because the athlete is unable to extend the distal phalanx actively.
75. **C.** Conservative treatment of mallet finger includes splinting the DIP joint in full slight hyperextension for 6–8 weeks.
76. **B.** The Jersey injury can occur at any finger, but most commonly, the ring finger is involved because of the longer length of the digit when grasping objects.
77. **A.** The flexor digitorum profundus (FDP) is isolated by blocking PIP joint motion while actively flexing the DIP joint. Inability to isolate and actively flex the DIP joint should raise suspicion for FDP injury.
78. **D.** Postoperative rehabilitation protocol of Jersey finger includes dorsal block splint, tendon gliding exercises, intrinsic and extrinsic compartment stretching, isometric and isotonic strengthening exercises, and sports-specific activities.
79. **C.** de Quervain tenosynovitis involves irritation of the extensor pollicis brevis and abductor pollicis longus tendons in the first dorsal extensor compartment of the wrist. It is seen most often in players of racquet sports, gymnasts, and golfers.
80. **A.** A positive Finkelstein test result indicates a strong possibility of de Quervain tenosynovitis.
81. **D.** Tendon gliding exercises involve making various types of fists with the digits in a progression that starts with full extension followed by a tabletop (intrinsic-plus) position, a flat fist, a full fist without the thumb, and finally, a hook (intrinsic-minus) position. These exercises are designed to facilitate the gliding of the FDS and FDP tendons through zone II and restore the balance between the intrinsic and extrinsic muscles.
82. **D.** Avulsion of the flexor digitorum profundus (FDP) ("Jersey finger") can occur in any digit but is most common in the ring finger. Lack of active flexion of the DIP joint (FDP function) must be specifically checked to make the diagnosis. Often the swollen finger assumes a position of extension relative to the other, more flexed fingers. The level of retraction of the FDP generally denotes the force of the avulsion.

83. **A.** In the gamekeeper's thumb, the ulnar collateral ligament's integrity is assessed by valgus stress testing with the MCP joint of the thumb in 30° of flexion.
84. **B.** Digital nerve compression, or Bowler's thumb, is a compression neuropathy of the ulnar digital nerve of the thumb.
85. **D.** Once pain-free ROM exercises are accomplished, strengthening exercises are begun by 3 months. Those exercises include weighted wrist curls, four-way diagonal upper extremity patterns using dumbbells or elastic tubing, Wall-falling, medicine ball throw.
86. **C.** "Place-and-hold" exercises by means of static muscle contractions to generate active tension of the finger flexors and impose controlled stress on the repaired tendon.
87. **B.** Rehabilitation programs initiate place-and-hold exercises of the repaired digit with the patient wearing either a dorsal blocking splint or a tenodesis splint.
88. **A.** Avoid finger extension combined with wrist extension for about 6–8 weeks, as this position places extreme tension on the repaired flexor tendon.
89. **D.** Exercises to reduce extensor lag of the fingers include: isolated MCP extension isolated PIP and DIP extension, terminal-range IP extension, differential gliding of the extensor digitorum tendons.
90. **D.** Sweater finger sign is positive for a ruptured flexor digitorum profundus tendon, which mostly occurs to the ring finger. This sign indicates the inability to flex the distal phalanx of one of the fingers while the patient is asked to make a fist.
91. **B.** The hallmark finding of a mallet finger is a flexed or dropped posture of the DIP joint and an inability to extend or straighten the DIP joint actively.
92. **D.** Apply a spiral strap from the anchor around the thumb (encompassing the MCP joint) & back to the anchor.
93. **C.** Trigger finger is an inability of the two flexor tendons of the finger (FDS and FDP) to slide smoothly under the A1 pulley, resulting in a need for increased tension to force the tendon to slide and a sudden jerk as the flexor tendon nodule suddenly pulls through the constricted pulley (triggering).

Chapter 8: Wrist and Hand Injuries

94. **D.** The mechanism of mallet finger injury is typically forced flexion of the fingertip, often from the impact of the thrown ball.
95. **B.** Digital nerve compression, or bowler's thumb, is a compression neuropathy of the ulnar digital nerve of the thumb.
96. **A.**
97. **A.** To stress the radial collateral ligament and lateral capsule of the wrist in order to detect pain and or laxity.
98. **B.** To establish the presence of abnormal movement of the lunate and triquetral bones indicating instability or subluxation.
99. **C.** Wrist Extension, MCP Flexion, IP Extension, and Thumb palmar abduction Rehabilitation can be achieved more quickly and easily from this so-called "safe" position.
100. **A.** The tendons receive their blood supply through synovial folds known as vincula, each tendon having two, vincula longa and vincula brevia.
101. **D.** It is a neuropathy of the hand generally caused by compression or trauma to the superficial branch of the radial nerve.
102. **A.** The mechanism of injury jamming the finger on the ground or another player in contact sports. Swelling and dorsal PIP joint tenderness to palpation.
103. **B.** Irritation of a ganglion depends on where it develops. A cyst on the dorsal wrist could be irritated with wrist extension, whereas a cyst that develops from the flexor tendon sheath could be irritated with finger flexion activity.
104. **C.** Power grips are primarily isometric functions. The fingers are flexed, laterally rotated, and ulnar deviated. The amount of flexion varies with the object held.
105. **D.** Putty tends to be more effective than a ball because it gives resistance throughout the entire range of motion. Putty can be used for gross grasp, pinch, or extension.
106. **C.** Wall push-ups encourage wrist motion and general upper-body strengthening. They also encourage weight-bearing and closed-chain activities.

107. **B.** Median nerve palsy shows the thumb falls back in line with the fingers as a result of the pull of the extensor muscles.
108. **A.** Extensor plus results in the inability of the patient to simultaneously flex the metacarpophalangeal and proximal interphalangeal joints, although they may be flexed individually.
109. **C.** Arm should be held at the patient's side with elbow flexed at approximately 90° when grip is measured.
110. **D.** The Detailed Assessment of Speed of Handwriting (DASH) is used to analyze the speed and legibility of a person's handwriting.
111. **B.** Paresthesia on the ulnar side of the ring finger and the entire little finger may be caused by pressure of the ulnar nerve at the elbow or in the palm.
112. **A.** Kaltenborn suggested ten tests to determine the mobility of each of the carpal bones. The movement of each of the bones is determined in a sequential manner, and both sides are tested for comparison.
113. **A.** Wrist arcs. Three arcuate lines can normally be constructed along the carpal articular surfaces: (1) Along the proximal margins of the scaphoid, lunate, and triquetrum; (2) along the distal aspects of these bones; (3) along the proximal margins of the capitate and hamate.
114. **C.** Inflammation in the knuckle joints and problems affecting the ligaments or muscles in the wrist and hand can result in ulnar deviation.
115. **A.** Colle's fracture is a complete fracture of the radius bone of the forearm close to the wrist resulting in an upward (posterior) displacement of the radius and obvious deformity.
116. **B.** Claw hand is a condition that causes curved or bent fingers.
117. **D.** Mobilization with movement (MWM) is the concurrent application of sustained accessory mobilization applied by a therapist and an active physiological movement to end range applied by the patient. Passive end-of-range overpressure, or stretching, is then delivered without pain as a barrier.
118. **A.** Wrist arthrodesis, also known as wrist fusion, is a procedure in which the wrist joint is immobilized by fusing the radius to the carpal bones.

CHAPTER 9

Injuries to the Groin and Hip

1. A violent muscle contraction or sudden passive stretch that results in severe immediate pain such that the athletes keep the hip and knee flexed is characteristic of:
   A. A pelvic avulsion
   B. A sacroiliac joint sprain
   C. Osteitis pubis
   D. A hip pointer
2. A direct blow to the buttock that results in pain or paralysis in the distribution of the nerve that innervates the posterior thigh is characteristic of which injury?
   A. Meralgia paresthetica
   B. Pudental nerve palsy
   C. Sciatic nerve injury
   D. Stress of the pubic rami
3. Which of the following studies is the most sensitive and specific for diagnosis of a femoral neck stress fracture?
   A. Bone scan
   B. MRI
   C. Radiography
   D. Arthrography
4. Severe pain in the anterior thigh with inability to extend the knee or ambulate is typical of which injury?
   A. Hamstring strain
   B. Myositis ossificans
   C. Quadriceps rupture
   D. Compartment syndrome
5. To improve strength and speed after a pelvis, hip or thigh injury which of the following rehabilitation techniques would likely be used?
   A. Proprioceptive neuromuscular facilitation
   B. Kinesthetics
   C. Plyometrics
   D. Functional exercises
6. The age related change in quadriceps tendon, which increase the chance of rupture under physiological loads is:
   A. Tendinosclerosis
   B. Fibroid and fatty degeneration
   C. Decreased strength of musculotendinous or tendo-osseous unit
   D. All of the above

7. **What is the extent of tissue involvement in acute compartment syndrome of 30 mmHg after 6 hours duration?**
   A. Capillary vessel damage occurs; full clinical recovery can be expected
   B. Permanent cell death and poor functional recovery
   C. Tissue damage noted to be completely reversible
   D. Irreversible tissue damage with incomplete clinical recovery

8. **Use of which special test has improved the accuracy and shortened the time to 2 weeks in the diagnosis of femoral stress fracture?**
   A. Distraction test   B. Fulcrum test
   C. Compression test   D. None

9. **What is the position of immobilization of hip following quadriceps contusion?**
   A. Flexion
   B. Extension
   C. External rotation with extension
   D. Internal rotation

10. **In the treatment protocol for quadriceps contusion in Phase I which exercise is more emphasized?**
    A. Abduction   B. Adduction
    C. Flexion   D. Extension

11. **What is the amount of active knee flexion that can be performed after moderate quadriceps contusion?**
    A. Greater than 90°   B. Less than 45°
    C. Between 45°–90°   D. Greater than 45°

12. **Groin pull is commonly referred to as:**
    A. Iliopsoas strain   B. Sartorius strain
    C. Rectus femoris strain D. Adductor strain

13. **Sprinter's fracture is avulsion fracture of:**
    A. Anterior superior iliac spine
    B. Posterior superior iliac spine
    C. Posterior inferior iliac spine
    D. Anterior inferior iliac spine

14. **In which position the sartorius muscle is placed on maximal tension leading to avulsion of anterior superior iliac spine?**

A. Knee extension, hip neutral
B. Knee flexion, hip extension
C. Knee extension, hip flexion
D. Knee flexion, hip neutral

15. Which movement increases pain following iliopsoas strain?
    A. Hip flexion, abduction
    B. Hip extension, adduction
    C. Hip flexion, external rotation
    D. Hip extension, internal rotation

16. Gilmore's groin refers to:
    A. Athletic pubalgia
    B. Osteitis pubis
    C. Inguinal hernia
    D. Prostatitis

17. Osteitis pubis results from increased shear forces at the symphysis pubis during which part of gait?
    A. Heel strike
    B. Mid stance
    C. Foot flat
    D. Heel off

18. In adductor strain which muscle is more often involved?
    A. Adductor magnus
    B. Adductor brevis
    C. Adductor longus
    D. All of the above

19. The mechanism of injury leading to adductor strain involves eccentric adductor muscle contraction along with:
    A. Hip external rotation and abduction
    B. Hip internal rotation and adduction
    C. Hip flexion and external rotation
    D. Hip extension and internal rotation

20. Medial hamstring is at more risk during which phase of the gait cycle?
    A. Mid-stance
    B. Swing phase
    C. Take-off portion
    D. Heel strike

21. Prevention strategies for hamstring strain is:
    A. Endurance training of the muscle
    B. Appropriate muscle warm up before athletic activity
    C. Muscle stretching before and after athletic activity
    D. All of the above

22. **Strengthening of which muscle is essential in case of athletic pubalgia?**
    A. Abdominals
    B. Hip adductors
    C. Hip flexors
    D. All of the above

23. **In adductor canal syndrome occlusion of superficial femoral artery takes place at which anatomical location?**
    A. Femoral triangle
    B. Obturator foramen
    C. Hunter's canal
    D. Inguinal ligament

24. **Which is the most common muscle strained in the body?**
    A. Triceps
    B. Tendon-Achilles
    C. Rectus femoris
    D. Long head of biceps femoris

25. **In Grade II hamstring strain loss of extension range of motion is:**
    A. Greater than 45°
    B. Less than 20°
    C. Greater than 60°
    D. Between 20°–45°

26. **Which movement is restricted in hip following slipped capital femoral epiphysis?**
    A. Abduction and internal rotation
    B. Adduction and external rotation
    C. Flexion and adduction
    D. Extension and adduction

27. **Hip pointer is:**
    A. Contusion of anterior superior iliac spine
    B. Contusion of iliac crest
    C. Contusion of anterior inferior iliac spine
    D. Contusion of symphysis pubis

28. **Nontraumatic trochanteric bursitis is commonly seen in which sports activity?**
    A. Running
    B. Volley ball
    C. Basket ball
    D. Tennis

29. **Freiberg's sign is used to detect which syndrome?**
    A. Iliotibial band syndrome
    B. Piriformis syndrome
    C. Adductor canal syndrome
    D. None of the above

Chapter 9: Injuries to the Groin and Hip

30. Mechanism of injury for an apophyseal separation in sports is most commonly due to:
    A. A sudden stop
    B. A sudden change in direction
    C. Sudden and unexpected eccentric muscle contraction
    D. All of the above
31. Skier's hip refers to:
    A. Head of femur fracture
    B. Shaft of femur fracture
    C. Neck of femur fracture
    D. Intertrochanteric and subtrochanteric fracture of femur
32. Cyclists usually complain of which nerve palsy?
    A. Sciatic nerve   B. Femoral nerve
    C. Pudental nerve   D. Obturator nerve
33. Exercises that are often used to determine if an athlete is ready to return to a higher level of activity or sports competition are called as:
    A. Functional exercises   B. Cardiovascular exercises
    C. Kinesthetic exercises   D. Plyometric exercises
34. A standing sign is indicative of which injury?
    A. Legg Calve Perthe's disease
    B. Pelvic floor myalgia
    C. Sacroiliac joint pain
    D. Pubic rami stress fracture
35. Which group of muscles should be strengthened in case of hip pointer?
    A. Back extensors   B. Hip abductors
    C. Abdominalis   D. Hip flexors
36. Avulsion fractures of the ischial apophysis is also called as:
    A. Jumper's fracture   B. Hurdler's fracture
    C. Runner's fracture   D. None of the above
37. Bench warmer's bursitis is referred to as:
    A. Trochanteric bursitis   B. Iliopectineal bursitis
    C. Iliac bursitis   D. Ischial bursitis

38. A sandstorm appearance on radiograph localized to middle one-third of femur identified by technetium and ultrasound indicates:
    A. Quadriceps contusion
    B. Femur fracture
    C. Myositis ossificans
    D. All of the above
39. Stretching and strengthening of which muscle is essential in the rehabilitation of osteitis pubis?
    A. Hip adductors
    B. Hip flexors
    C. Hip extensors
    D. Hip external rotators
40. Adductor tubercle avulsion fracture is caused by the pull of which muscle?
    A. Adductor magnus
    B. Adductor longus
    C. Adductor brevis
    D. All of the above
41. What is the most common complication expect in a femoral neck fracture?
    A. Avascular necrosis
    B. Delayed union
    C. Tendinopathies
    D. Neuritis
42. What type of fracture results from cyclic loads causing osteon debonding and microfractures?
    A. Fatigue
    B. Tension
    C. Stress
    D. Compressive
43. Which muscle can be isolated by doing resisted hip external rotation from a position of internal rotation?
    A. Gluteus medius
    B. Gluteus minimus
    C. Piriformis
    D. Sartorius
44. Name the condition causes catching and locking during hip injuries.
    A. Iliopsoas strain
    B. Labral tears
    C. Tendinopathy
    D. Loose bodies
45. What type of injury can occur in athletes, gymnastics, and aerobics trying to achieve more hip abduction?
    A. Gluteus medium tendinopathy
    B. Adductor tendinopathy
    C. Ligamentum teres tear
    D. Ganz lesions

46. Which one of the following clinical conditions causes pain in athletes recognized in activities that combine high running loads, rapid changes of direction, and kicking is _____?
    A. Pubic syndesmosis
    B. Longstanding groin pain syndrome
    C. Obturator neuropathy
    D. Synovitis
47. What is the most appropriate condition seen in ballet dancers, refers to a clicking or popping noise in the hip region?
    A. Femoral bossing   B. Snapping hip
    C. Pistol grip hip   D. Hip bursitis
48. If a player suffered a direct blow of ball to the anterior thigh and examination confirms an area of tenderness and swelling with worsening on active contraction and passive stretch. Which of the following diagnosis suitable for the above condition?
    A. Quadriceps contusion   B. Femoral torsion
    C. Adductor tendinopathy   D. Ischemic contracture
49. Intramuscular hematoma of the thigh after a blunt contusion may result in:
    A. Quadriceps muscle strain
    B. Quadriceps inhibition
    C. Compartment syndrome
    D. Myositis ossificans
50. What is the most common injury in sports among sprinters and long jumpers, especially at the muscle-tendon junction in the posterior thigh region?
    A. Piriformis syndrome
    B. Sciatica
    C. Iliotibial band strain
    D. Hamstring muscle strain
51. When an altered sensation over the lateral thigh symptoms reproduced by pressure or percussion just medial to the ASIS called as:
    A. OA hip   B. Meralgia paresthetica
    C. Iliopsoas strain   D. Tensor fascial lata strain

52. A clinical condition characterized by hip pain usually worsens with sitting on hard surfaces, cycling, and prolonged standing is known as:
    A. Ischiogluteal bursitis
    B. Subtrochanteric bursitis
    C. Vascular claudication
    D. Chondral lesion
53. Excessive external rotation of the leg, accompanied with toeing-out, occurs in:
    A. Femoral anteversion
    B. Femoral retroversion
    C. Coxa vara
    D. Coxa valga
54. What posture indicates on increased hip extension in relaxed standing?
    A. Lateral pelvic tilt
    B. Anterior pelvic tilt
    C. Sway back
    D. Vertical displacement
55. Lateral asymmetry in relaxed standing is characterized by a high iliac crest on one side is termed as:
    A. Tibial torsion
    B. Genu varum
    C. Genu valgum
    D. Trendelenburg sign
56. Which one of the following techniques can be used to assess for pain and any hypomobility at the hip joint?
    A. Traction
    B. Joint compression
    C. Joint distraction
    D. Stretching
57. Name the test that used extensively to evaluate the flexibility of the ITB and TFL.
    A. Ober
    B. FABER
    C. FADIR
    D. Scour
58. A type of exercise that is performed using cuff weights or to develop strength and endurance of all of the hip musculature is:
    A. Close-chain
    B. Open-chain
    C. Resisted
    D. Plyometrics
59. A 23-year-old female athlete presents a groin pain history due to strain or tear of any soft tissue in the lower abdomen area. Examination revealed groin pain that goes away with rest but returns during sports activity. What would be the most appropriate diagnosis?
    A. Enterocele
    B. Pelvic organ prolapses
    C. Hernia
    D. Abdominal tightness

60. What indicates the presence of serious pathology posterior to the axis of flexion and extension in the hip?
    A. Sign of buttock
    B. Avascular necrosis
    C. Compartment syndrome
    D. Varicose veins
61. Pain in the groin or medial thigh is reproduced with palpation over one side of the symphysis pubis is called as:
    A. Quadriceps contusion
    B. Myositis ossificans
    C. Osteitis pubis
    D. Pubalgia
62. How do you test the ligamentous laxity of the hip joint?
    A. Log roll
    B. Patrick
    C. Frieberg
    D. Pace
63. A 30-year-old sportsperson has a history of closed traumatic soft tissue degloving injury in the pelvis characterized by separation of the dermis from the underlying fascia. What would be the most appropriate diagnosis?
    A. Frank dislocation
    B. Morel–Lavallee lesion
    C. Hypertrophic ossification
    D. Gluteal nerve entrapment
64. Where is the pain typically felt with a femoral neck fracture?
    A. Lateral hip
    B. Groin
    C. Piriformis
    D. Greater trochanter
65. Which condition shows contusion of the lateral hip, usually results from a direct blow to the iliac crest?
    A. Iliopectineal bursitis
    B. Iliopsoas bursitis
    C. Oblique muscle strain
    D. Hip pointer

ANSWERS

1. **A.** The most common areas are anterior superior iliac spine where there is insertion of sartorius, anterior inferior iliac spine where there is insertion of rectus femoris and ischial tuberosity with insertion of hamstring.
2. **C.** Sciatic nerve courses through buttock and posterior thigh, so any direct blow may compress the nerve or injure the nerve leading to the symptoms.
3. **B.** Femoral neck stress fracture is classified into compression-side, tension-side and displaced types and usually results from overstraining and can occur in almost any sport. MRI is most sensitive and specific for diagnosis than a bone scan.
4. **C.** Rupture of quadriceps often results from an eccentric contraction of the muscle as the knee is flexed.
5. **C.** Plyometric exercises are those that allow a muscle to obtain its maximum strength or produce a maximum amount of force as rapidly as possible.
6. **D.**
7. **D.** The time interval is decreased when compartment pressure are greater, requiring urgency of diagnosis and treatment of acute compartment syndrome of the thigh.
8. **B.** Fulcrum's test: Examiner's arm is under the patient's distal thigh as gentle pressure is placed over the dorsum of the knee. The examiner's arm is moved proximally under the thigh until a point where maximal tenderness is found. (Ref: Orthopedics and sports physical therapy).
9. **A.** This position increases tension within the anterior compartment, theoretically reducing hemorrhage, swelling and inflammation.
10. **C.** Since the leg is immobilized in flexed position, flexion exercise is more emphasized to prevent disability and development of myositis ossificans.
11. **B.** Classification is based on the amount of pain, swelling and loss of knee flexion. In moderate quadriceps contusion, 45°–90° of knee flexion is possible.
12. **D.**

Chapter 9: Injuries to the Groin and Hip

13. **D.** Forceful eccentric and concentric contraction of rectus femoris tendon results in avulsion fracture of anterior inferior iliac spine.
14. **B.** With knee flexed and hip extended the sartorius is placed on maximal tension leading to the avulsion fracture of anterior superior iliac spine.
15. **D.** The position of hip extension and internal rotation increases strain of iliopsoas tendon thereby increasing pain.
16. **A.** European literature refers athletic pubalgia as "Gilmore's groin" or sportsman's hernia.
17. **B.** Shear forces are greatest during midstance when the unsupported pelvis attempts to drop. The increased shear at the pubis results in an inflammatory reaction and pain localized to symphysis.
18. **C.**
19. **A.** Mechanism of injury involves eccentric adductor muscle contraction with concurrent hip external rotation and abduction.
20. **B.** Electromyography evaluation has demonstrated that semimembranosus and semitendinosus are the most active during late swing phase of the gait cycle.
21. **D.** All these preventive strategies improve the elasticity of the muscle for taking up the forces during the sporting activities.
22. **D.** Strengthening these muscles will help them take up the forces or shock and prevent the strain to the pubic region.
23. **C.** Hunter's canal is located in the middle third of anterior thigh. Canal is bordered by vastus medialis laterally, sartorius medially and adductor longus posterolaterally.
24. **D.**
25. **D.** In Grade II hamstring strain, there is moderate pain with moderate amount of spasm, ecchymosis and swelling. Loss of motion is between 20°-45° and no palpable defect is noted.
26. **A.** The leg is externally rotated and adducted in the slipped capital femoral epiphysis with limited internal rotation and adduction.

27. **B.** Hip pointer is a contusion of the iliac crest due to a focused impact at some point between the iliac crest and the prominence of the greater trochanter.
28. **A.** Repetitive snapping of the tensor fascia over the prominent greater trochanter with the trochanteric bursa wedged between these two structures can lead to inflammation of the bursa.
29. **B.** Where pain is elicited with passive internal rotation of hip.
30. **D.**
31. **D.** It frequently occurs in alpine and cross-country skiers and also among athletes who participate in contact and high-speed sports.
32. **C.** Due to repeated pressure in the peroneal area, numbness is felt and in more severe cases mild urinary or bowel incontinence is found.
33. **A.** Functional activities include everything from walking to sport-specific drills. These are often timed and are only limited by the imagination.
34. **D.** It is the inability to stand on the affected limb without support. Pubic rami are most common bone in the region to be afflicted by stress fracture in long distance runners.
35. **C.**
36. **B.** This fracture occurs when the hamstrings strongly contract while the pelvis is fixed and flexed and the knee is extended.
37. **D.** Benchwarmer's bursitis occurs due to sitting for a prolonged period of time, especially with the leg crossed or on a hard surface leading to tenderness over the ischial bursa.
38. **C.** Myositis ossificans is a frequent complication after muscle contusion. In first three weeks there is an indurated tenderness localized to anterior compartment seen as sandstorm in the ultrasound and technetium.
39. **A.**
40. **B.** There will be palpable defect and muscle belly retraction.
41. **A.** Avascular necrosis of the hip is the destruction and death of bone in the hip region as a result of ischemia.
42. **B.** Tension fracture are extensional and leads to higher stresses and rapid failure of the bone, and displacement may occur.

43. **C.** The piriformis is a small muscle located deep in the buttock, behind the gluteus maximus. It helps the hip to rotate externally, turning the leg and foot outward.
44. **D.** Loose bodies in the hip are relatively rare but can present with catching and locking of the hip joint. Loose bodies may not appear on X-ray and usually need to be removed arthroscopically.
45. **C.** Ligamentum teres tear: Tears of the ligamentum teres leads to some instability of the hip joint. Scarring after the tear can cause a 'cyclops' lesion and catching/clunking of the hip.
46. **B.** Longstanding groin pain syndrome: The two most common sports associated with this syndrome are soccer and Australian football, which both require players to run fast and kick across the body. Longstanding groin pain is also a major concern in basketball, American football, rugby and field hockey.
47. **B.** Snapping hip: There are two forms of snapping hip. Lateral (or external) snapping hip is localized at the lateral aspect of the hip and is produced by the tensor fascia lata or the abducting fibers of gluteus maximus sliding over the greater trochanter and producing a characteristic sound.
48. **A.** Quadriceps contusion: Trauma to the muscle will cause primary damage to myofibrils, fascia and blood vessels. Localized bleeding may increase tissue pressure and cause relative regional anoxia that can result in secondary tissue damage.
49. **C.** Compartment syndrome: Trauma to the muscle will cause primary damage to myofibrils, fascia and blood vessels. Localized bleeding may increase tissue pressure and cause relative regional anoxia that can result in secondary tissue damage.
50. **D.** Hamstring muscle strain: The majority of hamstring muscle injuries occur in the biceps femoris muscle, mainly at the muscle-tendon junction. They are usually a non-contact injury and mostly occur during sprinting.
51. **B.** Meralgia paresthetica is a condition characterized by tingling, numbness and burning pain in the outer part of your thigh. The condition is caused by compression of the

lateral femoral cutaneous nerve, which supplies sensation to your upper leg.

52. **A.** Ishciogluteal bursitis: Inflammation of the fluid-filled sac, or bursa that lies between the ischial tuberosity. Examination of patients with bursitis reveals a soft tissue mass in the gluteal region of the affected hip.

53. **B.** Femoral retroversion is a rotational or torsional deformity in which the femur twists backward (outward) relative to the knee.

54. **C.** Sway back posture characterized by a posterior pelvic tilt and hyperextension of the knees, and results in a stretch on the anterior joint capsule of the hip and stress on the iliopsoas muscle and tendon.

55. **D.** Trendelenburg sign: The difference in height between the two crests must be greater than one-half inch to have clinical significance.

56. **C.** Joint distraction: The patient's thigh is grasped by the clinician as proximal as possible, and a distraction force is applied along the line of the femoral neck.

57. **A.** Ober test: The patient is placed in the side lying position, and with the hip extended and abducted and the knee flexed to 90°, the proximal part of the tested leg is released and allowed to drop passively.

58. **B.** Open-chain exercises are initially performed using concentric contractions and then advanced to eccentric contractions using a variety of speeds and resistance.

59. **C.** Sports hernia: The symptoms of a sports hernia are characterized by pain during sports movements, particularly twisting and turning during single-limb stance. The pain usually radiates to the adductor muscle region, although it is often difficult for patients to pinpoint.

60. **A.** Sign of buttock: To identify the presence of a lesion or pathology within the buttock, including the possibility of ischial bursitis, an abscess, or neoplasm within the buttock.

61. **C.** Osteitis pubis: Osteitis pubis is a condition in which there's inflammation where the right and left pubic bones meet at the lower front part of the pelvis. Abdominal and adductor muscle spasm may accompany pain, and gait may be antalgic with movement adapted to reduce pain.

62. **A.** Log roll test: Patient is positioned supine and the leg is passively rolled into internal rotation and external rotation. Clicking may be indicative of a labral tear, and increased external rotation range of motion may indicate iliofemoral ligament laxity.
63. **B.** The Morel-Lavallee lesion is a closed degloving injury in which the subcutaneous tissue is separated from the underlying fascia. The avascular tissue then undergoes necrosis, resulting in accumulation of liquefied fat and hematoma.
64. **C.** Piriformis: Microtrauma may result from overuse of the piriformis muscle, such as in long-distance walking or running or by direct compression.
65. **D.** Hip pointer: In most cases, the TFL muscle belly is impacted and presents with hematoma; however, the injury may involve tearing of the external oblique at its iliac insertion, periostitis of the iliac crest, or contusion to the greater trochanter.

Thigh and Leg Injuries

1. Off balance position from a long jump or from a basket ball rebound leads to the injury of:
   A. Quadriceps/patellar tendon
   B. Hamstrings
   C. Gastrosoleus
   D. Tendoachilles
2. In contact sports, in order to avoid knee injuries, the shoe surface interface should be:
   A. Low coefficient of friction
   B. High coefficient of friction
   C. Rubber soled shoes
   D. Shoes with long cleats
3. Among them which ligament in the knee joint gets injured while playing on the harder surface of the artificial turf?
   A. ACL
   B. PCL
   C. MCL
   D. LCL
4. Early complications of poorly treated contusion of the anterior thigh results in:
   A. Stiffness
   B. Poor quadriceps action
   C. Muscle wasting
   D. All of the above
5. Myositis ossificans occur as the late complication of the thigh injury might be due to:
   A. The thigh is reinjured before healing occur
   B. Massage or heat has been applied to the hematoma
   C. The hematoma has been poorly treated
   D. The bleeding is associated with hemophilia
   E. All of the above
6. Which of the following factors predisposes to quadriceps muscle strain?
   A. Tight quadriceps muscle
   B. An imbalance between the quadricep's power of the two legs
   C. Short leg
   D. Insufficient warm up at the beginning
   E. All of the above

7. Which is the most common muscle among the quadriceps group prone for strain?
   A. Vastus medialis   B. Vastus lateralis
   C. Rectus femoris   D. Sartorius
8. Hamstring pull is the most common injury among which group of sports players?
   A. Sprinters   B. Tennis players
   C. Ballistic players   D. Table tennis players
9. Factors that cause hamstring "pull" is:
   A. Lack of flexibility of the hamstring group
   B. Imbalance in the ratio of strength and power between the hamstring and quadriceps
   C. Inequality of strength of the left versus the right hamstring group
   D. Biceps muscle receive two nerve supply
   E. All of the above
10. Slow onset hamstring strain occurs particularly in which group of players?
    A. Sprinters   B. Long distance runners
    C. Cricketers   D. Tennis players
11. Rapid swelling of the knee within twelve hours of the injury indicates:
    A. Joint effusion   B. Synovitis
    C. Hemarthosis   D. Ecchymosis
12. The onset of swelling following meniscal tear is:
    A. Gradual   B. Rapid
    C. Sudden onset   D. Intermittent
13. Which point of history suggest indicative of retropatellar irritation?
    A. History of giving in
    B. History of locking
    C. History of pop
    D. History of pain on going up or downstairs
14. Pain under the patella and along the patellar tendon after jumping activities in basketball is indicative of:
    A. Retropatellar irritation   B. Patellar tendonitis
    C. Meniscal injury   D. ACL injury

15. A subluxing patella can produce a history of:
    A. Giving way
    B. Locking
    C. Swelling
    D. All of the above
16. Positive hyperextension test indicates which ligament injury?
    A. ACL
    B. PCL
    C. MCL
    D. LCL
17. The positive valgus or varus stress at 0° is the indication of:
    A. Medial stabilizing complex
    B. Lateral stabilizing complex
    C. Both medial and lateral stabilizing complex
    D. Both medial and lateral stabilizing complex along with PCL or ACL
18. Which is the best position for testing in order to identify the stability of medial and lateral stabilizing complex?
    A. Valgus or varus at 30°
    B. Valgus or varus at 0°
    C. Valgus or varus at 45°
    D. Valgus or varus at 60°
19. Which test is used to find out anteromedial rotatory instability?
    A. Anterior drawer's sign
    B. Anterior drawer's sign with foot in external rotation
    C. Anterior drawer's sign with foot in internal rotation
    D. Posterior drawer's sign
20. Anterior drawer sign with foot in internal rotation shows incompetency of:
    A. ACL
    B. LCL
    C. Posterolateral corner (posterior oblique ligament)
    D. All of the above
21. Pivot shift test is to demonstrate which of the following instabilities in the knee joint?
    A. Anterolateral rotatory instability
    B. Medial instability
    C. Lateral instability
    D. Anterior rotatory instability

Chapter 10: Thigh and Leg Injuries

22. Q angle is formed by:
    A. A line from ASIS to midpoint of patella and from there to the tibial tubercle
    B. Line from greater trochanter to midpoint of patella and from there to the tibial tubercle
    C. Line from midpoint of patella to tibial tubercle from there to the lateral malleolus
    D. Line through the shaft of femur to midpoint of patella from there to the tibial tubercle
23. Vastus medialis obliques can be tested in which position?
    A. Knees are held at 45° against resistance
    B. Knees are held at 60° against resistance
    C. Knees in full extension
    D. Knees in full flexion
24. In unhappy triad, which are all structures gets injured?
    A. Lateral ligament, ACL, medial meniscal tear
    B. Medial ligament, ACL, medial meniscal tear
    C. Medial ligament, ACL, lateral meniscal tear
    D. Medial ligament, PCL, medial meniscal tear
25. Which structure in knee joint is more prone for injury in wrestlers?
    A. LCL
    B. Medial meniscus
    C. MCL
    D. ACL
26. Why does medial meniscus injure more frequently than the lateral meniscus?
    A. Lack of freedom of movement of the medial meniscus
    B. Excess movement of medial meniscus
    C. Larger femoral condyle on medial part
    D. Large menisci on medial aspect
27. Painful arc sign in the knee joint indicates lesion in the:
    A. Posterior horn of meniscus
    B. Anterior horn of meniscus
    C. Mid portion of the meniscus
    D. Anterior edge of the meniscus

28. What is osteochondral fracture in knee joint?
   A. Avulsion fracture of patella
   B. Fracture of articular cartilage and the underlying bone of patella or lateral femoral condyle
   C. Articular damage of patella
   D. Fracture of lateral femoral condyle
29. The condition where articular cartilage can degenerate from recurrent impingement of the plica on the patella and the femoral condyles is known as:
   A. Synovial plica
   B. Infrapatellar fat pad lesion
   C. Bipartite patella
   D. Dislocation
30. Place the affected knee at 90° of flexion, then internally rotating the tibia and extending the knee, as the knee is extended, a valgus force is applied; pain at 30° of flexion indicates a positive sign for osteochondritis dissecans in knee joint. What is the test?
   A. Apprehension sign
   B. Apley's sign
   C. McMurray's sign
   D. Wilson's sign
31. Herniation of the synovium on the posterior medial aspect of the knee is:
   A. Baker's cyst
   B. Synovial plica
   C. Osteochondritis dissecans
   D. Dislocation of knee
32. Jumper's knee refers to tendonitis involving:
   A. Patellar tendon
   B. Quadriceps tendon
   C. Both A and B
   D. Quadriceps strain
33. Jumper's knee is commonly found in which group of people?
   A. Swimmers
   B. Basketball players
   C. Runners
   D. Cycling
34. In lateral view of knee, if the patellar tendon length exceeds the patellar length by 1 cm is considered as:
   A. Patella infera
   B. Patella baja
   C. Squinting patella
   D. Patella alta

35. For osteochondral fracture or osteochondritis dissecans, which view of X-ray is preferable?
    A. Tunnel view
    B. Anteroposterior view
    C. Lateral view
    D. Tangential view
36. The X-ray view in which the knee is bent nearly in to full flexion to see the inferior surface of the patella?
    A. Laurin view
    B. Merchant view
    C. Hughston view
    D. Sunrise view
37. In Hughston view the knee is bent approximately-degrees with the X-ray tube angle at-degrees?
    A. 45°, 30°
    B. 20°, 30°
    C. 45°, 10°
    D. 60°, 45°
38. Which X-ray view gives an accurate estimation of the intercondylar notch, the congruency angle, and the situation of the patella?
    A. Laurin view
    B. Merchant view
    C. Sunrise view
    D. Hughston view
39. Sudden, violent muscle contraction (eccentric or concentric) or an increased muscular stretch across an open epiphysis leads to _____ injury?
    A. Tear
    B. Sprain
    C. Strain
    D. Avulsion fracture
40. What are the causes of getting IT band syndrome?
    A. Sudden increase in distance, speed, work, hill running
    B. Leg length discrepancy
    C. Biomechanical faults
    D. All of the above
41. How can we distinguish gluteal medius tendonitis and trochanteric bursitis?
    A. Gluteus medius tendonitis-resisted hip abduction is painful and in trochanteric bursitis-resisted hip abduction is painless
    B. Gluteus medius tendonitis-resisted hip abduction is painless and in trochanteric bursitis-resisted hip abduction is painful
    C. Resisted hip abduction is painful in both conditions
    D. Resisted hip abduction is painless in both conditions

42. How can we differentiate gracilis syndrome from osteitis pubis?
    A. Resisted abduction is painful in gracilis syndrome
    B. Painful resisted adduction with no radiologic changes
    C. Painless resisted adduction in gracilis syndrome
    D. Radiological changes in gracilis syndrome

43. Select the symptoms of a quadriceps strain from the following:
    A. Pain down the entire length of the rectus femoris
    B. Localized tenderness
    C. Pain with an active quadriceps contraction and passive stretching
    D. All of the above

44. Position of hip in posterior dislocation:
    A. Flexed, adducted, internally rotated
    B. Flexed, abducted, externally rotated
    C. Extended, adducted, externally rotated
    D. Extended, abducted, internally rotated

45. How can we identify the femoral anteversion or retroversion?
    A. Telescopic test   B. Galeazzi test
    C. Craig test   D. Ortolani's test

46. What are the differential diagnoses of a traumatic hemarthosis?
    A. Meniscal/ligamentous tear
    B. Osteochondral fracture
    C. Patellar dislocation
    D. All of the above

47. Significance of fat globules found in the knee indicates the presence of which of the following?
    A. Meniscal tears   B. Osteochondral fracture
    C. Patellar dislocation   D. Ligamentous injury

48. What is the most common cause of knee injury?
    A. Compression
    B. Distortion
    C. Internal and external rotation
    D. Shear

49. What is the differential diagnosis of a locked knee?
    A. Bucket-handle meniscal tear
    B. Loose body/suprapatellar plica
    C. ACL tears
    D. All of the above
50. What is the primary function of ACL?
    A. Restraint posterior displacement of tibia
    B. Restraint anterior displacement of tibia
    C. Restraint internal rotation of tibia
    D. Restraint external rotation of tibia
51. What are the mechanisms of injury for ACL?
    A. Hyperextension
    B. Varus or internal rotation
    C. Extremes of valgus and external rotation
    D. All of the above
52. The allografts used for ACL reconstruction surgery are:
    A. Patellar tendon   B. Achilles tendon
    C. Posterior tibialis tendon   D. All of the above
53. Which is the primary function of PCL?
    A. Restraint internal rotation of tibia
    B. Restraint anterior displacement of tibia
    C. Restraint posterior displacement of tibia
    D. Restraint external rotation of tibia
54. What are the common causes of PCL injury?
    A. Valgus injury to the knee
    B. Fall on the flexed knee with forces directed posteriorly
    C. Dash board injuries to the knees
    D. All of the above
55. The bucket handle tear of the meniscus involves:
    A. Vertical tear at the periphery where meniscus remain intact anteriorly and posteriorly
    B. Horizontal tear at the periphery
    C. Vertical tear at the periphery where the meniscus separated anteriorly and posteriorly
    D. Tear of posterior horn of meniscus

56. In housemaid's knee which bursa gets inflamed?
    A. Prepatellar bursa
    B. Intrapatellar bursa
    C. Suprapatellar bursa
    D. Semitendinosus bursa
57. Which is the muscle insertion that forms pesanserinus?
    A. Sartorius, rectus femoris, semimembranosus
    B. Sartorius, gracilis, semimembranosus
    C. Sartorius, gracilis, semitendinosis
    D. Sartorius, rectus femoris, semitendinosus
58. The common condition relatively in knee joint for down hill runners and bicyclists is:
    A. Quadriceps tendinitis
    B. Iliotibial band friction syndrome
    C. Hamstring tendinitis
    D. Patellar tendinitis
59. An inflammatory condition in which pain is increased by flexing the knee to 90° and resisting internal rotation of tibia is:
    A. Semimembranosus tendinitis
    B. Bicipital tendinitis
    C. Hamstring tendinitis
    D. Rectus femoris tendinitis
60. What are the differential diagnoses of chronic exertional leg pain?
    A. Medial tibial stress syndrome
    B. Exertional compartment syndrome
    C. Stress fracture
    D. All of the above
61. Descriptive term for an inflammatory condition of one or more musculotendinous units of the leg.
    A. Stress fracture
    B. Medial tibial stress syndrome
    C. Referred discogenic leg pain
    D. Shin splints
62. Inflammatory condition involving the periosteum of the deep posterior compartment of lower leg is known as:

Chapter 10: Thigh and Leg Injuries 193

    A. Referred discogenic leg pain
    B. Chronic exertional compartment syndrome
    C. Medial tibial stress syndrome
    D. Stress fracture

63. Most common location for stress fracture in the leg is:
    A. Proximal third of tibia
    B. At the junction of the middle and distal third of tibia
    C. Along the posterior medial margin of tibia
    D. All of the above

64. A clinical syndrome in which the athletes typically have pain in the involved compartment during exercise session, numbness in the top of the foot and weakness of ankle dorsiflexion, symptoms may slowly subside after cessation of exercise, what will be the condition?
    A. Exertional compartment syndrome
    B. Acute compartment syndrome
    C. Vascular claudication
    D. Stress fracture

65. The first case report of a thigh injury was described by:
    A. Petit   B. Fleming
    C. Alexander   D. Blecker

66. Stress fracture of the femur was first described by:
    A. Fleming   B. Blecker
    C. Alexander   D. Pavlou

67. In athletic population, which muscle among the hamstring group is more prone for strain?
    A. Semitendinosis   B. Semimembranosus
    C. Long head of biceps   D. Short head of biceps

68. Why does the strains are twice as found to occur in the second half of play compared with the first half?
    A. Fatigue   B. Lack of stretching
    C. Lack of warm up   D. All of the above

69. Complete hamstring rupture without bony avulsion is best imaged with-magnetic resonance imaging?
    A. Both T1 and T2 weighted   B. T1 weighted
    C. T2 weighted   D. None of the above

70. In athletic pubalgia where will be the location of pain with regard to the adductor tubercle?
    A. Above the adductor tubercle
    B. Medial to the adductor tubercle
    C. At the adductor tubercle
    D. Below the adductor tubercle
71. In which players the adductor strain is more common?
    A. Rugby
    B. Track and field
    C. Tennis
    D. Hockey
72. What is the mechanism of ASIS avulsion fracture?
    A. Knee flexed and the hip extended
    B. Knee extended and hip flexed
    C. Knee flexed and hip flexed
    D. Knee extended and hip extended
73. What are the anthropomorphic risk factors for the development of stress fractures in lower leg?
    A. Broad tibial width
    B. Planus foot
    C. Higher degree external rotation of hip
    D. All of the above
74. Why stress fracture is common in female athletes?
    A. Narrow tibial width
    B. Osteoporosis
    C. Cavus foot
    D. Planus foot
75. What is the most common site of tibial stress fracture?
    A. Posteromedial cortex
    B. Anterolateral cortex
    C. Posterolateral cortex
    D. Anteromedial cortex
76. How does pneumatic brace helps in stress fractures?
    A. Unloading the tibia
    B. Act as a venous tourniquet
    C. Shifting electrolytes into the interstitial fluid
    D. All of the above
77. What is the clinical significance of anterior cortex tibial stress fracture?
    A. Infection
    B. Malunion
    C. Nonunion
    D. Tibial varus

78. What type of athletes is more prone for tension tibial stress injuries?
    A. Jumpers
    B. Runners
    C. Footballers
    D. Cricketers
79. What type of athletes is more prone for compression tibial stress fractures?
    A. Jumpers
    B. Runners
    C. Volleyball players
    D. Tennis players
80. Which is the most common site of anterior cortex tibial stress fracture?
    A. Upper third
    B. Lower third
    C. Middle third
    D. All of the above
81. Distal fibular stress fracture will occur in which type of athletes?
    A. Distance runners
    B. Swimmers
    C. Divers
    D. Footballers
82. Proximal fibula stress fractures are common in which group of people?
    A. Athletes
    B. Sedentary individuals
    C. Adults
    D. Children
83. In what type of sports, the fractures of the tibia and fibula are common?
    A. Table tennis
    B. Distance runners
    C. Tennis
    D. Soccer
84. What are the other names of medial tibial stress syndrome?
    A. Shin splints
    B. Shin soreness
    C. Soleus syndrome
    D. All of the above
85. Which muscle plays a major role in the genesis of MTSS?
    A. Soleus
    B. Flexor digitorum longus
    C. Tibialis posterior
    D. Tibialis anterior
86. What is the predisposing factor for the development of MTSS?
    A. Excessive dorsiflexion
    B. Excessive plantar flexion
    C. Excessive pronation
    D. Excessive supination
87. What is the bone inclination at the proximal tibiofibular joint leads to proximal tibiofibular instability?

A. Lesser than 20 degrees   B. 20 degrees
C. Greater than 20 degrees   D. All of the above

88. Among the proximal tibiofibular instability injuries which of the following is more common?
    A. Superior dislocation   B. Posteromedial dislocation
    C. Inferior dislocation   D. Anterolateral dislocation

89. What is the mechanism of anterolateral dislocation of the proximal fibula?
    A. Fall on an everted and dorsiflexed foot with the knee extended and the leg abducted
    B. Fall on an inverted and plantar flexed foot with the knee flexed and the leg abducted
    C. Fall on an everted and plantar flexed foot with the knee extended and the leg adducted
    D. Fall on the inverted and plantar flexed foot with the knee extended and the leg adducted

90. Posteromedial dislocation of the fibula is associated with contraction of which muscle?
    A. Biceps femoris   B. Gastrocnemius
    C. Soleus   D. Popliteus

91. Following are the causes of entrapment of the common peroneal nerve, *except*:
    A. Compression of peronial musculature
    B. Genuvarum
    C. Posterolateral knee reconstruction
    D. Genuvalgum

92. A nerve, which is often compressed from high boots with tight laces is:
    A. Common peroneal nerve   B. Superficial peroneal nerve
    C. Deep peroneal nerve   D. Sural nerve

93. What is the cause of acquired tibiofibular synostosis?
    A. Intrauterine trauma
    B. Infection
    C. Developmental arrest after joint cavitation
    D. Leg length discrepancy
    E. All of the above

Chapter 10: Thigh and Leg Injuries

94. What is the possible mechanism of injury leads to tibiofibular synostosis?
    A. Internal rotation or inversion force
    B. Internal rotation or eversion force
    C. External rotation or inversion force
    D. External rotation or eversion force

95. The mechanism of adductor strain is:
    A. Eccentric adductor muscle contraction with concurrent hip internal rotation and adduction
    B. Eccentric adductor muscle contraction with concurrent hip internal rotation and abduction
    C. Eccentric adductor muscle contraction with concurrent hip external rotation and abduction
    D. Concentric adductor muscle contraction with concurrent hip external rotation and abduction

96. What is the possible mechanism of getting injury for medial gastrocnemius?
    A. Simultaneous knee flexion and ankle plantar flexion
    B. Simultaneous knee flexion and ankle dorsiflexion
    C. Simultaneous knee extension and ankle dorsiflexion
    D. Simultaneous knee extension and ankle plantar flexion

97. Who described the clicking or snapping hip first?
    A. Nunzaiata   B. Binnie
    C. Blumend   D. Quirk

98. Following group of athletes is more prone for clicking or snapping hip, *except*:
    A. Tennis players
    B. Cheer leaders
    C. Recreational athletes
    D. Triathletes

99. Which test is used to identify anterolateral rotatory instability?
    A. Jerk test
    B. Extended rotation recurvatum test
    C. Jacob test
    D. Posterolateral drawer test

100. **Which test is used to identify posterolateral rotatory instability?**
    A. Reverse pivot shift
    B. Lateral pivot shift test
    C. Flexion rotation drawer test
    D. Anterolateral drawer test

101. **The mechanism of ACL injury in noncontact sports is:**
    A. Skiing injuries
    B. Deceleration injuries with increased quadriceps contraction
    C. Hyperextension
    D. All of the above

102. **What is known as Segnod fracture?**
    A. Avulsion # of PCL
    B. Avulsion # of ACL
    C. Avulsion # of the inferior lateral capsule adjacent to the tibia
    D. Avulsion # of the patellar tendon

103. **Calcification adjacent to the adductor tubercle signifies an old collateral ligament injury of longer than 6 weeks is known as:**
    A. Pellegrini-Stieda lesion
    B. Segond fracture
    C. Grade III injury of MCL
    D. Posterolateral ligament instability

104. **What activities typically aggravate the patellofemoral joint pain?**
    A. Ascending stairs
    B. Squatting
    C. Sitting with the knees flexed to 90°
    D. All of the above

105. **During 'Screw Home' mechanism what motion of tibia helps to stabilize the knee in full extension from flexed position?**
    A. External rotation of tibia during last 30° of extension
    B. External rotation of tibia during last 20° of extension
    C. Internal rotation of tibia during last 20° of extension
    D. Internal rotation of tibia during last 30° of extension

106. The most common cause for patellofemoral joint pain is:
    A. Extensor mechanism malalignment
    B. Internal derangements of knee
    C. Insufficiency of quadriceps muscle
    D. Recurrent dislocation
107. For rehabilitation after a posterior cruciate ligament injury, strengthening of which muscle group should be emphasized early?
    A. Quadriceps
    B. Hamstrings
    C. Pes anserine group
    D. Popliteus
108. Which is the common area of pain in iliotibial band friction syndrome during palpation?
    A. Lateral femoral epicondyle
    B. Lateral knee joint line
    C. Tibial tubercle
    D. Lateral tibial condyle
109. A 13-year-old girl discusses the possibility of anterior cruciate reconstruction with her orthopedic surgeon. The girl injured her knee while playing soccer and is concerned about the future impact of the injury on her athletic carrier. Which of the following factors would have the greatest influence on her candidacy for surgery?
    A. Anthropometric measurements
    B. Hamstrings/quadriceps strength ratio
    C. Skeletal maturity
    D. Somatotype
110. A therapist examines a patient diagnosed with an Achilles tendon injury, which clinical finding is not indicative of a ruptured Achilles tendon?
    A. Negative Thompson test
    B. Absent Achilles reflex
    C. Lack of toe-off during gait
    D. A palpable defect in the musculotendinous unit
111. Which of the following conditions lead to the locking of knee?
    A. Meniscal Injury
    B. Loose bodies within the joint
    C. A and B
    D. Prepatellar bursitis

112. Name the most sensitive test to detect an anterior cruciate ligament (ACL) tear that involves a relaxed patient and relaxed lower extremity.
    A. Lachman test
    B. McMurray test
    C. Posterior drawer test
    D. Apley compression test
113. While applying Apley compression test, medial pain with the tibia in external rotation indicates:
    A. Lateral meniscus tear
    B. Medical meniscal tear
    C. Inner tear
    D. None of the above
114. _____ can be used safely during ACL rehabilitation because they appear to generate low anterior shear force and tibial displacement through most of the knee flexion range.
    A. Open-chain extension exercises
    B. Closed-chain exercises
    C. Both A and B
    D. Leg extension machine
115. In case of anterior knee pain, activities increasing the patellofemoral joint reaction forces should be avoided and those includes:
    A. Deep squats
    B. Stairmaster
    C. Jogging
    D. All of the above
116. Which type of exercise generates minimal or no force in the posterior cruciate ligament (PCL)?
    A. Open-kinetic chain flexion exercises
    B. Open-kinetic chain extension exercises from 60°-90°
    C. Open-kinetic chain extension exercises from 0°-60°
    D. Hamstring resisted exercises
117. The Ober test is used to assess the flexibility of:
    A. Quadriceps
    B. Iliotibial band
    C. Hamstrings
    D. Adductors
118. _____ refers to a sharp jump of the patella into the trochlear groove that raises the suspicion of patellar instability.
    A. J-sign
    B. Posterior sag sign
    C. Hoover's sign
    D. McMurray test

119. What are the positional relationships that are evaluated statically and dynamically by Quadriceps sets in McConnell taping?
    A. Glide and tilt component   B. Rotational component
    C. Anteroposterior tilt   D. All of the above
120. Rehabilitation of the patellar tendinitis or Jumper's knee include:
    A. Use of a chopat "counterforce" strap
    B. Closed-chain kinetic exercises
    C. Balance training
    D. All of the above
121. Which one of the following is not a potential risk factor related to a quadriceps strain?
    A. Flexibility
    B. Previous history of strains
    C. Inadequate warm-up routine
    D. Muscle weakness or fatigue
122. Immediate management of an athlete suffering a muscle strain is:
    A. Progressive resistance exercises
    B. Rest, Ice, Compression, and Elevation (RICE)
    C. Agility drills
    D. Endurance exercises
123. Which of the following exercises is not observed under the chronic stage (maturation and remodeling phase) of quadriceps strain rehabilitation?
    A. Plyometric exercises
    B. Agility drills
    C. Isometric quadriceps exercises
    D. Endurance training
124. _____ is a condition marked by an audible snapping sound that may be associated with hip pain during activity.
    A. Coxa saltans
    B. Iliotibial band syndrome
    C. Coxa vara
    D. Osteitis pubis

125. What are the contributing factors to the onset of an extra-articular snapping hip?
    A. Repetitive overuse of hip flexors
    B. Trauma
    C. Anatomic factors
    D. All of the above

126. Physiotherapy interventions for snapping hip include:
    A. Rest and therapeutic modalities
    B. Hip flexor and tensor fascia latae flexibility exercises
    C. Strengthening of the lower quadrant
    D. All of the above

127. In distance runners, iliotibial band syndrome often occurs due to the:
    A. Poor footwear
    B. Lack of muscle flexibility
    C. Poor training
    D. All of the above

128. The occurrence of adductor strains is high in sports such as:
    A. Ice hockey
    B. Soccer
    C. Swimming
    D. All of the above

129. Name the adductor muscle, which is most often strained?
    A. Adductor longus
    B. Adductor magnus
    C. Pectineus
    D. Gracilis

130. Which one of the following is not an injury risk factor for hip adductor muscle strain in sportspersons?
    A. Decreased hip adduction strength
    B. Excessive hip abduction range of motion
    C. A previous hip adductor injury
    D. Breaststroke swimming

131. Which one of the following is the injury risk factor for hamstring muscle strain?
    A. Hamstring weakness (eccentric)
    B. Previous history of a hamstring injury
    C. Failure to properly warm up before a sport
    D. All of the above

132. Which one of the following is the eccentric exercise for the hamstrings?
    A. Inverted hamstring
    B. Romanian deadlift
    C. Nordic or Russian hamstring curl
    D. All of the above
133. Females with patellofemoral pain syndrome (PFPS) generally have significant weakness in following muscles:
    A. Gluteus medius
    B. Gluteus maximus
    C. Hip external rotators
    D. All of the above
134. _____ assess the presence of patellofemoral dysfunction.
    A. Clarke's sign
    B. Indentation test
    C. Bohler's sign
    D. Bragard's sign
135. The key aspects to emphasize while rehabilitating patients with patellofemoral pain syndrome (PFPS) are:
    A. Overcoming any VMO inhibition
    B. Addressing the biomechanical abnormalities
    C. Increasing the functional load tolerance through the joint
    D. All of the above
136. A 22-year-old male runner diagnosed with iliotibial band syndrome complains of pain along his right knee when he runs on a banked track or when he runs distances greater than three miles. Which of the following would be the MOST appropriate intervention?
    A. Initiate a lower extremity flexibility program
    B. Implement short-arc knee extension exercises
    C. Perform cycling for 20 minutes at 80 revolutions per minute or greater
    D. Wear a neoprene sleeve over the knee during all running activities
137. A 26-year-old male marathon runner is referred to physical therapy for the management of left lateral knee pain. While taking history, the marathon runner states that the pain began approximately four weeks ago after increasing his running mileage. Physical examination reveals normal lower

extremity strength, a positive Ober test (knee extended), and moderate abduction during the modified Thomas test on the left. The marathon runner's above clinical presentation is MOST consistent with:

A. Greater trochanteric bursitis
B. Iliotibial band syndrome
C. Chondromalacia patella
D. Tibial plateau fracture

138. While examining a patient diagnosed with a grade III posterior cruciate ligament sprain, the most consistent description of a positive posterior sag test is:

A. Static positioning reveals a posterior position of the tibia in relation to the femur
B. Static positioning reveals an anterior position of the tibia in relation to the femur
C. Manual resistance to the tibia in a posterior direction reveals excessive posterior translation
D. Manual resistance to the tibia in an anterior direction reveals excessive posterior translation

139. Which one of the following is the MOST likely outcome of the valgus test applied to a sprinter two days status of the grade I medial collateral ligament sprain?

A. Pain with no discernable laxity when compared to the contralateral limb
B. Pain with discernable laxity when compared to the contralateral limb
C. No pain with discernable laxity when compared to the contralateral limb
D. No pain with no discernable laxity when compared to the contralateral limb

140. A sports physical therapist attempts to select an appropriate intervention to treat an athlete who sustained an injury, immobilized his knee, and is recovering with a 10-degree limitation in knee extension. Which of the following mobilization techniques would be indicated?

A. Lateral glide of the patella   B. Caudal glide of the patella
C. Posterior glide of the tibia   D. Anterior glide of the tibia

141. A physical therapist examines a 26-year-old male elite soccer player diagnosed with piriformis syndrome. The player indicates he has experienced pain in his lower back and buttock region for three weeks. Which motions would you expect to be weak and painful during muscle testing based on the elite soccer player's diagnosis?
    A. Abduction and lateral rotation of the thigh
    B. Abduction and medial rotation of the thigh
    C. Adduction and lateral rotation of the thigh
    D. Adduction and medial rotation of the thigh

142. A physical therapist examines an 18-year-old male diagnosed with right knee anterior cruciate ligament insufficiency. During the examination, the therapist performs the Lachman test. Ideally, the therapist should perform the test with the knee in:
    A. Complete extension
    B. 20–30° flexion
    C. 30–40° flexion
    D. 40–50° flexion

143. A physical therapist examines a 14-year-old school boy diagnosed with Osgood–Schlatter disease. The patient reports limiting the intensity and duration of activities due to a progressive increase in pain over the last month. The MOST likely objective finding based on the diagnosis is:
    A. Patella crepitus
    B. Increased lateral tibial rotation
    C. Inability to extend the knee against gravity
    D. Tenderness to palpation over the tibial tubercle

ANSWERS

1. **A.** Complete rupture of the quadriceps or patellar tendon is a major injury which occurs when the athlete lands in an off-balance position from a long jump or from a basketball rebound.
2. **A.** If athlete is wearing a shoe with a low coefficient of friction, there is a definite chance the foot will move with the blow, thereby eliminating the force on the ligaments.
3. **B.** PCL injury is common while playing on the harder surface of the artificial turf, which occur when the tibial tubercle comes into contact with the unrelenting surface, forcing the tibia backwards.
4. **D.** Poorly treated contusion of the anterior thigh can result in a prolonged recovery, with stiffness, poor quadriceps action and muscle wasting.
5. **E.** Myositis ossification is a feared complication and is particularly apt to occur if (a) the athlete reform to participation to soon (b) thigh is reinjured before healing occurs (c) massage or heat has been applied to the hematoma (d) the hematoma has been poorly treated or (e) the bleeding is associated with hemophilia.
6. **E.** The predisposing factor for quadriceps strain includes tight quadriceps muscle, insufficient warm up, an imbalance between the quadriceps power of two legs and a short leg.
7. **C.**
8. **A.** An acute hamstring pull is a common and frustrating injury occurring particularly in sprinters.
9. **D.** Hamstring pull related to some of the following factors: lack of flexibility of the hamstring group, imbalance in the ratio of strength and power between the hamstrings and the quadriceps, inequality of strength of the left versus the right hamstrings group, biceps muscle receives two nerve supply and poor running style.
10. **B.** Slow onset hamstring strain occurs particularly in the long-distance runners, progressive tightness and discomfort are noted in the upper most third of the posterior aspect of the leg.

Chapter 10: Thigh and Leg Injuries

11. **C.** Rapid swelling of the knee with in twelve hours of the injury indicates bleeding into the joint (i.e., Hemarthosis).
12. **A.** Swelling of the joint with relatively gradual onset, occurring more than twelve hours after an injury is indicative of synovial irritation and a joint effusion. A meniscal tear might be the causative factor.
13. **D.** Pain on going up or down stairs, particularly on walking down, is indicative of retropatellar irritation.
14. **B.** Pain under the patella and along the patellar tendon after such jumping activities as basketball, is indicative of patellar tendonitis.
15. **D.** A subluxing patella can produce vague symptoms like giving way, locking and swelling.
16. **A.** If hyperextension is excessive on the affected side, it may indicate rupture or incompetence of the ACL, with or without a tear of PCL.
17. **D.** Valgus and varus stress at 0 degree indicates involvement not only of the stabilizing complex but also of the ACL and PCL.
18. **A.** Valgus or varus stress at 30° localizes the stress to the medial or lateral stabilizing complex.
19. **B.** Anterior drawers sign with foot in external rotation (15°) is the Slocum test for anterior medial rotatory instability.
20. **D.** Anterior drawers sign with foot in internal rotation with anterior stress, the lateral tibial plateau moves anteriorly and rotates medially from the lateral side when there is incompetency of either or both the ACL or the LCL and the posterior lateral corner.
21. **A.** Pivot shift tests are designed to demonstrate anterolateral rotatory instability and can be used in both acute and chronic situation.
22. **A.** Measure the Q angle by taking a line from ASIS down to the thigh to the midpoint of the patella, and from there to the tibial tubercle.
23. **A.**
24. **B.**
25. **A.** Frequently flexed attitude of the knee with the foot in external rotation causes lateral ligament injuries occurring relatively more often in wrestlers.

26. **A.** Medial meniscus appears to be injured more frequently than lateral meniscus may be due to relative lack of freedom of movement of medial meniscus, since the lateral meniscus can move out of the way of the lateral femoral condyle as it rotates.
27. **C.** Pain through the mid range of knee movement, with the extremes of flexion and extension being pain free, indicates a tear of the midportion of the meniscus and is called painful arc sign.
28. **B.**
29. **A.** Synovial plica—the athlete usually complains of pain and swelling, accompanied by a catching or snapping sensation. The articular cartilage can degenerate from recurrent impingement of the plica on the patella and the femoral condyle diagnosed arthroscopically.
30. **D.** Wilson's sign is positive for osteochondritis dissecans and this test can be negative although osteochondritis dissecans is present.
31. **A.** Baker's cyst—actually a herniation of the synovium, this swelling is usually found on the posteromedial aspect of the knee. The herniation forms a sac and fills with synovial fluid.
32. **C.** Jumper's knee refers to tendinitis involving either the patellar tendon, the quadriceps tendon or both.
33. **B.** Jumper's knee is peculiar to athletic activities, particularly those involving constant repetitive jumping and landing, such as basketball, the long and high jump and the triple jump.
34. **D.** If the patellar tendon length exceeds the patellar length by 1 cm or more it is considered as patella alta.
35. **A.** Tunnel view is used to visualize the femoral condyles particularly when looking for osteochondral fractures or osteochondral dissecans.
36. **D.** Sunrise view—views of the inferior surface of the patella can be obtained in cases of a suspected osteochondral fracture.
37. **A.** In Hughston view—the knee is bent approximately 45° with the X-ray tube angle at 30°.

38. B. The merchant view gives an accurate estimation of the intercondylar notch, the congruency angle, and the situation of the patella.

39. D. Avulsion fracture is caused by a sudden violent contraction (eccentric or concentric) or an increased muscular stretch across an open epiphysis.

40. D. IT band syndrome is due to training errors, such as sudden increase in distance, speed, work, hill running, leg length discrepancy or biomechanical faults.

41. A. Gluteus medius insertional tendinitis demonstrates maximum tenderness proximal to the gluteal tendon and has pain on resisted hip abduction. Trochanteric bursitis demonstrates pain over the lateral aspect of the trochanter and no pain with resisted hip abduction.

42. B. The gracilis syndrome involves the gracilis muscle at its origin on the pubic symphysis. There is sharp pain with resisted hip adduction followed by a dull ache. Radiographs often are negative unless injury was traumatic. Osteitis pubis is an inflammatory lesion of the bone with well-defined radiologic changes.

43. D. Symptoms of the quadriceps strain are pain down the entire length of the rectus femoris, localized tenderness, pain with an active quadriceps contraction and pain with passive stretching.

44. A. The leg is aligned in posterior dislocation is flexion, adduction, internal rotation with prominent trochanter and buttock.

45. C. Craig test or Ryder method will help to identify the anteversion and retroversion of femur.

46. D. The differential diagnosis of the traumatic hemarthrosis are meniscal tear, ligamentous tear, and osteochondral fracture and patellar dislocation.

47. B. The presence of fat globules found in the knee signifies osteochondral fracture, with the fat globules originating from the marrow components.

48. C. Internal and external rotation is the most common cause of knee injuries.

49. **D.** The differential diagnosis of a locked knee is bucket handle meniscal tear, loose body, ACL tear and suprapatellar plica.
50. **B.** ACL is the prime restraint to anterior displacement of the tibia.
51. **D.** Mechanism of injury for ACL is hyperextension, varus or internal rotation and extremes of valgus and external rotation.
52. **D.** For ACL reconstruction, allografts can be used from frozen or freeze-dried patellar tendon bone, Achilles tendon and tibialis tendon.
53. **C.** PCL is the primary restraint to posterior subluxation of the tibia on the femur.
54. **D.** The common mechanism of PCL injury is valgus injury to the knee; fall on the flexed knee with forces directed posteriorly and dash board injuries.
55. **A.** A bucket handle tear of the meniscus is a vertical tear at the periphery. The meniscus remains intact anteriorly and posteriorly.
56. **A.** Prepatellar bursitis is otherwise known as housemaid's knee.
57. **C.** The tendons of sartorius, gracilus, semitendinosus together form pes anserinus.
58. **B.** IT band friction syndrome is an acute inflammatory condition that occurs when the IT band repeatedly rubs over the lateral femoral epicondyles. It is commonly seen in runners who incorporate excessive downhill running into their training as well as in bicyclist who are not conditioned for long ride.
59. **A.** In semimebranous tendinitis, the pain is usually increased by flexing the knee to 90° and resisting internal rotation of the tibia. It is necessary to rule out intra articular pathology.
60. **D.** The differential diagnosis of chronic exertional leg pain are medial tibial stress syndrome, chronic exertional compartment syndrome, stress fracture, vascular claudication, referred discogenic leg pain, true shin splints.
61. **D.** Shin splint is a descriptive term for an inflammatory condition of one or more of the musculotendinous units of the leg.

Chapter 10: Thigh and Leg Injuries

62. **C.** Medial tibial stress syndrome is an inflammatory condition involving the periosteum of the deep posterior compartment of leg.
63. **D.** Stress fractures of tibia are more common in the proximal third or at the junction of the middle and the distal thirds along the posterior medial margin.
64. **A.** In exertional compartment syndrome, athletes typically have pain in the involved compartment that begins at a consistent time into their exercise session. Symptoms may then slowly subside after cessation of exercise. They may note numbness in the top of foot and weakness of ankle dorsiflexion.
65. **A.** The first case report of a thigh injury was described by Petit in 1722.
66. **B.** Stress fracture of the femur was first described by Blecker in 1905.
67. **C.** In athletic population, the most common muscle strained in the body is the hamstring; specifically, the long head of the biceps is most often injured, making this the most common muscle strained in the body.
68. **D.** NCAA soccer statistics support fatigue; lack of stretching and lack of warm up as major factors; as twice as many strains are found to occur in the second half of play compared with the first half.
69. **C.** Complete hamstring rupture without bony avulsion is best imaged with T2 weighted magnetic resonance imaging (MRI).
70. **A.** Pathology in the groin region is best categorized by location of symptoms with regard to the adductor tubercle. Pain below the adductor tubercle is frequently associated with strain injury. Pain at the adductor tubercle is usually a result of avulsion fracture of inferior ramus, stress fracture and pain above the adductor tubercle is common to athletic pubalgia. Pain at the tubercle or just medial to the adductor tubercle is frequently found with osteitis pubis.
71. **D.** Adductor strains are more common strain injuries in hockey, with a reported injury rate as high as 0.43/1000 hours.
72. **A.** With the knee flexed and the hip extended, the sartorius is placed on maximal tension leads to avulsion fracture of ASIS.

73. **C.** Anthropomorphic risk factors for stress fractures were identified by Giladi and colleagues is that a narrow tibial width, higher degree of external rotation of the hip and a cavus foot.
74. **B.** A high incidence of stress fractures has been reported in women. The "female athlete triad" refers to a female athlete with an eating disorder, amenorrhea and osteoporosis.
75. **A.** Tibial stress fracture are most frequently encountered in the posteromedial cortex or compression side.
76. **D.** The pneumatic brace has been proposed to work similarly to a functional weight-bearing cast. By unloading the tibia at the site of the stress fracture, the brace theoretically hastens the healing time. Alternatively, the pneumatic brace may act as a venous tourniquet, shifting electrolytes into the interstitial fluid space. This creates an electronegative charge that stimulates osteoblastic bone formation.
77. **C.** Anterior cortex tibial stress fractures exhibit poor healing properties because of poor blood supply.
78. **A.** Tension tibial stress injuries occur in athletes performing repetitive jumping and leaping activities.
79. **B.** Compression tibial stress fractures which usually occur in distance runners.
80. **C.** Location of tibial stress fractures is the anterior cortex of the middle third of the tibia.
81. **A.** The usual site of fibular stress fracture is just proximal to the inferior tibiofibular ligaments at the junction of cortical and cacellous bone. This injury predominantly occurs in distance runners who train on hard surface.
82. **B.** Proximal fibula stress fracture occur in sedentary individuals who abruptly begin a vigorous exercise program.
83. **D.** Fracture of the tibia and fibula can occur in any sport, soccer players are at high risk due to the high energy associated with the kicking maneuver.
84. **D.** Numerous terms, such as shin splints, shin soreness, soleus syndrome and MTSS has been used to describe activity related pain along the middle to distal aspect of the posteromedial tibia.
85. **A.** Based on the strength and location of the soleus bridge in cadaveric specimens, the authors concluded that the soleus is the major contributory to the development of MTSS.

Chapter 10: Thigh and Leg Injuries

86. **C.** The runner with excessively pronated feet has been shown to be predisposed to the development of overuse syndrome.
87. **C.** Ogden proposed that the oblique inclination greater than 20°, is inherently less stable than the horizontal articulation.
88. **D.** Ogden divided proximal tibiofibular instability injuries into four types; subluxation, anterolateral dislocation, posteromedial dislocation and superior dislocation. In his review anterolateral dislocation was the most common type accounting for 67.4%.
89. **B.** The classic mechanism of anterolateral dislocation of proximal fibula involves a fall on an inverted and plantar flexed foot with the knee flexed and the leg abducted.
90. **A.** Posteromedial dislocation are caused by direct high energy trauma or by a twisting motion associated with a strong biceps femoris contraction.
91. **D.** The mechanism of injury of common peroneal nerve involves contraction of the peroneal musculature when the foot is in a plantar flexed and inverted position. Other factors that may be responsible for peroneal nerve irritation include genuvalgum, posterolateral knee reconstruction and mechanical pressure from proximal tibiofibular instability.
92. **B.** Superficial peroneal nerve compression may be caused by the fascial hernia, fibula fracture, direct trauma, a space-occupying lesion, stretching of the nerve secondary to recurrent ankle sprains; or compression from high boots with tight laces.
93. **E.** Acquired synostosis may occur in association with leg length discrepancy, exostosis, tibia and/or fibular fractures and posterolateral tibial bone grafting.
94. **C.** The mechanism of injury either involves an external rotation or inversion force to the foot.
95. **C.** The mechanism of adductor strain is eccentric adductor muscle contraction with concurrent hip external rotation and abduction.
96. **C.** Gastrocnemius injuries occur during explosive sprinting, jumping, or change of direction of activities. There is usually simultaneous knee extension and ankle dorsiflexion, placing the muscle- tendon unit under stress.

97. **B.** Binnie first described an entity called the snapping hip in 1913.
98. **A.** Clicking or snapping hip is unique to dancers due to excessive turn out; although this problem has subsequently been noted in runners, cheer leaders, triathletes and other recreational athlete.
99. **A.** The tests used to identify the anterolateral rotatory instability are Jerk test (Hugston and Losec), lateral pivot shift test (Macintosh), flexion rotation drawer test (Noyer), anterolateral drawer test.
100. **A.** The tests used to identify the posterolateral rotatory instability are external rotation recurvatum test, Reverse pivot shift (Jacob), posterolateral drawer test, tibial external rotation test.
101. **D.** Skiing injuries in downhill skiers, a forward fall in which the inside edge of the ski is caught in the snow, placing the knee in external rotation and valgus stress. Deceleration injuries with increased quadriceps contraction anterior force on the proximal tibia is caused by tremendous quadriceps contraction. Hyperextension noncontact ACL injuries also are seen with hyperextension injury in basketball players (e.g., in rebounding) and in gymnastic during the dismount.
102. **C.** A Segond fracture is an avulsion fracture of the inferior lateral capsule adjacent to the tibia. It is highly suggestive of an injury to the ACL but it is seen in only about 6% of the cases.
103. **A.** The Pellegrini-Stieda lesion is seen on the anteroposterior radiograph. Calcification adjacent to the adductor tubercle signifies an old collateral ligament injury of longer than 6 weeks.
104. **D.** Activities that load the patellofemoral joint or create high compressive forces, such as ascending and descending stairs, squatting, and sitting with the knee flexed to 90° for prolonged periods of time, cause significant patellofemoral pain.
105. **B.**
106. **C.**
107. **A.**

Chapter 10: Thigh and Leg Injuries

108. A.
109. C.
110. A.
111. C. Locking is typically indicative of a meniscal injury or loose body within the joint. A "locked" knee typically still has flexion, but the patient has difficulty getting the last 5 to 20° of full extension.
112. A. The most sensitive test for an ACL tear is a Lachman test with a relaxed patient and relaxed lower extremity.
113. B. Apley compression test (meniscal test) involves the prone knee is flexed to 90°. The knee is compressed (pushed downward) while the knee is alternately externally and internally rotated at the foot. Medial pain on external rotation suggests a medial meniscal tear. Lateral pain on internal rotation suggests a probable lateral meniscal tear.
114. B. Closed-chain exercises can be used safely during the rehabilitation of the ACL because they appear to generate low anterior shear force and tibial displacement through most of the flexion range, although some evidence now exists that low flexion angles during certain closed-kinetic chain activities may strain the graft as much as open-chain activities and may not be as safe as previously thought.
115. D. For a patient who begins to show signs of anterior knee pain, the rehabilitation program should be modified to eliminate exercises that may place undue stress on the patellofemoral joint. Activities that increase the patellofemoral joint reaction forces (PFJRFs) should be avoided; these include: deep squats, Stairmaster use, jogging, and excessive weight during leg presses. Terminal knee extension exercises also often elicit anterior knee pain.
116. C. With open-kinetic chain activities, there appears to be a tremendous force exerted on the PCL during flexion exercises. However, with open-kinetic chain extension, minimal or no force appears to be generated in the PCL from 0 to 60°, but from 60 to 90°, significant stress is produced in the PCL.
117. B. The Ober test is used to assess iliotibial band flexibility.

118. **A.** A sharp jump of the patella into the trochlear groove, sometimes referred to as the J-sign or late centering of the patella, should raise the suspicion of patellar instability.
119. **D.** In McConnell taping, four positional relationships are evaluated statically (sitting with the legs extended and quadriceps relaxed) then dynamically by doing a quadriceps set. They are glide component, tilt component, rotational component, and anteroposterior tilt.
120. **D.** Rehabilitation of the patellar tendinitis or Jumper's knee includes use of a chopat "counterforce" strap, flexibility exercises, closed-chain kinetic exercises, four-position hip strengthening, endurance training, and balance training.
121. **A.** Potential risk factors associated with a quadriceps strain include: muscular fatigue, lack of flexibility, previous history of strains, muscular weakness, muscular imbalance, or inadequate warm-up routine.
122. **B.** Immediate treatment of an athlete suffering a strain is rest, ice, compression, and elevation (RICE).
123. **C.** In chronic stage (maturation and remodeling phase) of the quadriceps strain rehabilitation, exercises prescribed are cardiovascular fitness (stationary bicycle, Stairmaster), return to running program, endurance training, progressive resistance exercises, strength training (squats, lunges, step-downs, knee extension machine), plyometrics, agility drills, and sports-specific training.
124. **A.** Coxa saltans, also known as a snapping hip, is a condition marked by an audible snapping sound that may be associated with hip pain during activity. Coxa saltans may be of either intra articular or extra articular origin.
125. **D.** Repetitive overuse (specifically hip flexion greater than 90°), trauma, and anatomic factors may contribute to the onset of an extraarticular snapping hip.
126. **D.** Physical therapy interventions should address asymmetries in flexibility and core dysfunction. Standard treatments include rest, modalities, lower extremity flexibility exercises [specifically for the hip flexors and the tensor fasciae latae (TFL)/ITB], and strengthening exercises for the lower quadrant.

Chapter 10: Thigh and Leg Injuries

127. **D.** Frequently experienced by distance runners, ITBS is often the result of poor training, poor footwear, anatomic factors, muscular inflexibility, muscle weakness, or any combination of these factors.
128. **D.** The incidence of adductor strains is high in sports such as ice hockey, soccer, swimming, American football, and Australian Rules football.
129. **A.** Among the adductor muscles, the adductor longus is the most frequently strained.
130. **B.** Injury risk factors for hip adductor muscle strain in sportspersons include decreased hip abduction range of motion (preseason) (Soccer); decreased hip adduction strength (preseason), muscular imbalance between the hip adductors and abductors, previous hip adductor injury, athletes who did not practice during the off season (ice hockey); previous history of groin strain (Australian Rules football); those who compete in the breaststroke (swimming).
131. **D.** Injury risk factors associated with a hamstring strain include hamstring weakness (eccentric), muscular imbalances, previous history of a hamstring injury, muscular inflexibility, muscular fatigue, failure to warm up before a sport properly, athlete's age, and athlete's position in a sport.
132. **D.** Eccentric exercises for the hamstrings include inverted hamstring, Romanian deadlift, and nordic or Russian hamstring curl.
133. **D.** Femoral internal rotation contributes significantly to patellofemoral joint (PFJ) kinematics. Females with patellofemoral pain syndrome (PFPS) usually have significant weakness in the gluteus medius, gluteus maximus, and hip external rotators.
134. **A.** Clarke's sign (patellar grind test) is the special test used to assess the presence of patellofemoral dysfunction.
135. **D.** The key areas to focus on for PFPS rehabilitation are overcoming any quadriceps (VMO) inhibition and addressing all main contributing biomechanical abnormalities (such as decreasing an excessive Q-angle), and increasing the functional load tolerance through the joint. This may require specific quadriceps training, gluteus medius work (such as

incorporating squat training with resistance bands around the knees), releasing all tight lateral thigh structures and attending to any foot-related issues.

136. **A.** The iliotibial band drops posteriorly behind the lateral femoral condyle with knee flexion and then snaps forward under the epicondyle during extension. Improving the flexibility of the hip abductors, hip flexors, and lateral thigh muscles can be helpful while treating this condition.

137. **B.** The lateral location of the knee pain and positive Ober test are indicative of iliotibial band tightness. When abduction occurs during the modified Thomas test, it often indicates tightness of the tensor fasciae latae and iliotibial band syndrome.

138. **A.** The posterior sag test is performed with the patient positioned in supine with the knee flexed to 90° and the hip flexed to 45°. A positive test is indicated by the tibia sagging back on the femur and may be indicative of a posterior cruciate ligament injury.

139. **A.** The medial collateral ligament (MCL) connects the medial epicondyle of the femur to the medial tibia and as a result resists medially directed force at the knee. The MCL is the primary stabilizer of the medial side of the knee against valgus force. A grade I MCL sprain is characterized by mild pain and swelling with little to no disruption of the ligament. Valgus stress testing will likely be painful given the acuity of the injury, however, rarely reveals detectable instability.

140. **D.** The tibiofemoral articulation consists of a concave tibial plateau articulating with the convex femoral condyles. An anterior glide of the tibia on the femur is indicated to increase knee extension.

141. **A.** Piriformis syndrome is caused by hypertrophy or spasm of the piriformis muscle, causing pressure on the sciatic nerve. Abduction and lateral rotation would likely be weak and painful since the motions serve as the prime function of the piriformis. The piriformis muscle originates on the anterior surface of the sacrum and the sacrotuberous ligament and inserts on the greater trochanter of the femur. The muscle is innervated by sacral nerves S1 and S2.

Chapter 10: Thigh and Leg Injuries

142. **B.** The Lachman test is perhaps the most common ligamentous instability test designed to assess the integrity of the anterior cruciate ligament. It is most commonly performed with the patient in a supine position and the knee flexed 20–30°.

143. **D.** Osgood-Schlatter disease or osteochondrosis of the tibial tuberosity is characterized by swelling and tenderness over the tibial tubercle that is exacerbated by exercise or any activity requiring active use of the quadriceps. The condition is most commonly observed in muscular adolescent boys. Patients with Osgood-Schlatter disease often present with an extremely prominent tibial tubercle.

Ankle and Foot Injury

1. The patients who excessively supinate and under pronate during gait commonly encounter which metatarsal stress fracture?
   A. 1st metatarsal
   B. 2nd metatarsal
   C. 4th metatarsal
   D. 5th metatarsal
2. Which nerve is compressed in Ski-boot syndrome?
   A. Medial plantar nerve
   B. Superficial peroneal nerve
   C. Lateral plantar nerve
   D. Deep peroneal nerve
3. Distal tarsal tunnel syndrome is otherwise called as:
   A. Jogger's foot
   B. Dancer's foot
   C. Jumper's foot
   D. Hopper's foot
4. Snowboarder's injury results in the fracture of:
   A. Fracture of anterior lateral process of calcaneum
   B. Fracture lateral talar process
   C. Fracture posterior talus
   D. Fracture anterior talus
5. Which fracture is detected by pinch test?
   A. Talus stress fracture
   B. Calcaneal stress fracture
   C. Cuboid stress fracture
   D. None of the above
6. A condition called painful pump-bump means:
   A. Fat pad syndrome
   B. Painful os trigonum
   C. Tarsal coalition
   D. Posterior lateral calcaneal exostosis
7. In tennis leg which plantar flexor is more commonly involved?
   A. Lateral head of gastrocnemius
   B. Plantaris
   C. Soleus
   D. Medial head of gastrocnemius

8. The generally accepted guidelines for the diagnosis of chronic exertional compartment syndrome are the following, *except*:
   A. Pre-exercise muscle tissue pressure more than 0–8 mm Hg
   B. A 1-minute post-exercise muscle tissue pressure more than 30 mm Hg
   C. A prolonged return of muscle tissue pressure to baseline levels (15 minutes post-exercise >20 mm Hg)
   D. Pre-exercise muscle tissue pressure more than 15 mm Hg
9. Chronic plantar heel pain can be caused by impingement of which nerve to abductor quinti muscle?
   A. Baxter's nerve
   B. Peroneal nerve
   C. Sural nerve
   D. Posterior tibial nerve
10. Rupture of which muscle leads to trigger toe?
    A. Abductor hallucis
    B. Flexor digitorum
    C. Flexor hallucis longus
    D. Flexor hallucis brevis
11. The medial head of gastrocnemius is more commonly involved in tennis leg because it presents all features, *except*:
    A. Originate more superiorly
    B. Slow twitch fibers
    C. Larger muscle mass
    D. Oblique fiber orientation
12. The major site of the transmission of ground reaction forces is:
    A. Subtalar joint
    B. Ankle joint
    C. Transverse tarsal joint
    D. Distal tibiofibular joint
13. In runners, strong shearing forces results across the calcaneal apophysis caused by plantar fascia and triceps surae leading to:
    A. Kohler's disease
    B. Sever's disease
    C. Freiberg's disease
    D. None of the above
14. In tarsal coalition there is an abnormal fusion taking place between:
    A. Forefoot and midfoot
    B. Midfoot and hindfoot
    C. Joints of hindfoot
    D. Joints of midfoot

15. Radiologically, calcaneonavicular bars involving superior calcaneal process projecting towards the middle of the tarsal navicular is called as:
    A. Grasshopper deformity
    B. Parrot beaking deformity
    C. Ant eater nose deformity
    D. None of the above

16. Abnormal course of popliteal artery that runs medial to the head of gastrocnemius is which type of popliteal artery entrapment syndrome?
    A. Type IV
    B. Type II
    C. Type III
    D. Type I

17. Treatment options for preventing black toe are the following, *except*:
    A. Trimming toenails within 2 mm of the nailbed
    B. Smoothing the edges of nails
    C. Proper shoeing with narrow toe box
    D. Wearing nonseamed socks

18. In Freiberg's infarction, avascular necrosis of which metatarsal is usually encountered?
    A. 2nd
    B. 1st
    C. 5th
    D. 4th

19. A bunion like enlargement of which metatarsophalangeal joint is called tailor's bunion?
    A. 4th
    B. 2nd
    C. 3rd
    D. 5th

20. The extrinsic factor contributing to overuse injury are:
    A. Training progression too rapid/inadequate rest
    B. Inappropriate footwear/equipment
    C. Incorrect sport technique
    D. All of the above

21. In syndesmosis ankle sprain or high ankle sprains, the athlete complains of inability to perform which part of gait cycle?
    A. Push-off
    B. Heel strike
    C. Swing through
    D. Midstance

22. Describe the Type III tibiofibular instability as classified by Ogden:
    A. Subluxation
    B. Superior dislocation
    C. Anterolateral dislocation
    D. Posterolateral dislocation

23. The diagnostic sign to detect interdigital neuroma is:
    A. Steve's click test
    B. Mulder's click test
    C. Peter's click test
    D. Clanton and Ford compression test
24. What are the factors that contribute to the development of "Turf Toe"?
    A. Hyperextension injury   B. Artificial playing surface
    C. Flexible lightweight shoes   D. All of the above
25. Blue or black painless discoloration can occur under the nail of the longest toe from repetitive trauma called as:
    A. Tennis toenail   B. Runner's toenail
    C. Kicker's toenail   D. Climber's toenail
26. Hallux saltans is the tendinosis of which tendon?
    A. Extensor digitorum longus
    B. Extensor hallucis longus
    C. Flexor hallucis longus
    D. Flexor hallucis brevis
27. In the entrapment of medial hallucal nerve due to hypertrophy of abductor hallucis muscle, pain is experienced:
    A. Under the lateral surface of 1st metatarsophalangeal joint
    B. On the dorsal surface of 1st metatarsophalangeal joint
    C. Under the medial surface of 1st metatarsophalangeal joint
    D. On the plantar surface of 1st metatarsophalangeal joint
28. The most common area of involvement for Achilles tendonopathy in runners is:
    A. 1-2 cm proximal to the insertion site
    B. 2-6 cm proximal to the insertion site
    C. 6-8 cm proximal to the insertion site
    D. 8-10 cm proximal to the insertion site
29. Nutcracker fracture is:
    A. Compression of lateral border of cuboid
    B. Avulsion fracture of dorsal lip of navicular
    C. Fracture dislocation of cuneiforms
    D. Fracture of body of talus

30. Which tendon is used for reconstruction of Achilles tendonosis?
    A. Hamstring
    B. Quadriceps
    C. Tensor fascia lata
    D. Flexor hallucis longus
31. Painful loss of motion at the great toe metatarsophalangeal joint often caused by arthrosis is referred to as which of the following?
    A. Turf toe
    B. Sesamoiditis
    C. Hallux rigidus
    D. Hallux valgus
32. Which of the following tests is used to assess calcaneofibular ligament integrity?
    A. Talar tilt test
    B. Squeeze test
    C. Anterior drawer test
    D. External rotation stress test
33. After an ankle injury, the athlete can usually begin which of the following exercises within 24 hours?
    A. Isokinetics
    B. Forward walking
    C. Gentle range of motion
    D. Proprioceptive training
34. Which is the strongest of the lateral ligamentous complex of ankle joint?
    A. Anterior talofibular ligament
    B. Posterior talofibular ligament
    C. Calcaneofibular ligament
    D. Middle talofibular ligament
35. The posterior tibial tendon is subjected to great amount of stress during which part of gait cycle leading to its rupture?
    A. After toe-off
    B. After midstance
    C. After heel-off
    D. After heel-strike
36. The most common stress fractures in athletes affect which of the following areas?
    A. Tibia
    B. Fibula
    C. Talus
    D. Navicular
37. The Thompson–Hamilton test is used to assess the instability of which joint?
    A. Talocalcaneal joint
    B. Calcaneocuboid joint
    C. Tarsometatarsal joint
    D. Metatarsophalangeal joint

38. Conservative management for corns is:
    A. Ball and ring stretching device to relieve pressure from shoe wear
    B. Doughnut-shaped pad over the area to reduce pressure
    C. Shoe wears modification, adequate width and depth in toe box
    D. All of the above
39. Pinky toe sling is used to stabilize which toe fracture?
    A. 2nd
    B. 4th
    C. 3rd
    D. 5th
40. All are the functions of sesamoids at metatarsophalangeal joint, *except*:
    A. Provides static plantar flexion force at metatarsophalangeal joint
    B. Acts as shock absorber to dissipate forces acting on the head of 1st metatarsal
    C. Decreases the moment arm of flexor hallucis brevis
    D. Protection for the tendon of flexor hallucis longus
41. Haglund's deformity is one of the important causes of:
    A. Posterior hindfoot pain
    B. Anterior hindfoot pain
    C. Lateral midfoot pain
    D. Plantar midfoot pain
42. Entrapment neuropathy of the sural nerve is caused due to:
    A. Recurrent ankle sprain
    B. Calcaneal fractures
    C. Ganglion cyst or fibrous tissue around ankle
    D. All of the above
43. Normal calcaneal inclination angle is:
    A. 5°
    B. 10°
    C. 15°
    D. 20°
44. Helbing's sign indicates:
    A. Fallen medial longitudinal arch
    B. Fallen lateral longitudinal arch
    C. Fallen transverse arch
    D. None of the above

45. One of the most common findings in the athletes who develop plantar fascitis is:
    A. Tight hamstring
    B. Tight tibialis anterior
    C. Tight tibialis posterior
    D. Tight tendoachilles
46. Cyma line is the line of articulation between which of the following joints:
    A. Tarsometatarsal and metatarsophalangeal joints
    B. Talonavicular and calcaneocuboid joints
    C. Intercuneiform joints
    D. Ankle and subtalar joints
47. Push-up test is used to determine the flexibility of:
    A. Hammer toe
    B. Claw toe
    C. Mallet toe
    D. Trigger toe
48. Which movement of ankle is restricted following tibiofibular synostosis?
    A. Inversion
    B. Eversion
    C. Dorsiflexion
    D. Plantar flexion
49. One of the primary factors contributing to recurrent ankle injuries and disability is inadequate restoration of which motion?
    A. Eversion
    B. Plantar flexion
    C. Dorsiflexion
    D. Inversion
50. Tibial stress fracture differs from medial tibial stress syndrome because:
    A. The area is usually more proximal
    B. Pain develops gradually
    C. Only positive in delayed images
    D. Both A and B
51. Homan's sign indicates:
    A. Thrombophlebitis of posterior tibial vein
    B. Tarsal tunnel compression syndrome
    C. Achilles tendon ruptures
    D. 1st ray mobility
52. Metatarsus primus elevatus deformity leads to which pathological condition?

A. Hallux limitus B. Metatarsalgia
C. Plantar fascitis D. Interdigital neuroma

53. All are the mechanical factors associated with plantar fascitis, *except*:
    A. Forefoot varus strength B. Prolonged pronation
    C. Tight Achilles tendon D. Increased first ray mobility

54. Foot orthosis should provide the following functions, *except*:
    A. Distribute the weight bearing stresses and pressures acting on plantar surface of foot
    B. Balance intrinsic deformities using appropriate postings
    C. Increase stresses acting on the proximal structures of lower extremity and spine secondary to excessive foot pronation or supination
    D. Control excessive foot pronation by reducing both the magnitude and rate of foot pronation

55. The problem associated with supinatory or limited foot types is:
    A. Increased shock absorption
    B. Decreased plantar pressures
    C. Increased plantar pressures over forefoot
    D. Hypermobile foot

56. Syndactyly means:
    A. Absence of toes B. Webbing of toes
    C. Presence of extra toes D. Underdeveloped toes

57. Duchenne test is positive in case of lesion of which nerve?
    A. Superficial peroneal nerve
    B. Tibial nerve
    C. Common peroneal nerve
    D. None

58. Hooked forefoot is otherwise called as:
    A. Pes planus B. Pes cavus
    C. Metatarsus adductus D. Hallux valgus

59. A female distance runner complains of recurrent friction blister whenever she increases the intensity of her training, managing blisters includes all of the following, *except*:

A. Pad the blister with a pressure pad
B. Use of skin tougheners
C. Soak regularly in ice water after activity
D. Make a large incision along the periphery of the blister with a sterile instrument

60. The tuberosity of the 5th metatarsal may be avulsed during violent eversion of the foot by the tendon of which muscle?
    A. Posterior tibialis   B. Peroneus longus
    C. Peroneus brevis   D. Peroneus tertius

61. An athlete with a ruptured tibialis posterior tendon presents with pain in the region of:
    A. Sustentaculum talus   B. Navicular tubercle
    C. Medial malleolus   D. Lateral malleolus

62. Which one of the following is the most stable position of the ankle?
    A. Dorsiflexion   B. Plantar flexion
    C. Inversion   D. Eversion

63. Which test is used to assess the height of the medial arch using the navicular position?
    A. Matles test   B. Feiss line
    C. Dimple sign   D. Heel-thump test

64. Which one of the following pulses can be palpated just lateral to the tendon of the extensor hallucis longus over the posterior aspect of the foot?
    A. Femoral   B. Popliteal
    C. Dorsalis pedis   D. Posterior tibial

65. Name the supportive device plays an important role in both the initial intervention and prevention of ankle injuries?
    A. Braces   B. Splints
    C. Tubigrip   D. Bandages

66. What is the most effective treatment method in restricting the motion of the ankle and has also been proved to decrease the incidence of ankle sprains?
    A. Mobilization   B. Stretching
    C. Strengthening   D. Taping

67. Which one of the following orthotic supports used to help redistribute the forces through the heel better and improve the natural shock-absorptive ability?
    A. Modified shoes
    B. Arch support
    C. Heel cups
    D. Heel straps
68. Sprain of the first MTP joint is called as:
    A. Os trigonum
    B. Turf toe
    C. Metatarsus varus
    D. Hallux valgus
69. Subtalar joint with injury to the talocalcaneal interosseous ligament leads to:
    A. Onychomycosis
    B. Talocrural subluxation
    C. Sinus tarsi syndrome
    D. Cuboid syndrome
70. The foot condition usually presents with redness or itchiness but can also appear as dry and flaky skin is known as:
    A. Tinea pedis
    B. Subungual hematoma
    C. Subungual exostosis
    D. Blisters
71. A traction apophysitis of the tuberosity of the fifth metatarsal causes:
    A. Sever disease
    B. Iselin's disease
    C. Plantar fascitis
    D. Fat pad syndrome
72. Which one of the following stress tests is performed to estimate the stability of the anterior talofibular ligament (ATFL)?
    A. Calcaneal tilt
    B. Talar tilt
    C. Anterior drawer
    D. Posterior drawer
73. What is the term used to describe the pain arising from the insertion of plantar fascia, with or without heel spur?
    A. Calcaneal apophysitis
    B. Retrocalcaneal bursitis
    C. Achilles tendon rupture
    D. Plantar heel pain
74. What is the most appropriate glide of the talocrural joint that can be used to increase ankle joint dorsiflexion?
    A. Posterior
    B. Anterior
    C. Medial
    D. Lateral

75. Sudden hyperextension of the forefoot causes fracture neck is so called:
    A. Essex-Lopresti
    B. Bohler's angle
    C. Hawkin's fracture
    D. Aviators astralagus
76. In running, how much foot loading during gait?
    A. 1.2 times the body weight
    B. 2 times the body weight
    C. 4 times the body weight
    D. 5 times the body weight
77. Which one of the following diagnostic methods is the most appropriate to detect stress fractures in the ankle and foot?
    A. MRI
    B. Arthrogram
    C. Bone scans
    D. Ultrasonography
78. Persistent pain during weight-bearing and long-term unsatisfactory functional results following ankle surgery lead to:
    A. Arthrodesis
    b. Osteotomy
    C. Total joint arthroplasty
    d. Excision arthroplasty
79. Overuse of the anterior tibialis muscle is the most common type of:
    A. Tibiofibular syndesmosis
    B. Plantar fasciitis
    C. Talar tilt
    D. Shin splints
80. Which of the following nerve injury leading to altered sensitivity of the lateral border of the foot?
    A. Tibial
    B. Popliteal
    C. Sural
    D. Common peroneal
81. When a patient uses weight-bearing exercises to stretch the plantar flexor muscles, choose one of the following methods to be adopted:
    A. Shoes with medial arch support
    B. No supports to be placed in the foot
    C. Silicon gels pads to place in the foot
    D. Shoes with heel pads

Chapter 11: Ankle and Foot Injury

82. Self-stretching of the foot into inversion by pulling on the towel through which side of the foot?
    A. Lateral
    B. Medial
    C. Anterior
    D. Posterior
83. Which phase of the gait cycle shows extension of the great toe at the metatarsophalangeal (MTP) joint?
    A. Heel strike
    B. Toe-off
    C. Push-off
    D. Heel-off
84. Which one of the following treatment methods is effective for Achilles' tendinopathy?
    A. Stretching
    B. Strengthening
    C. Infrared radiation
    D. Extracorporeal shockwave therapy
85. A fracture affecting one or more of the malleoli is known as:
    A. Pott's
    B. Maisonneuve
    C. Chondral
    D. Subchondral
86. A physical therapist examines a patient with an acute grade II lateral ankle sprain. Which one of the following injury mechanisms predisposes to anterior talofibular ligament sprain?
    A. Inversion and dorsiflexion
    B. Inversion and plantar flexion
    C. Inversion
    D. Eversion and dorsiflexion
87. While selecting an assistive device for a patient rehabilitating from an ankle injury, which of the following would serve as the most significant obstacle to independent ambulation with axillary crutches?
    A. Cognitive impairment
    B. Weight-bearing restrictions
    C. Architectural barriers
    D. Unilateral lower extremity weakness

88. A sports physical therapist performs the talar tilt test on a 21-year-old male athlete rehabilitating from an inversion ankle sprain. Which ligament does the talar tilt test examine?
    A. Anterior tibiofibular
    B. Calcaneofibular
    C. Deltoid
    D. Posterior tibiofibular
89. A 29-year-old baseball player rehabilitating from ankle surgery has consistent difficulty with functional activities that emphasize the frontal plane. Which of the following would be the most difficult for the patient?
    A. Anterior lunge
    B. Six-inch posterior step up
    C. Six-inch lateral step down
    D. Eight-inch posterior step down
90. During the examination of a patient diagnosed with Achilles tendonitis, it is observed that the patient's foot and ankle appear to be pronated in standing. Which of the following motion combinations create pronation?
    A. Adduction, dorsiflexion, inversion
    B. Abduction, dorsiflexion, eversion
    C. Abduction, plantar flexion, eversion
    D. Adduction, plantar flexion, inversion
91. The application of a ventral glide mobilization technique of the distal tibiofibular articulation would be most beneficial to improve:
    A. Ankle plantar flexion
    B. Subtalar inversion
    C. Ankle dorsiflexion
    D. Subtalar eversion
92. A 19-year-old male sustained a grade I ankle sprain two days after participating in a collegiate level marching band practice session. Based on the narration of the history, the mechanism of injury is consistent with inversion and plantar flexion. Which of the following ligaments would most likely be affected?

A. Anterior talofibular ligament
B. Calcaneofibular ligament
C. Tibiofibular ligament
D. Deltoid ligament

93. An 18-year-old collegiate basketball player who sustained a grade III inversion ankle sprain is examined in a physiotherapy department. The player prone to this injury approximately 36 hours ago. The most appropriate treatment is:
    A. Whirlpool (29° Celsius) and passive exercise
    B. Ice pack and intermittent compression
    C. Ultrasound and electrical stimulation
    D. Ice massage and mobilization

94. While taking the history of a 21-year-old female collegiate student, she completely tore one of the ligaments in her ankle. If the patient's comment is accurate, the injury to the ligament is most likely to be classified as a:
    A. Grade I sprain   B. Grade I strain
    C. Grade III strain   D. Grade III sprain

95. A physical therapist administers an ultrasound treatment using water immersion on a patient rehabilitating from ankle surgery. During the session, the therapist notices that air bubbles tend to accumulate on the sonated area of the skin and face of the soundhead. The MOST appropriate therapist action is:
    A. Wipe off the air bubbles on the skin periodically
    B. Wipe off the air bubbles on the face of the soundhead periodically
    C. Wipe off the air bubbles on the skin and face of the soundhead periodically
    D. Avoid wiping off any of the air bubbles

ANSWERS

1. **D.** About 55% of lower extremity fractures are metatarsal stress fractures. For patients who excessively supinate and underpronate during gait, the maximum weight bearing force falls over the lateral border of the fifth metatarsal bone leading to stress fracture.
2. **D.** Compression of the deep peroneal nerve occurs at the inferior edge of the extensor retinaculum, is commonly seen in football and basketball players, runners and athletes who wear tight fitting shoes or boots.
3. **A.** In jogger's foot, the plantar nerve may be compressed by osteophyte from the talonavicular joint or fibrosis at the master knot from repeated trauma, such as running and jumping.
4. **B.** Fracture of lateral beak or lateral talar process is known as Snowboarder's injury caused by eversion loading injury or inversion dorsiflexion mechanism.
5. **B.** Calcaneal stress fracture is seen in patients who perform repetitive jumping or running exercises. Pinch test is used to detect the fracture by squeezing the medial and lateral portion of midheel which elicits discomfort.
6. **D.** Posterior lateral calcaneal exostosis is a bony prominence found posterior and lateral to the achilles insertion and produces discomfort when rubbing against the heel counter causing posterior heel pain.
7. **D.** Injury to the gastrocnemius musculotendinous complex has often been referred to as tennis leg because of its frequency in tennis participants who presents with a history of sharp pain in posterior calf.
8. **A.** It is the normal resting compartment pressure. Levels greater than 30–40 mm Hg is associated with microcirculatory disturbances leading to muscle and nerve ischemia.
9. **A.** Chronic plantar heel pain medially and laterally is caused by impingement of Baxter's nerve to abductor quinti muscle at the edge of deep abductor hallucis fascia where it turns the corner and produces sharp burning heel pain.
10. **C.**

Chapter 11: Ankle and Foot Injury

11. **B.** Medial head of gastrocnemius is fast twitch fibers in contrast to soleus. Additionally, it crosses two joints making it vulnerable to injury during eccentric contraction.
12. **A.** During heel strike the subtalar joint is supinated, in stance phase it is pronated and during toe-off again supinated absorbing all the forces when contact with the ground.
13. **B.** Calcaneal apophysitis represents an inflammation of the open calcaneal growth plate, which is thought to occur due to traction on the apophysis of the os calcis.
14. **B.** In tarsal coalition, union between the bones may be fibrous, cartilagenous or osseous. The cause of union could be accessory ossicles within the foot or autosomal dominant inheritance or failure of segmentation involving the primitive mesenchyme of foot.
15. **C.** The appearance of calcaneonavicular bars involving superior calcaneal process on lateral radiographs represents a tubular elongation of the anterior portion of the superior calcaneum as a 'nose' which projects forwards into the middle of the tarsal navicular known as 'ant eater nose deformity'.
16. **B.** Popliteal artery entrapment syndrome occurs due to intermittent compression of the popliteal artery. The underlying cause has classically been described as anatomic in origin.
17. **C.** Wide toe boxes should be used to avoid friction at the medial and lateral borders of foot.
18. **A.** In Freiberg's infarction, avascular necrosis of second metatarsal is occasionally seen as a cause of metatarsalgia, in later stages leading to degenerative arthritis of the joint.
19. **D.** Tailor's bunion is a painful bursitis overlying the lateral aspect of foot in relation to fifth metatarsal head, associated with abnormal weight on the foot.
20. **D.**
21. **A.** This injury happens as tibia and fibula is forced apart, injuring the ligament that binds these bones together as in forced dorsiflexion. Instability in the syndesmosis area makes the athlete to walk on toes and unable to push-off during gait.

22. **D.** Posteromedial dislocation are caused by direct high energy trauma or twisting motion associated with a strong biceps femoris contraction.
23. **B.** Mulder's test: Compression of the web space will usually reproduce the pain and a click may be felt on compression of the foot as the web space is pressed.
24. **D.** All these factors cause trauma to plantar capsuloligamentous sprains affecting the push-off strength of the first metatarsophalangeal joint required in athletic competition.
25. **A.** Blue or black painless discoloration under the nail is caused by trauma or acute subungal hematoma, resolves with shoe modification with metatarsal pad, tighter vamps, warm soaks and rest.
26. **C.** Hallux saltans or trigger toe is common in dancing athlete affecting flexor hallucis longus starting as tenosynovitis and progressing to tendinosis.
27. **C.** Medial hallucal nerve is a branch of tibial nerve, which provides sensation to the medial aspect of the great toe.
28. **B.** Because it is the area of diminished blood supply during propulsion where microtrauma more likely happens from repetitive forces at subthreshold level in an abusive fashion.
29. **A.** Nutcracker fracture is the compression of the lateral border of cuboid that shortens the lateral column of foot and is treated by open reduction and restoration of length with bone grafting.
30. **D.**
31. **C.** Sporting events that require jumping, cutting and acceleration are dependent on dorsiflexion of the first metatarsophalangeal joint and push-off from the hallux. Synovitis→dorsal callus→bunion deformity→limited range of motion at first metatarsophalangeal joint leading to the development of hallux rigidus.
32. **A.** Talar tilt test: The examiner stabilizes the tibia by supporting the medial aspect of the distal tibia in one hand and placing the opposite hand on the lateral aspect of the heel. With ankle in neutral dorsiflexion, talar tilt is determined by turning the heel inward. The degree of tilt is determined.
33. **C.** Depending on the severity of injury, gentle range of motion exercises to restore dorsiflexion may be initiated within

Chapter 11: Ankle and Foot Injury

24 hours after injury. This allows for early, painfree ambulation during walking, which is the key to accelerating the recovery time.

34. **B.** The posterior talofibular ligament is the strongest of the lateral ligamentous complex. It is 30 mm long, 5 mm wide and 8 mm thick and runs from the lateral malleolus to the posterior talus.

35. **D.** The posterior tibial tendon is subjected to great amount of stress just after heel strike because it controls hindfoot movement from a position of eversion into inversion producing rigid foot necessary for toe-off.

36. **A.** Tibia bears 80% of the body weight during running and jumping activities, so can lead to stress fracture which develop from repetitive loads on bone that cause an imbalance of bone resorption over formation.

37. **D.** Thompson–Hamilton test: The test is performed by stabilizing the metatarsal head and the proximal phalanx of toe. The thumb is used to apply pressure to the toe. Symptoms of pain are typically reproduced when instability is present. Laxity in the dorsal-plantar plane appreciated.

38. **D.** Hard corn develops at a callous, typically over the PIP joint of fifth toe. Soft corn on the lateral aspect of fourth toe. Conservative management is to relieve pressure or friction that takes place between the toe and shoe wear.

39. **D.**

40. **C.** Sesamoids increase the moment arm by which flexor hallucis brevis acts upon the hallux, therefore providing a mechanical advantage in much the same fashion that the patella affects the extensor apparatus at the knee.

41. **A.** Haglund's deformity is the prominence of posterior superior calcaneum, which is a cause of posterior hindfoot pain.

42. **D.** All these conditions cause compression of the sural nerve between the heads of gastrocnemius proximally and just posterior to the peroneal tendons distally.

43. **C.** Calcaneal inclination angle is formed by plane of support and the calcaneal inclination axis and helps to evaluate whether pronation or supination of foot is excess.

44. **A.** Helbing's sign indicates fallen medial longitudinal arch where the Achilles tendon curves out.

45. **D.** Very tight Achilles (especially the soleus) leads to the development of plantar fascitis in athletes. Proper stretching is the key to recovery.
46. **B.** In pronated foot: Talus slides anteriorly creating an anterior break in the cyma line with talonavicular joint distal to calcaneocuboid joint. In supinated foot: Talus slides posteriorly into the ankle mortise creating posterior break in the cyma line with talonavicular joint proximal to calcaneocuboid joint.
47. **B.** Push up test: Performed by placing dorsal pressure underneath the metatarsal heads of foot. Claw toe deformity is considered flexible when the toes straighten and clawing corrects.
48. **C.**
49. **C.** Dorsiflexion range for normal ambulation is approximately 10° during walking and 20° during running. Any restriction in this range suggests not only ankle pathology but also heel cord tightness.
50. **D.** The tibial stress fracture is reflected in a positive bone scan in all three phases with more localized uptake whereas medial tibial stress syndrome is only positive in delayed images.
51. **A.** Homan's sign: Patient sits with legs off the edge of the table and both feet in a slight plantarflexed position. Examiner compresses or squeezes calf muscle and the patient complains of pain in case of thrombophlebitis.
52. **A.** Hallux limitus is defined as a restriction in 1st metatarsophalangeal extension. The cause could be trauma to fore foot, degenerative changes, congenital variation in shape of 1st metatarsal head and dorsiflexed first ray deformity (metatarsus primus elevatus)
53. **D.** Decreased first ray mobility and plantar flexion contribute to the development of plantar fascitis.
54. **C.** Foot orthoses decreases the stress acting on the proximal joints of lower extremity and spine.
55. **C.** The problems associated with supinatory foot are decreased shock absorption, increased plantar pressures and also limited mobility of foot.
56. **B.**

Chapter 11: Ankle and Foot Injury 239

57. **A.** Duchenne test: Examiner pushes upon the head of 1st metatarsal through the sole, pushing the foot into dorsiflexion. The patient is asked to plantarflex the foot. Medial border dorsiflexes and offers no resistance while the lateral border plantarflexes.
58. **C.** Foot appears to be adducted and supinated and hindfoot may or may not be in valgus.
59. **D.**
60. **C.**
61. **B.** Navicular tubercle: Examination reveals thickening or absence (less frequent) of the tibialis posterior tendon and inability to raise the heel. A flattened medial arch is a classic sign but this may not be evident immediately.
62. **A.** Dorsiflexion: As the foot moves into dorsiflexion, the talus glides posteriorly and the widest portion of the talus becomes wedged into the ankle mortise.
63. **B.** Feiss is a line from the medial malleolus to the plantar aspect of the first metatarsophalangeal joint, used to measure pronation of the foot during weight bearing.
64. **C.** Dorsalis pedis is a blood vessel of the lower limb that carries oxygenated blood to the dorsal surface of the foot. It is located 1/3 from medial malleolus. It arises at the anterior aspect of the ankle joint and is a continuation of the anterior tibial artery.
65. **A.** Braces are used to compress, protect, and support the ankle. It also functions to limit ROM of the injured ankle, most importantly plantar flexion and inversion, which is a precarious position for the sprained ankle.
66. **D.** Ankle tape can provide stability, support, and compression for the ankle joint. It can help reduce swelling after an ankle injury and prevent reinjury.
67. **C.** Heel cups provide immediate heel pain relief by cushioning the area of pain and elevating the heel bone.
68. **B.** Turf toe: Football players are at higher risk of this injury, if they are tackled while landing from a jump or if another player lands on the back of their heel, forcing the first MTP joint into hyperdorsiflexion.

69. **C.** Sinus tarsi syndrome: The mechanism of injury involves an inversion sprain in a plantar flexed position that injures both the talocrural and subtalar joint and is sometimes difficult to distinguish from a routine ankle sprain.
70. **A.** Athlete's foot (tinea pedis) is a fungal infection that usually begins between the toes. It commonly occurs in people whose feet have become very sweaty while confined within tightfitting shoes.
71. **B.** Iselin's disease: The patient is usually involved in sports with running, cutting, and jumping. Resisted eversion typically reproduces the pain.
72. **C.** Anterior drawer test: Patient's tested leg bent to about 90° of flexion. The examiner should sit on the foot of the patient's leg. Place a hand along each side of the patients.
73. **D.**
74. **A.** Posterior glide of the talocrural joint can be used to increase ankle joint dorsiflexion.
75. **D.** Aviator astragalus is an antiquated reference to a pattern of isolated fracture/dislocation injury of the talus.
76. **B.** During movement, the foot is subjected to high loading (i.e., two times the body weight), and pathology may cause the gait to be altered.
77. **C.** A bone scan is a nuclear imaging test that helps diagnose and track several types of bone disease.
78. **A.** Arthrodesis also known as artificial ankylosis or syndesis, is the artificial induction of joint ossification between two bones by surgery.
79. **D.** A hypomobile gastrocnemius-soleus complex and weak anterior tibialis muscle as well as foot pronation are associated with anterior shin splints.
80. **C.** The sural nerve is a cutaneous nerve, providing only sensation to the posterolateral aspect of the distal third of the leg and the lateral aspect of the foot, heel, and ankle.
81. **A.** Shoes with arch supports should be worn or a folded washcloth placed under the medial border of the foot to minimize the stress to the arches of the foot.

Chapter 11: Ankle and Foot Injury

82. **B.** Medial side: Long-sitting with a towel or belt looped under the foot. Have the patient pull on the medial side of the towel to cause the heel and foot to turn inward.
83. **C.** Extension of the great toe at the MTP joint is critical during the push-off phase of gait.
84. **D.** Extracorporeal shock wave therapy is a noninvasive method that uses pressure waves to treat various musculoskeletal conditions. High-energy acoustic waves (shock waves) deliver a mechanical force to the body's tissues.
85. **A.** Pott's fracture is a fracture affecting one or both of the malleoli. During activities, such as landing from a jump (volleyball, basketball) or when rolling an ankle, a certain amount of stress is placed on the tibia and fibula and the ankle joint.
86. **B.** The anterior talofibular ligament runs from the anterior portion of the lateral malleolus to the lateral aspect of the talar neck. The ligament is placed under stress with inversion and plantar flexion. The anterior talofibular, calcaneofibular, and posterior talofibular ligaments make up the lateral collateral ligaments of the ankle complex.
87. **A.** A significant cognitive impairment may result in a patient being unable to safely use axillary crutches.
88. **B.** The talar tilt test can be used to identify the presence of a calcaneofibular ligament sprain.
89. **C.** The frontal plane divides the body into front and back halves. Movements in the frontal plane occur as side-to-side movements, such as abduction or adduction. Rotary motion in the frontal plane occurs around an anterior-posterior axis.
90. **B.** Pronation of the foot consists of eversion of the head, abduction of the forefoot, and dorsiflexion of the subtalar and midtarsal joints.
91. **C.** Ventral and dorsal glides of the distal tibiofibular articulation increase the mobility of the ankle mortise and therefore are used to improve ankle dorsiflexion.
92. **A.** The anterior talofibular ligament is the first ligament of the lateral ankle complex to stretch during plantar flexion and inversion. The calcaneofibular ligament and the posterior

talofibular ligament are not typically involved in a grade I sprain.

93. **B.** A grade III inversion ankle sprain involves a severe disruption of the lateral ligaments of the ankle complex. Since the injury occurred only 36 hours ago, the patient is in the acute phase of inflammation and, as a result, should be treated with rest, ice, compression, and elevation.

94. **D.** A third-degree sprain involves a complete rupture or a break in the continuity of a ligament. The injury usually results in significant joint play hypermobility.

95. **C.** The air bubbles on the skin and the face of the soundhead should be periodically removed to promote maximum transmission of the ultrasound energy.

CHAPTER 12

Spine and Chest Injuries

A. CERVICAL SPINE INJURIES

1. According to "Laws of Freyette" in the atlantoaxial joint:
   A. Rotation and side bending occurs together
   B. Rotation and side bending does not occur together
   C. Only side bending takes place
   D. Only rotation takes place

2. If an athlete is down on the field but is conscious, which of the following signs or symptoms may be associated with a spinal cord injury?
   A. Upper extremity neurologic signs and symptoms
   B. Mild neck pain
   C. Abnormal neurologic signs in a non-dermatome distribution
   D. Cervical spine point tenderness

3. Stinger's or Burner's syndrome is more commonly seen in which players?
   A. Basketball
   B. Tennis
   C. Cricket
   D. Football

4. Which of the following motion can cause a hypomobile facet?
   A. Flexion
   B. Extension
   C. Side bending
   D. Axial compression

5. How much upper extremity strength should an athlete recovering from a stinger's syndrome regain before returning to play?
   A. 100%
   B. 75%
   C. 50%
   D. 25%

6. For hypomobile segment, which glide is commonly used?
   A. Transverse glide
   B. Posteroanterior glide
   C. Anteroposterior glide
   D. None of the above

7. Contact sports are an absolute contraindication for which condition?
   A. Atlanto-occipital fusion
   B. Odontoid anomalies
   C. Klippel-Feil anomaly
   D. All of the above
8. Locked facet is typically more painful during:
   A. Movement
   B. Rest
   C. Sitting
   D. Standing
9. What should an athletic trainer do first when evaluating an unconscious athlete on the playing field?
   A. Check for vital signs and airway
   B. Remove the helmet
   C. Log roll the athlete into a supine position while stabilizing the cervical spine
   D. Arrange for transport to the emergency department
10. In cervical cord neuropraxia-transient quadriplegia, the complete sensory and motor recovery usually occurs in:
    A. Less than 5 minutes
    B. By 10-15 minutes
    C. 1 month
    D. Does not occur at all
11. How many millimeters of translatory displacement is normal in cervical spine?
    A. 2 mm
    B. 5 mm
    C. 10 mm
    D. 4-6 mm
12. Which of the following treatment is more effective for an athlete with a dysfunctional spinal segment?
    A. Manual therapy
    B. Cryotherapy
    C. Diathermy
    D. Ultrasound
13. The Torg ratio in the cervical spine that is indicative of cervical stenosis is:
    A. Between 1 and 2
    B. Less than 2
    C. Less than 0.8
    D. Between 0.8 and 1
14. Sharp-purser test is used to detect:
    A. Subluxation of atlanto-axial joint
    B. Lax tectorial membrane
    C. Integrity of alar ligament
    D. Tear of transverse ligament

15. Type II odontoid fractures are more prone to develop:
    A. Malunion
    B. Vascular injuries
    C. Nerve injuries
    D. Nonunion
16. The characteristic of "Spear Tackler's" spine is:
    A. Developmental stenosis of cervical spine
    B. Persistent straightening of cervical lordotic curve on radiograph
    C. Pre-existing post-traumatic radiographic abnormalities of cervical spine
    D. All of the above
17. Cervical cord neuropraxia results from:
    A. Spinal stenosis
    B. Congenital fusion of vertebra
    C. Cervical instability
    D. All of the above
18. Which of the following exercises is given first after surgical treatment of disc disease?
    A. Strengthening
    B. Isometrics
    C. Active range of motion
    D. Stabilization
19. Injury to the subscapular nerve can be detected by:
    A. Weakness of supraspinatus and infraspinatus muscle
    B. Loss of sensation on lateral aspect of shoulder
    C. Both A and B
    D. None of the above
20. What type of special test is "Bakody's sign"?
    A. Provocation test
    B. Relief test
    C. Aggravation test
    D. None of the above
21. Which of the following muscle group is tight in upper crossed syndrome?
    A. Deep neck flexors
    B. Pectoralis major, trapezius
    C. Rhomboids
    D. Serratus anterior, lower trapezius
22. Contusion of the anterior neck usually result as:
    A. Severe distress
    B. Aphonia
    C. Dyspnea
    D. All of the above

23. **Cow boy collar worn by players who have experienced Burner's syndrome limits which movement of cervical spine?**
    A. Extreme hyperextension
    B. Extreme lateral bending
    C. Extreme rotation
    D. Both A and B
24. **Klippel-Feil anomaly refers to as:**
    A. Congenital fusion of ring of atlas
    B. Inherent instability between C1 and C2
    C. Congenital fusion of two or more vertebra
    D. Absence of axis vertebra
25. **Upper limb tension test 3 (ULTT3) is used to determine which nerve pathology?**
    A. Radial
    B. Ulnar
    C. Median
    D. Musculocutaneous
26. **Absolute contraindication to further participation in contact sports exists in the presence of which of the following fractures?**
    A. Comminuted fracture of vertebral body with displacement into spinal canal
    B. Vertebral body fracture with a sagittal component
    C. Fracture of vertebral body with or without associated arch fractures or ligamentous laxity
    D. All of the above
27. **Close packed position of the cervical spine is:**
    A. Slight extension
    B. Full extension
    C. Slight flexion
    D. Full flexion
28. **Reverse Spurling's sign indicates:**
    A. Ligament sprain
    B. Vertebral artery compression
    C. Nerve root compression
    D. Muscle spasm
29. **To find the pathology of vertebral artery, which test is performed?**
    A. Soto Hall test
    B. Romberg's test
    C. Quadrant test
    D. Dizziness test

Chapter 12: Spine and Chest Injuries

30. Each link of the head and neck chain has how many degrees of freedom?
    A. 2°
    B. 6°
    C. 8°
    D. 10°

31. A 35-year-old wrestler having sudden and violent blow with lateral flexion of the neck may compress one of the following structures, causing a burning sensation on the side opposite to the blow?
    A. Ligaments
    B. Intervertebral disc
    C. Nerve roots
    D. Vertebral arteries

32. A 25-yer-old rugby player is suspected when there is a lack of alignment of the vertebral bodies, or facet joints in the cervical spine, which may reflect subluxation. What would be the most appropriate diagnosis present with that player?
    A. Stability of the cervical spine
    B. Instability of the cervical spine
    C. Neck stiffness
    D. Myofascial syndrome

33. Which one of the following diagnoses is defined as an encroachment on either the spinal cord (through narrowing of the spinal canal) or the nerve roots (through narrowing of the intervertebral foramina) in the cervical spine sports injuries?
    A. Impingement
    B. Stenosis
    C. Subluxation
    D. Dislocation

34. What is the term indicating loss of function, ranging from pain to paraplegia?
    A. Disability
    B. Contracture
    C. Stiffness
    D. Impairment

35. A 20-year-old female high jumper has a history of spinal cord compression during forced cervical hyperextension, diminishing the anteroposterior diameter of the spinal canal. Which one of the following diagnoses is relevant to the above-mentioned sports injury scenario?
    A. Cervical spondylolisthesis
    B. Vertebral artery compression
    C. Neuropraxia of the cervical spinal cord with transient quadriplegia
    D. Disc protrusion

36. What is the most common cervical injury in contact sportspersons, which characterizes a transient loss of function (weakness) with burning pain, numbness, or tingling irradiating down one arm following a collision?
    A. Whiplash injury
    B. Burner injury
    C. Stinger injury
    D. Both B and C

37. A 43-year-old male baseball player having the most severe nerve injury in the neck and leads to complete disruption of the endoneurium. What is the type of nerve injury confirming the above condition?
    A. Neurotmesis
    B. Axonotmesis
    C. Neuropraxia
    D. Neurolysis

38. A 30-year-old man was injured in a cross-country motorcycle racing accident. MRI scan revealed a dural tear, through which CSF leakage occurs to form a pseudomeningocele. Which of the following nerve root and plexus lesions associated with the above complaint?
    A. Spinal cord injury
    B. Traumatic brachial plexus avulsion
    C. Craniocervical dislocation
    D. Atlantoaxial dislocation

39. Which one of the following structures operates as an osmotic system, holding neighboring vertebral bodies together while simultaneously pushing them apart?
    A. Apophyseal joint
    B. Mammillary bodies
    C. Intervertebral disc
    D. Unicate process

40. A 35-year-old motorcyclist is having a limited cervical range of motion. As part of the examination, the therapist attempts to screen the patient for possible vertebral artery involvement, but is unable to position the patient's head and neck in the recommended test position. The most appropriate action is to:
    A. Complete the vertebral artery test with the head and neck positioned in approximately 50% of the available cervical range of motion
    B. Complete the vertebral artery test as far into the available cervical range of motion as tolerated

C. Avoid completing the vertebral artery test until the patient has full cervical range of motion

D. Avoid all direct cervical treatment techniques until the vertebral artery test can be assessed at the limits of normal cervical range of motion

41. A physical therapist develops a chart detailing expected functional outcomes for a variety of spinal cord injuries. Which is the highest spinal level at which independent transfers with a sliding board would be feasible?

   A. C4
   B. C6
   C. T1
   D. T3

42. A 40-year-old female sprinter was diagnosed with a cervical spine injury reports to physical therapy for a scheduled treatment session. While walking with the patient to the treatment area the physical therapist notices that the patient's cervical orthosis is very loose. In such a scenario, what would be the most appropriate action taken by that physical therapist?

   A. Document the observation in the medical record
   B. Reapply the orthosis correctly at the conclusion of the treatment session
   C. Remind the patient of the donning instructions for the orthosis
   D. Contact the referring physician

43. A 27-year-old male patient is referred to physical therapy with a C6 nerve root injury. Which of the following clinical findings would not be expected with this type of injury?

   A. Diminished sensation on the anterior arm and index finger
   B. Weakness in the biceps and supinator
   C. Diminished brachioradialis reflex
   D. Paresthesia's of the long and ring fingers

44. A 50-year-old female shuttle player is having a history of cervical pain with giddiness for the past 3 months. On examination, the physical therapist completes a vertebral artery test on a patient diagnosed with a cervical strain. Which component of the vertebral artery test is most likely to assess the patency of the intervertebral foramen?

A. Rotation B. Lateral flexion
C. Flexion   D. Extension

45. A physical therapist performs goniometric measurements on a patient rehabilitating from injuries sustained in a motor vehicle accident. When measuring the rotation of the cervical spine, which of the following landmarks would be the most appropriate for the axis of the goniometer?
    A. Centered over the external auditory meatus
    B. Centered over the center of the cranial aspect of the head
    C. Centered over the C7 spinous process
    D. Centered over the midline of the occiput

46. A 40-year-old cricket player diagnosed with an acute cervical strain is referred to physical therapy. During the examination, the physical therapist asks the patient to bend his head to the right and then proceeds to apply a downward compressive force to the patient's head. Which of the following subjective findings would be indicative of a positive test?
    A. Pain radiates into the right arm
    B. Pain radiates into the left arm
    C. Pain radiates into the arms bilaterally
    D. Pain radiates into the arms and legs bilaterally

47. A 38-year-old female tennis player having a complaint of weakness on his right forearm and wrist. On examination, the physical therapist completes an upper quarter screening examination on a patient with a suspected cervical spine lesion. Which objective finding is not consistent with C5 involvement?
    A. Muscle weakness in the supinator and wrist extensors
    B. Diminished sensation in the deltoid area
    C. Muscle weakness in the deltoid and biceps
    D. Diminished biceps and brachioradialis reflex

48. A 42-year-old car racer is diagnosed with "whiplash" following a motor vehicle accident. The accident occurred approximately two months ago. Before initiating a trial of manual traction, the therapist attempts to determine if the patient is an appropriate candidate. Which of the following

findings would be considered a contraindication for the specified intervention?
A. Rheumatoid arthritis
B. Cervical hypomobility
C. Headaches
D. Neck pain

49. A male rugby player complains of cervical pain that radiates to the deltoid area and anterior aspect of the entire arm to the base of the thumb. Which of the following tests is performed by the physical therapist to assess for C5 radiculopathy?
A. The patient pushes his arm away from the chest against resistance.
B. The patient holds his extended fingers together against the therapist's attempts to open the fingers.
C. The patient holds his shoulders in abduction against the downward force applied by the examiner.
D. The patient lifts his arm against resistance by the examiner.

50. A 42-year-old javelin thrower with decreased range of motion of the cervical spine secondary to pain and muscle spasm is assessed for signs that may support the diagnosis of cervical spondylosis. The physical therapist notes that nipping of the middle finger elicited reflex contraction of the thumb and index fingers. Based on this finding, which of the following signs is positive in that patient?
A. Hoffman sign
B. Lhermitte sign
C. Spurling sign
D. Yergason sign

ANSWERS

1. **B.** Rotation and side bending occur to opposite sides at the occipito-atlanto articulation; the only segment in the spine where rotation and side bending do not occur together is the atlanto-axial articulation because the ring-like structure of atlas allows only rotation to occur.
2. **D.** There are four indications for spinal cord injury:
   1. Severe neck pain
   2. Point tenderness in the cervical spine
   3. Abnormal neurologic signs secondary to dermatome and myotome check
   4. Neurologic signs and symptoms, such as numbness or weakness in the lower limb along a dermatome or myotome distribution
3. **D.** It leads to brachial plexus stretch, which occurs after contact about head or neck and can produce sensory and motor, or both the symptoms.
4. **C.**
5. **A.** The athlete should have normal strength in the upper extremities before returning to play. Without normal strength the athlete would be unable to protect him or herself and would be highly susceptible to further injury.
6. **B.** Central posterior anterior glide is performed with thumb and minimal pressure directly over the spinous process.
7. **D.** Odontoid anomalies lead to inherent instability between C1 and C2 is contraindicated for contact sports because any violent impact can lead to a catastrophic injury to cervical spinal cord.
8. **B.**
9. **C.** This is done to prevent further injury to the spinal cord.
10. **B.** It includes sensory changes like burning pain, numbness tingling and loss of sensation whereas motor changes range from weakness to complete paralysis involving upper and lower extremities.
11. **A.** White and Punjabi have defined clinical instability and established 3.5 mm translation and 11° of rotation as two factors to be used in determining indications for surgical stabilization.

Chapter 12: Spine and Chest Injuries

12. **A.**
13. **C.** Torg ratio is the ratio of spinal canal diameter to the vertebral body diameter in the cervical spine. The normal ratio is 1. It is an indication of possible cervical stenosis.
14. **A.** This test is used to determine subluxation of the atlas on the axis, which happens in case of torn transverse ligament.
15. **D.** Type II odontoid fracture occurs through the base either at or slightly below the level of superior articular surface. It is more prone to develop nonunion. Healing is based on age of patient and degree of displacement.
16. **D.**
17. **D.** Undergoing cause associated with these conditions decreases the anteroposterior diameter of the spinal canal and cause neuropraxia to the nerves that exists from the foramen.
18. **C.** Immediately after surgery, there should be a period of maximal protection followed by a period of deliberate active range of motion with moderate protection followed by isometrics.
19. **A.**
20. **B.** Otherwise called as shoulder abduction test. The patient actively elevates the arm through abduction so that the hand or forearm rests on the top of the head. Relief or decrease in symptoms indicate cervical extradural compression like herniated disc, nerve root compression.
21. **B.** Cervical upper crossed syndrome shows the effect of poking chin posture on the muscles. Where deep neck flexors, rhomboids, serratus anterior, lower trapezius are weak and pectoralis major, minor and upper trapezius are tight.
22. **D.**
23. **D.** Extreme hyperextension and lateral bending provide maximum traction to the brachial plexus thereby producing symptoms of pain and numbness and inability to move the involved extremity.
24. **C.** Leads to short neck, lower posterior hairline, limited neck range of motion, scapular anomalies leading to dangerous changes and contraindicate to participate in sports.

25. **A.** ULTT is a sensitizing test. It places stretch of the specified nerve root to find the pathology. ULTT3 is done to find the radial nerve compression.
26. **D.**
27. **B.** Full extension is the close packed position of cervical spine where all the structures are taut and the movement is restricted.
28. **D.** Foraminal compression or Spurling's test is done to find nerve root compression if the patients complain of pain in opposite side of neck. It indicates muscle spasm.
29. **C.** Patient's head and neck is taken into extension and side flexion and held for 30 seconds if dizziness or nystagmus occurs it indicates compressed vertebral arteries.
30. **B.**
31. **C.** Nerve roots: Typically, the player experiences a sharp burning pain in the shoulder with paraesthesia or dysesthesia radiating into the arm, thumb, and index finger.
32. **B.** Instability of the cervical spine. Stability of the cervical spine is essential element in sports. Instability of the cervical spine indicates damage to one or several of structural elements including the intervertebral disc, the ligaments, the osseous structures (vertebral bodies, facet joints) and the facet joint capsule.
33. **A.** Impingement is a painful syndrome caused by the friction of joint tissues, which is both the cause and the effect of joint biomechanics.
34. **D.** Impairment can be due to structural causes (e.g., disc herniation, fracture-luxation, ligament injury) or to mild functional causes.
35. **C.** Patients can become quadriplegic after a minor trauma to the spine, even without suffering a spinal fracture dislocation.
36. **D.** Stinger or burner injury: These lesions are often under-diagnosed or inadequately assessed. Symptoms usually resolve within a few minutes; however, recurrences are common and can lead to permanent neurologic deficits.
37. **A.** Neurotmesis: This injury is associated with the most unfavorable prognosis.

Chapter 12: Spine and Chest Injuries

38. **B.** Traumatic brachial plexus avulsion: Traditionally cervical myelography, followed by CT myelography, has been the gold standard for demonstration of these lesions, showing both complete and incomplete traction injuries.
39. **C.** Intervertebral disc is a dynamic structure that responds to stresses applied from vertebral movement or from static loading.
40. **B.** The therapist should perform the test and clear the patient's vertebral artery for their available range of motion. As the patient gains additional range of motion, the test can be readministered. It is possible to observe findings such as nystagmus and slurring of speech prior to achieving full rotation, extension and lateral flexion.
41. **B.** Key muscles that are partially or fully innervated at the C6 level include the brachialis, biceps, trapezius, deltoids, rhomboids, latissimus dorsi, rotator cuff, serratus anterior, and extensor carpi radialis.
42. **C.** Reminding the patient of the donning instructions for the orthosis provides the patient with the best opportunity to learn the correct technique. Although reapplying the orthosis correctly at the conclusion of the treatment session is appropriate, the action does not provide any specific feedback to the patient.
43. **D.** Paresthesia's of the long and ring fingers are commonly associated with the C7 nerve root, while the thumb and index finger are associated with C6.
44. **B.** Lateral flexion, extension, and rotation are all components of the vertebral artery test. Extension is the most likely motion to assess the integrity of the intervertebral foramen, while lateral flexion and rotation have a greater effect on the vertebral artery.
45. **B.** The axis of the goniometer should be positioned over the center of the cranial aspect of the head. The stationary arm should be parallel to an imaginary line between the two acromial processes, while the moving arm should be aligned with the tip of the nose.
46. **A.** A foraminal compression test or Spurling's test is considered to be positive if pain radiates into the arm toward the side of

head flexion during compression. The provocative test can be administered in progressive stages.
47. **A.** Muscle weakness of the supinator and wrist extensors is associated with C6 involvement.
48. **A.** Rheumatoid arthritis could cause instability of the alar and/or transverse ligaments, and as a result traction could potentially be detrimental.
49. **B.** Weakness in shoulder abduction tests for C5 radiculopathy.
50. **A.** The patient is positive for Hoffman sign. This finding is evidence of an upper motor neuron lesion.

B. CHEST AND THORACIC SPINE INJURIES

1. The most common type of injury leading to fractures in athletes is:
   A. Compression injury
   B. Distraction injury
   C. Translation injury
   D. Avulsion injury
2. Which of the following methods can be used effectively to treat lack of motion in a facet joint?
   A. Stabilization
   B. Bracing
   C. Manipulation
   D. Posture correction
3. Which technique is used to centralize the pain in thoracic disc herniation?
   A. Mulligan
   B. McKenzie
   C. Maitland
   D. None of the above
4. How many weeks of bed rest is indicated for the initial non-surgical treatment of a stable thoracic spine fracture?
   A. 6-8 weeks
   B. 4-6 weeks
   C. 2-4 weeks
   D. 1-2 weeks
5. Instability of the thoracic spine can be treated with:
   A. Bracing
   B. Stabilization exercises
   C. Postural education
   D. All of the above
6. Which type of thoracic spine fracture usually requires surgical treatment?
   A. Distraction injuries affecting anterior and posterior elements
   B. Compression injuries involving vertebral body
   C. Multidirectional injuries with translation of anterior and posterior elements
   D. Both A and B
7. An athlete with a thoracic disc herniation experiences pain in which of the following areas?
   A. Lower extremity
   B. Anterior chest
   C. Retroperitoneal area
   D. None of the above
8. Bracing following compression fracture of thoracic spine is used to prevent which movement of the spine?
   A. Flexion
   B. Rotation
   C. Extension
   D. All of the above

9. Indirect signs of thoracic spine injury are:
   A. Sternal fracture
   B. Rib fracture
   C. Cervical spine fracture
   D. Both A and B
10. What is the best method for imaging the thoracic spine following spinal cord pathology?
    A. MRI scan
    B. CT scan
    C. Ultrasound
    D. Radiograph
11. Which structure plays an important role in stabilizing the thoracic spine during loading and resist anterior shear loads?
    A. Costovertebral joints
    B. Ligamentum flavum
    C. Facet joints
    D. Supraspinous and interspinous ligament
12. Which muscle is frequently tense and tender in the presence of rib dysfunction?
    A. Transversocostalis
    B. Iliocostalis
    C. Longismus
    D. Spinalis
13. With which type of structural rib dysfunction is intercostal neuralgia often noted?
    A. Rib subluxation
    B. Laterally flexed rib
    C. Rib torsion
    D. Rib compression
14. Superiorly subluxated first rib may present with hypertonicity of which muscle?
    A. Rhomboids
    B. Trapezius
    C. Sternocleidomastoid
    D. Scalene
15. Which type of fracture is commonly seen in the floating ribs?
    A. Communited fracture
    B. Avulsion fracture
    C. Transverse fracture
    D. Oblique fracture
16. Biomechanical function of rib cage related to thoracic spine is to:
    A. Increase the mobility of the spine
    B. Protect the spine
    C. Allow displacement during trauma
    D. Decrease the transverse diameter of the thoracic spine

17. Which rib commonly encounters stress fracture?
    A. 1st   B. 5th
    C. 7th   D. 9th
18. Cause for hypermobility in a thoracic segment is:
    A. Adjacent hypomobile segment
    B. Individual's genetic make-up
    C. Response to repeated stress
    D. All of the above
19. Mechanism of injury leading to sternal fracture is:
    A. Rotation injury   B. Thoracic extension injury
    C. Thoracic flexion injury D. None of the above
20. Patient with myocardial contusion will experience chest pain that:
    A. Increases with breathing
    B. Decreases with breathing
    C. Does not increase or decrease with breathing
    D. Both A and B
21. Stretching of which muscle is essential in case of Scheuermann's disease?
    A. Quadriceps   B. Hamstring
    C. Gluteus maximus   D. Back extensors
22. In type II chance fracture, fracture travels through:
    A. Vertebral body and spinous process
    B. Vertebral body and asymmetrically through posterior elements of vertebra
    C. Vertebral body and between the spinous processes
    D. Vertebral body
23. Long thoracic nerve palsy leads to:
    A. Winging of scapula
    B. Anterior tipping of scapula
    C. Posterior tipping of scapula
    D. All of the above
24. Which of the following sports activity is commonly seen with Kissing spines?
    A. Sky diving   B. Swimming
    C. High jump   D. Gymnastics

25. Lonstein developed an expression to calculate the progression of scoliosis, which is:
    A. Cobb angle/Chronologic age
    B. Cobb angle - (5 × Risser's sign)/Chronologic age
    C. Cobb angle- (10 × Risser's sign)
    D. Cobb angle- (3 × Risser's sign)/Chronologic age
26. What is the degree of pelvic inclination angle observed in round back deformity?
    A. 10°   B. 20°
    C. 30°   D. 40°
27. Passive scapular approximation test is indicative of which nerve root pathology?
    A. T1   B. T3
    C. T4   D. T8
28. Forestier's bowstring sign indicates:
    A. Anterior wedging of 1 or 2 bodies of thoracic vertebra
    B. Severe rotation deformity of thoracic vertebra
    C. Ipsilateral paraspinal muscle tightness
    D. Mild rib hump
29. In which condition does a barrel chest deformity develop?
    A. Asthma   B. Emphysema
    C. Cystic fibrosis D. Bronchiectasis
30. Tietze's syndrome means inflammation of:
    A. Costovertebral junction   B. Manubriosternal junction
    C. Costochondral junction   D. All of the above
31. A 28-year-old male swimmer had a burst fracture of a thoracic vertebra secondary to a hyperflexion injury. The physician's note indicates the fracture is stable. Which of the following would not be considered appropriate immediate physical therapy management?
    A. Bed mobility exercises
    B. Active spinal range of motion exercises
    C. Postural education
    D. Instruction in donning and doffing a spinal brace
32. A 34-year-old rugby player had an injury in the thoracic spine. Physical therapy status post spinal fusion is referred for chest

physical therapy. The physical therapist instructs the patient in diaphragmatic breathing exercises. The instructions are given to the patient to place his dominant hand over the midrectus abdominis area and his nondominant hand over the midsternal area. As the patient inhales slowly through the nose, the therapist encourages the patient to?

A. Direct air so that a nondominant hand rises during inspiration
B. Direct air so that the dominant hand rises during inspiration
C. Direct air so that both hands rise equally during inspiration
D. Direct air so that both hands do not move during inspiration

33. A physical therapist examines a patient with an injury to the thoracodorsal nerve. Which of the following finding would be consistent with this injury?
    A. Shoulder medial rotation weakness
    B. Shoulder extension weakness
    C. Paralysis of the rhomboids
    D. Forward displacement of the lateral end of the clavicle

34. A physical therapist treats a 13-year-old female diagnosed with idiopathic scoliosis. The patient exhibits a right thoracic curve that measures 30° and a left lumbar curve measuring 15°. The MOST likely form of medical management is:
    A. Spinal orthosis and a home exercise program
    B. Bone growth generators and postural awareness exercises
    C. Electrical stimulation and a home exercise program
    D. Surgery and postoperative physical therapy intervention

35. A 61-year-old male at home following thoracic surgery under the care of a physical therapist. As part of treatment, the therapist designs a general exercise program for the patient. The patient is extremely eager to begin the exercise program, however his spouse expresses serious doubt about the program's importance. The most appropriate therapist action is to:
    A. Explain to the patient and spouse why the exercise program is an essential part of rehabilitation
    B. Redesign the exercise program to address the spouse's concerns

C. Ask the spouse to leave the room during treatment sessions

D. Discharge the patient from physical therapy

36. A 29-year-old boxer has been described as a consequence of fracture of the scapula, and mechanical irritation who work with arms above their head or abduct and rotate them externally. Which one of the following syndromes has often been associated with sporting activities?

    A. Suprascapular nerve entrapment
    B. Subdeltoid nerve entrapment
    C. Supraspinatus impingement
    D. Subcoracoid impingement

37. A 27-year-old sportsperson who reports the onset of mid-back pain and rib cage pain after competing in a tug-of-war contest at a company picnic 2 weeks ago. He complains of pain when laying supine and taking a deep breath. Radiographs were negative for fracture. He appears to have motion impairments, including limited thoracic extension and right rotation, rib asymmetry on the right with palpation, and restricted mobility of the rib cage on the right with deep inspirations. What would be the most appropriate diagnosis?

    A. Interspinous ligament sprain
    B. Sprained facet/costovertebral joint
    C. Spondylosis
    D. IVDP

38. The thoracic spine tends to have less mobility than the cervical and lumbar regions due to:

    A. Kyphosis   B. Intercostal muscles
    C. Rib cage and disc height   D. Ligament attachments

39. Which type of disorders tend to present as throbbing or pounding symptoms in the thoracic spine?

    A. Neural   B. Articular
    C. Structural   D. Vascular

40. Which one of the following structures is a frequent source of dysfunction in patients with thoracic and lumbar region pain?

    A. Facet joint   B. Thoracolumbar junction
    C. Intervertebral bodies   D. Intervertebral disc

41. Which one of the following thoracic spine movement is necessary for most overhead functional activities?
    A. Flexion
    B. Extension
    C. Side flexion
    D. Rotation
42. A 35-year-old basketball player had an injury on his thorax region. On examination, he is complaining of pain on inspiration, palpable tenderness, and possible crepitation. What is the most appropriate diagnosis for the above condition?
    A. Vertebral body fracture
    B. Dislocation
    C. Subluxation
    D. Rib fracture
43. A 65-year-old male has had chronic thoracic and low back pain. In the past 6 months, the patient has noted the onset of bilateral radiating leg pain, numbness, and tingling. Standing erect and walking make his symptoms worse; sitting in a flexed position completely alleviates his symptoms. His deep tendon reflexes in the lower extremities are hyperactive, and he has a positive Babinski test. What would be the most appropriate diagnosis?
    A. Sciatica
    B. Thoracic spine spondylolisthesis
    C. Thoracic spine central canal stenosis
    D. Cauda equina syndrome
44. What type of activities will take the stress off of the posterior spinal ligaments?
    A. Extension-based
    B. Flexion-based
    C. Rotation-based
    D. Combined motion
45. A 31-year-old female gymnast who presents with a 2-month history of pain in the right upper back, shoulder, and arm. She also felt paresthesia's in all digits of her right hand, glove-like numbness of the hand and forearm, weakness, hand clumsiness, and deep aching pain in her upper thoracic spine and right shoulder. The springing of the upper thoracic spine was deemed hypomobile and exactly reproduced her symptoms. What is the most suitable condition that affects the gymnasts?
    A. T10 syndrome
    B. T8 syndrome
    C. T6 syndrome
    D. T4 syndrome

46. Which one of the following tests to detect possible restriction of the movement of the first rib in patients with brachialgia?
    A. Lateral shear test
    B. Anterior shear test
    C. Upper cervical quadrant test
    D. Cervical rotation lateral flexion (CRLF) test
47. Name the three sets of thoracic articulations.
    A. Costotransverse joint, costovertebral joint, and apophyseal joint
    B. Costosternal joint, costoclavicular joint, costotransverse joint
    C. Costovertebral joint, costosternal joint, apophyseal joint
    D. Apophyseal joint, costoclavicular joint, costotransverse joint
48. During rib movements, ribs 7–10 mainly increase in lateral or transverse dimension. The above-mentioned rib movement is termed as:
    A. Caliper action
    B. Pump handle movement
    C. Bucket handle movement
    D. Anteroposterior direction
49. A mechanism involving pull of the serratus anterior and external oblique muscles on the rib has been proposed as the cause of repetitive bending of the rib, leading to:
    A. Stress fracture
    B. Avulsion fracture
    C. Winging of scapula
    D. Scapula tipping
50. A 35-year-old male javelin thrower had an injury in the chest. On examination he is complaining of pain occurs at the joints between the sternum and ribs. What would be most appropriate diagnosis?
    A. Costochondritis
    B. Costochondral dislocation
    C. Sternoclavicular dislocation
    D. Rib fracture

Chapter 12: Spine and Chest Injuries

ANSWERS

1. **A.** Most thoracic spine injuries in athletes result from high velocity sports, such as racing and skiing. Most fractures seen in athletic field are compression fracture with or without associated disruption of the surrounding soft tissues.
2. **C.** Joint manipulation is a skilled passive movement of a joint either within or beyond its active range of motion. It restores normal joint motion, increases tolerance to further insult, decreases pain, restores nutrition and repairs joint structures.
3. **B.** McKenzie technique uses repetitive motion for centralization of pain. In thoracic disc herniation, prone press-ups and prone on elbows with the use of breathing is practiced for centralization of pain.
4. **D.** In case of stable thoracic spine fracture, treatment usually entails bed rest for 1-2 weeks, appropriate bracing, ambulation as exercise followed by strengthening spinal musculature, postural education and body mechanics is taught.
5. **D.** Instability means looseness, unsteadiness or an inability to withstand normal physiological loading without mechanical deformation of which all the techniques help stabilize the part.
6. **C.** Type C thoracic spine fracture-multidirectional injuries with translation that also affects anterior and posterior elements. It is an unstable fracture and has the greatest degree of deficit and surgical treatment.
7. **B.** Common signs and symptoms are dull, deep retrosternal or retrogastric pain, "band-like" anterior chest pain, interscapular pain, lower extremity paresthesia, muscle weakness, backpain and bowel and bladder dysfunction.
8. **A.** Treating an athlete for compression fracture of thoracic spine involves bracing to prevent flexion and reduces the chance of an increased kyphosis.
9. **D.** The athletic trainer should be aware of the indirect signs of the possible thoracic spine injury. Sternal fracture and rib fracture not only indicate the presence of thoracic spine fracture but also an increased risk of instability.

10. A.
11. C. Facet joints are direct source of pain and are important stabilizing structures and resist anterior shear loads while the disc carries the remaining and contributes to the overall stability of the spine.
12. B. Iliocostalis muscle attaches to the rib angle and is the intermediate layer of back muscles and is tender and tense in the presence of rib dysfunction.
13. A. Rib subluxation is referred to as positional fault, can occur in the anterior or posterior direction with frequent complaints of intercostal neuralgia at the adjacent interspace and marked decrease in motion of the rib cage on inhalation and exhalation.
14. D. Scalene muscle is attached to the 1st rib and is at a state of contraction in the subluxation of 1st rib superiorly leading to hypertrophy.
15. B. The fracture of the floating ribs is unique. These ribs have only one articulation as opposed to the typical three articulations of the 3rd -10th pairs. Fracture of the floating ribs is usually an avulsion fracture of the attachments to the external oblique muscle of the abdominal wall.
16. B. Rib cage protects the spine, stiffens and strengthens the spine, increases resistance to displacement, increases thoracic spine transverse dimension and adds to the spines strength and energy absorbing capacity during trauma.
17. A. Fracture of 1st rib is more often caused by the mechanism of throwing; the theory being that sudden powerful contraction of the scalene muscle may cause the rib to fracture at its thinnest part. Repetitive contractions of these muscles during athletic performance may also cause a fatigue stress fracture of the 1st rib.
18. D. Hypermobility is increase in normal motion. Treatment is not to manipulate it, but to stabilize it.
19. C. Severe flexion injuries of the thoracic vertebra may produce sternal fracture particularly to upper and middle body of the sternum.
20. C.

Chapter 12: Spine and Chest Injuries

21. **B.** Scheuermann's disease is a postural deformity. Some adults will compensate for tight lumbodorsal fascia and hamstring by developing this round back deformity.
22. **C.** Chance fracture results from a seat-belt flexion distraction injury.
23. **A.** Injury to long thoracic nerve causes neurogenic back pain. The nerve is unprotected at the inferior margin of scapula.
24. **D.** Kissing spines commonly found in female gymnasts, refers to interspinous bursitis wherein the interspinous ligament develops a pseudobursa and there is chronic inflammation and even osteophyte formation on the adjacent spinous process.
25. **D.** The progression factor does not take into account the patient's sex, female's menarchal status and location of the curve.
26. **C.** Pelvic inclination angle decreases in round back deformity. The normal angle is 30°.
27. **A.** Patient is prone while examiner passively approximates the scapula by lifting the shoulder up and back. Indicative of T1 or T2 nerve root problem on the side on which the pain is experienced.
28. **C.** Forestier's bowstring sign is evident in ipsilateral paraspinal muscle tightness which indicates hypomobility/hypermobility at a specific segment.
29. **B.** In barrel chest deformity, the sternum projects forward and upward so that the anteroposterior diameter is increased.
30. **C.** Tietze's syndrome is inflammation and painful, tender non-suppurative swelling of a costochondral junction.
31. **B.** There is not enough information presented to determine if active spinal range of motion exercises are appropriate for the patient. The remaining options offer valuable treatment alternatives that are considerably less aggressive.
32. **B.** In diaphragmatic breathing, the patient's hand placed over the midrectus area should rise during inspiration and fall during expiration.
33. **B.** The latissimus dorsi is innervated by the thoracodorsal nerve. Weakness in this muscle would produce impaired strength during shoulder extension.

34. A. Spinal curves that measure between 20 and 40 degrees and remain flexible are best treated with a spinal orthosis and exercise. Based on the patient's age and size of the scoliotic curve, the patient would be a good candidate for a spinal orthosis and a home exercise program.

35. C. A supportive spouse can be extremely helpful to a patient completing a home exercise program. In order for the spouse to be an asset, she must first recognize the value of the program.

36. A. Suprascapular nerve entrapment. Boxers, tennis players, and weight lifters are athletes who frequently suffer from this syndrome.

37. B. This patient most likely sprained a facet joint and/or a costovertebral joint, which is causing the pain with movement and breathing. Some treatment approaches advocate treating the rib impairments first, then focusing on the thoracic spine any rib impairments.

38. C. Articulations with the rib cage and the fact that the ratio of the height of the disc to the vertebral body is 1:5, compared to 1:3 in the lumbar spine and 2:5 in the cervical spine.

39. D. Vascular disorders present in the thoracic spine leads thoracic aortic aneurysm may present with pain in the thoracic spine and a palpable pulse in the abdomen.

40. B. Thoracolumbar junction: Thoracolumbar spine is the transitional zone between the stiff thoracic cage and the mobile lumbar spine. Therefore, it is a vulnerable region for injury, including fracture and dislocation.

41. B. Extension: Impairments in thoracic motion may predispose the patient to injury in the neck and shoulder.

42. D. Rib fracture: Stress fractures of the first rib are common in overhead activities.

43. C. The most likely cause of his symptoms is central canal stenosis in the thoracic spine. Symptoms of stenosis typically get worse with extension and better with flexion. The fact that the reflexes are elevated and the fact that he has a positive Babinski test suggest that the cord compression is proximal (above L1 or L2) and most likely represents an upper motor neuron lesion.

Chapter 12: Spine and Chest Injuries

44. **A.** Extension-based activities. Pathologies eased by extension include posterior disc herniations, disc-related radiculopathy, and ligament strains.
45. **D.** T4 syndrome refers to a clinical pattern that involves upper extremity pain and paranesthesia's with or without symptoms into the neck and/or head. Passive movement of an upper thoracic vertebrae (commonly T4) may reproduce the symptoms. The sympathetic nervous system may provide a pathway for referral from the thoracic spine to the head and arms, so thoracic manual therapy should be considered.
46. **D.** In the presence of a hypomobile first rib, passive lateral flexion is restricted when the cervical spine is maximally rotated passively away from the hypomobile side due to the first thoracic transverse process bumping against the elevated first rib. This test has excellent intertester reliability as well as validity based on cineradiographic examination.
47. **A.** Costotransverse joint, costovertebral joint and apophyseal joint
48. **C.** Bucket handle movement, is a movement of ribs that results in change in transverse diameter of the thorax.
49. **A.** Stress fracture: A modified technique using less reach, pull-through, and layback should decrease the forces transmitted to the rib by these muscles, and decrease the risk for stress fractures.
50. **A.** Costochondritis occurs at the plane joints between the sternum and ribs. It is characterized by activity-related pain and tenderness localized to the costochondral junction. This condition is sometimes known as Tietze's syndrome.

C. LUMBAR SPINE INJURIES

1. In the rehabilitation of athletes with spondylolisthesis which type of exercise is contraindicated?
   A. Flexion exercise
   B. Extension exercise
   C. Side-bending exercise
   D. Rotation

2. Which technique can be used effectively to treat hemipelvic asymmetry?
   A. Muscle energy technique
   B. Combined movement
   C. McKenzie approach
   D. Neural mobilization

3. The primary stabilizer of the lumbar vertebra is:
   A. Rotators
   B. Multifidus
   C. Trunk oblique muscles
   D. All of the above

4. A nutated sacrum should be treated with a:
   A. Medial force on the sacrum
   B. Posteroanterior force on the superior sacrum to the sacral promontory
   C. Posteroanterior force on the lower sacrum between the two inferior lateral angles
   D. Medial force on the sacral promontory

5. Which of the following statements about a 'locked' facet is true?
   A. It is usually more painful with movement than at rest
   B. It may have resulted from forward flexion
   C. It often produces radiating sensory pain
   D. It can cause significantly restricted range of motion

6. Sacralization of the vertebra means:
   A. 5th lumbar vertebra fuses with sacrum and ilium
   B. S1 segment may be mobile
   C. The 5 sacral segments function as independent vertebrae
   D. All the lumbar vertebra are fused

7. Which movement in the lumbar spine is a coupled osteokinematic movement?
   A. Extension
   B. Side bending
   C. Flexion
   D. Gliding

Chapter 12: Spine and Chest Injuries

8. Following acute herniated nucleus pulposus, in which position is an athlete treated with McKenzie regimen?
   A. Prone
   B. Supine
   C. Standing
   D. Sitting
9. Which treatment can be best opted for facet dysfunction?
   A. Rocking the supine athlete's knee from side to side
   B. Passive rotation of hypomobile segment
   C. Mobilization of facet joint
   D. All of the above
10. The special test that is used to assess the passive intervertebral motion in the lumbar spine is:
    A. Quadrant test
    B. Pheasant test
    C. Spring test
    D. Milgram's test
11. In lumbosacral tunnel syndrome, L5 nerve root is compressed under which structure?
    A. Inguinal ligament
    B. Adductor canal
    C. Iliolumbar ligament
    D. None of the above
12. According to Meyerdling's Grade III classification of spondylolisthesis, what is the percentage of slippage?
    A. 85%
    B. 75%
    C. 95%
    D. 100%
13. Name the pathology which is assessed using the Stoop test?
    A. Segmental instability
    B. Neurogenic intermittent claudication
    C. Neuropathy
    D. Radiculopathy
14. Cafe au lait spots indicates:
    A. Neurofibromatosis
    B. Spina bifida occulta
    C. Diastematomyelia
    D. Spina bifida cystica
15. Deyerle's sign indicates irritation of the sciatic nerve in which region?
    A. Foot
    B. Above knee
    C. Buttock
    D. Below knee
16. Lumbar lordosis decreases with which sacral movement?
    A. Nutation
    B. Counternutation
    C. Both A and B
    D. None of the above

17. Rupture of supraspinous ligament following acute flexion injury of the spine is termed as:
    A. Dowager's hump
    B. Round back
    C. Sprung back
    D. Flat back
18. Normal lumbosacral angle is:
    A. 140°
    B. 120°
    C. 100°
    D. 80°
19. 'Greyhound' is the term used to represent the radiographic appearance of what type of defect in pars interarticularis?
    A. Lytic pars interarticularis
    B. Acute fracture of pars interarticularis
    C. Congenital deficiency of pars interarticularis
    D. Elongated pars interarticularis
20. Swayback increases the risk of which condition in lumbar spine?
    A. Spondylosis
    B. Disc herniation
    C. Spondylolysis
    D. All of the above
21. Tenderness over Baer's point indicates:
    A. Acute appendicitis
    B. Sprain of sacroiliac ligament
    C. Spasm of iliacus
    D. Both B and C
22. In athletes with lumbar canal stenosis, which of the following activities aggravates pain?
    A. Running downhill
    B. Running uphill
    C. Running in plains
    D. None of the above
23. Which level of lumbar spine involves in Maigne's syndrome?
    A. L3–L4
    B. T10–L1
    C. T12–L2
    D. L4–L5
24. Entrapment of L5 nerve root between the transverse process of L5 and the ala of the sacrum is called as:
    A. Radicular pain syndrome
    B. Quadratus lumborum syndrome
    C. Far out syndrome
    D. Complex regional pain syndrome

Chapter 12: Spine and Chest Injuries

25. Abnormal contraction of which muscle initiates posterior joint syndrome?
    A. Erector spinae
    B. Transverse abdominis
    C. Multifidus
    D. Obliques externus
26. Gillet's test designed to detect dysfunctional sacroiliac joint motion; the posterior superior iliac spine moves in which direction?
    A. Laterally
    B. Medially
    C. Inferiorly
    D. Superiorly
27. How many degrees of torsion can a degenerative disc withstand before failure?
    A. 14.3°
    B. 22.6°
    C. 5.8°
    D. 31.7°
28. Chronic low back pain syndrome can result from which of the following causes?
    A. Atrophy of muscle
    B. Fibrosis within and around the muscle
    C. Degeneration of facet joints
    D. All of the above
29. What type of stress leads to changes in posterior facet joints?
    A. Flexion
    B. Rotational
    C. Axial compression
    D. Extension
30. Principle of proper body mechanics includes all, *except*:
    A. Use of neutral spine
    B. Use small muscles of upper and lower body to do work
    C. Keep shoulder and hip parallel
    D. Maintain wide base of support
31. A 14-year-old female gymnastics referred to physical therapy with a complaint of pain, following the activity of unable to tolerate the intensity of training. Based on the presented X-ray (Scottie dog decapitated), the therapist would expect the patient's medical diagnosis to be:
    A. Spondylitis
    B. Spondylolysis
    C. Spondylolisthesis
    D. Spondyloarthropathy
32. A 28-year-old female athlete referred to the physical therapist was diagnosed with facet impingement in the lumbar spine.

The athlete appears to be somewhat fixed in side bending to the right and rotation to the left. When assessing a lumbar range of motion, which motions would you expect to be most restricted?
A. Side bending to the right and rotation to the left
B. Side bending to the left and rotation to the right
C. Side bending to the right and rotation to the right
D. Side bending to the left and rotation to the left

33. A physical therapist discusses the importance of proper posture with a patient rehabilitating from back surgery. Which body position would place the most pressure on the lumbar spine?
A. Standing in the anatomical position
B. Standing with 45° of hip flexion
C. Sitting in a chair with reduced lumbar lordosis
D. Sitting in a chair

34. A 27-year-old football player had an injury in his lower back. On examination, the physical therapist attempts to assess the integrity of the L4 spinal level. Which deep tendon reflex would provide the therapist with the most useful information?
A. Lateral hamstrings
B. Medial hamstrings
C. Patellar reflex
D. Achilles' reflex

35. A 50-year-old athlete calls to ask for advice after injuring his lower back. The patient explains that he cannot bend down and touch his toes with severe pain and has muscle spasms throughout the entire lower back. The physical therapist works in a state without direct access but would like to help the patient. The most appropriate response would be:
A. Explain to the patient you would be happy to treat him, however, since you have not completed a formal examination, it would be unfair to prescribe treatment over the phone
B. Arrange a time for the patient to come into your clinic for immediate treatment
C. Refer the patient to a qualified physician
D. Prescribe flexion exercises and ice every three hours

Chapter 12: Spine and Chest Injuries

36. A physical therapist completes a positional assessment of the sacrum with a patient lying prone. The examination results reveal a deep sacral sulcus on the left and a posterior and caudal inferior lateral angle on the left when the patient moves into a prone on elbow position. This finding is most indicative of:
    A. Bilateral sacral flexion dysfunction
    B. Bilateral sacral extension dysfunction
    C. Unilateral left extended sacrum
    D. Unilateral left flexed sacrum

37. A physical therapist completes a standing flexion test to identify possible innominate distortion in a patient referred to physical therapy with chronic back pain. The most appropriate structure to palpate while completing the test is:
    A. The spinous process of L5
    B. Anterior superior iliac spines
    C. Pubic tubercles
    D. Posterior superior iliac spines

38. A 40-year-old male basket player with low back pain. He describes pain radiating down the outer thigh and leg, stiffness in the low back region, and increased pain with attempted movement of the spine. Which of the following would be the MOST likely cause of the patient's symptoms?
    A. Microtears of the ligamentum flavum and posterior longitudinal ligament
    B. L3-L4 lumbar facet joint arthropathy
    C. Soft tissue strain of the lumbar extensors
    D. Posterolateral protrusion of the lumbar intervertebral disc at L5-S1

39. Low back pain is frequently caused by lumbar disc disease, which is influenced by aging and degenerative cascade. What is the nomenclature specific to lumbar disc disease that involves breaking off of the disc fragment from the nucleus pulposus?
    A. Disc bulge
    B. Disc protrusion
    C. Disc sequestration
    D. Disc extrusion

40. A physical therapist conducts a thorough physical assessment on a 24-year-old long jumper suspected of the sacral spine and pelvis dysfunction. The following tests are used to test the sacral spine and pelvis, *except*:
    A. Approximation test
    B. Quadrant test
    C. Supine-to-sit test
    D. Gillet test

41. A 45-year-old female athlete is evaluated for chronic pain in the lower back, weakness, and numbness in the legs during walking. The symptoms are usually resolved by rest. Bending forward diminishes the pain. On physical examination, the patient is noted for wide-based gait, abnormal Romberg test, and thigh pain after 30 seconds of lumbar extension. The patient is positive for the stoop test and negative for the straight leg raise test. Based on these assessment findings, the patient is most likely diagnosed with:
    A. Lumbar spinal stenosis
    B. Lumbar disc herniation
    C. Arthritis of the spine
    D. Intermittent claudication due to arterial disease

42. A 36-year-old female hockey player is having a complaint of lower back pain with severe lumbar movement limitation. After examination, the physical therapist plans a treatment program for a recently diagnosed patient with lumbar spinal stenosis. The program would consist of conservative treatment modalities, including exercise and activity. Which of the following is least likely included in the exercise program?
    A. Lumbar extension exercises
    B. Spinal flexion exercises
    C. Abdominal muscle strengthening
    D. Inclined treadmill testing

43. A 34-year-old male football player is having a chronic low back problem for the past 3 months. A physical therapist prepares a home exercise program for a patient rehabilitating from a disc protrusion in the lumbar spine. Assuming the patient successfully completes the pictured exercises (prone on hands), which activity would be next to occur in the extension progression?

A. Single knee to chest
B. Double knee to chest
C. Prone on elbows
D. Extension exercises in standing

44. A football player referred to physical therapy with chronic low back pain has failed to progress toward meeting established goals in over three weeks of treatment. The physical therapist has employed various treatment techniques but has yet to observe any sign of subjective or objective improvement in the patient's condition. The most appropriate action would be to:
    A. Transfer the patient to another therapist's schedule
    B. Re-examine the patient and establish new goals
    C. Continue to modify the patient's treatment plan
    D. Alert the referring physician to the patient's status

45. Which muscle is considered to have the greatest potential to provide dynamic control to the trunk motion segment, particularly in its neutral zone?
    A. Lumbar multifidus
    B. Transverse abdominis
    C. Rectus abdominis
    D. Internal oblique

46. Which surgical procedure is designed to decompress neural tissues by removing the IVD material causing the compression and irritation of the nerve root?
    A. Laminectomy
    B. Microdiscectomy
    C. Disc implantation
    D. Lumbar fusion

47. Which diagnostic tool can be used as an indirect method of measuring correct activation of the spinal segment stabilization coactivation contraction?
    A. Electromyography
    B. Sphygmomanometer
    C. Pressure biofeedback
    D. Abdominal pressure test

48. When the anterior tip of sacral promontory moves posteriorly and superiorly and anterior ilium on sacrum rotation. What is the above mechanism stated for?
    A. Upslip
    B. Down slip
    C. Counternutation
    D. Nutation

49. Which exercises should be used cautiously or avoided in most cases of acute disc prolapse and when a laterally shifted posture is present?
    A. Extension
    B. Flexion
    C. Side bending
    D. Rotation

50. An athlete is scheduled for decompressive lumbar laminectomy due to significant lumbar radiculopathy. After the surgery, the physical therapist encourages the following activities, *except*:
    A. Basic mobility activities
    B. Proper body mechanics
    C. Immobilization
    D. Back safety techniques

Chapter 12: Spine and Chest Injuries

ANSWERS

1. **B.** Extension exercises prevent further slippage of the vertebra holding the segments in extended position whereas flexion exercises aggravate the condition.
2. **A.** Muscle energy technique attempts to realign structures by using the athlete's own muscle strength.
3. **D.** These muscles bring about the segmental stability to the lumbar vertebra.
4. **C.** With a nutate sacrum, the sacral sulci will be relatively deep and the inferior lateral angles will be more superficial.
5. **D.** In locked facet joint:
   1. Pain is more at rest
   2. Results from backward bending, side bending and rotation
   3. No radiating pain experienced
6. **A.**
7. **B.** Flexion and extension motion of lumbar spine are pure motions. Lateral flexion and rotation are coupled motion, which facilitates motion.
8. **A.** Prone position allows normal lumbar lordosis and some degree of spinal extension.
9. **D.** All these techniques alleviate pain by releasing the locked facet.
10. **C.** Spring test: Posteroanterior glide over the spinous process is performed with the athlete in prone position. Done to confirm hypomobility or hypermobility at a segment.
11. **C.** Iliolumbar ligament is in the iliolumbar canal, underneath passes the L5 nerve root, which can be compressed in case of trauma, osteophytes or tumor.
12. **B.**
13. **B.** Stoop test: Indicates neurogenic intermittent claudication. Patient is asked to walk briskly; pain ensures in the buttock and lower limb within a distance of 50 m. To relieve the pain, the patient flexes forward.
14. **A.** Unusual skin marking or presence of skin lesions in the midline. Indicates underlying neural and mesodermal anomalies.

15. **B.** Deyerle's sign: With the patient seated, examiner extends the patient's affected leg to point of pain then flexes knee and gives strong pressure into the popliteal fossa, radicular symptom increases above knee.
16. **B.** In counternutation the lumbar spine is flexed decreasing the lumbar lordosis.
17. **C.** Sprung back is a term coined by Newman to describe the rupture of supraspinous ligament following sudden flexion strain applied to spine with pelvis fixed leading to segmental instability.
18. **A.**
19. **D.** MacEwen have described the 'Greyhound' to represent the radiographic appearance of the elongated pars interarticularis.
20. **D.** Swayback, i.e., hyperlordotic posturing of the low back may be flexible or fixed which increases the shear load in the facet joints and disc leading to the related pathologies.
21. **D.** Baer's point is located in the right iliac fossa anterior to the right sacroiliac joint and slightly medial to McBurney's point.
22. **B.** Running uphill will cause the lumbar spine to extend and decrease the space in the canal and thereby aggravate the radicular pain.
23. **C.** Maigne's or thoracolumbar syndrome is associated with facet joint dysfunction at T12-L2 levels. The mechanism of pain is mediated by the posterior primary rami that innervate these facet joints.
24. **C.**
25. **C.** Torsional injury caused by abnormal contraction of multifidus initiates lesions in the posterior facet joints and disc. Each recurrent strong contraction tends to cause further injury leading to degenerative changes in facet joints.
26. **D.** In Gillet's test, the examiner palpates the posterior superior iliac spine and ask the patient to raise the respective leg, the posterior superior iliac spine moves inferior in relation to sacrum but in case of dysfunction it moves superiorly.
27. **A.** According to Farfan's work, normal disc withstands 22.6° and degenerative disc 14.3° of torsion before failure, beyond which peripheral circumferential tears in the annulus results leading to disc herniation.

Chapter 12: Spine and Chest Injuries

28. D. Lack of use or immobilization of the back results in atrophy, fibrosis of muscles and degeneration of facet joints. This process enhanced by emotional status and stress leads to long-standing symptoms and signs.

29. B.

30. B. Use large muscles of upper and lower body to do the work. Proper body mechanics will reduce the forces imposed on the lower back muscles and joints thereby prevent injury.

31. C. Spondylolisthesis refers to the forward displacement of one vertebra over another. The X-ray involves spondylolisthesis at the L_5-S_1 level. Individuals involved in physical activities, such as weightlifting, gymnastics or football are particularly susceptible to this condition. The severity of the spondylolisthesis is classified on a scale of 1–5 based on how much a given vertebral body has slipped forward over the vertebral body beneath it.

32. B. Facet impingement often results in a patient being locked in a selected position. In the thoracic and lumbar spine, the position involves side bending and rotation occurring in opposite directions. The patient will experience the greatest discomfort and restriction of movement when moving away from the locked position.

33. C. According to a study performed by Nachemson, intradiscal pressure is greatest when sitting in a chair with reduced lumbar lordosis.

34. C. Lateral hamstrings reflex (S1-S2), medial hamstrings reflex (L5-S1), patellar reflex (L3-L4), Achilles' reflex (S1-S2).

35. C. The most appropriate response is to refer the patient to a qualified physician. This action will allow the patient to receive a thorough examination, and if indicated, a referral to physical therapy.

36. D. If the inferior lateral angle on the same side as the deep sacral sulcus becomes more caudal in prone on elbows, it may be indicative of a unilateral flexed sacrum.

37. D. The standing flexion test is designed to identify innominate distortion. The physical therapist should palpate the inferior portion of the posterior superior iliac spine as the patient actively flexes the spine.

38. **D.** Acute low back pain that radiates down the posterolateral aspect of the thigh and leg is often caused by a posterolateral protrusion of the lumbar intervertebral disc at the L5-S1 level. The lumbar region of the vertebral column often becomes rigid and movement is painful due to muscle spasm.
39. **C.** Disc sequestration is the separation of the disc fragment from the nucleus pulposus. In a disc bulge, the annular fibers are intact. Protrusion of the disc involves localized bulging of the disc with damaged annular fibers. Disc extrusion involves an extended bulge with destroyed annular fibers; the disc is intact.
40. **B.** The quadrant test is used to assess for nerve-root irritation or facet pathology.
41. **A.** The patient is most likely diagnosed with lumbar spinal stenosis. Lumbar stenosis is the narrowing of the vertebral canal and vertebral foramina. This condition typically demonstrates signs of neurogenic claudication, which is caused by increased metabolic demands of compressed nerve roots due to the stenosis. In contrast to vascular claudication, neurogenic claudication is not aggravated by biking and lumbar flexion and is not alleviated by standing. Diminished lumbar extension is the most significant finding in lumbar spinal stenosis.
42. **A.** Lumbar extension exercises are avoided. This type of exercise encourages spinal extension and increased lumbar lordosis, which may aggravate the pain. Spinal flexion exercises should be emphasized because they reduce the lordosis and the stress applied to the lumbar spine. Strengthening of the abdominal muscles would increase lumbar spine support. Inclined treadmill testing causes longer walking times, due to spinal flexion.
43. **D.** The traditional progression from lowest to highest level is: lie in prone on a firm surface, prone on elbows, prone press-up, extension exercises in standing.
44. **D.** The physician should be informed about the patient's lack of progress. The patient may be discharged from physical therapy or referred back to the physician.
45. **A.** Lumbar multifidi are responsible for more than two-thirds of the stiffness at the L4-5 segmental level.

46. **B.** Microdiscectomy: Following a discectomy, patients are generally able to return to their previous levels of activity, including participation in recreational sports.
47. **C.** Pressure biofeedback: The stabilizer is inflated to 40 mm Hg pressure and placed under the patient's abdomen, or back. The patient should be instructed to contract the transversus in a way that does not make the pressure in the cuff start to rise or fall.
48. **C.** Counternutation describes when the sacrum is rotated backwards relative to the iliac bones.
49. **B.** In patients recovering from disc-related back pain, flexion exercise should not be commenced immediately after a flat-lying rest interval longer than 30 minutes.
50. **C.** Immobilization: After the surgery, it is essential that the patient is encouraged to ambulate as soon as possible. Basic mobility exercises, proper body mechanics, and back safety exercises are also encouraged. A short course of physical therapy is recommended. The program consists of lower back and abdominal muscle strengthening exercises.

Chapter 13

Stress Fracture

1. Stress fractures occur among sportspersons such as:
   A. Runners
   B. Elite gymnasts
   C. World-class ice skaters
   D. All of the above
2. The classic location of stress fractures occurs among athletic populations, mainly running and field sports is:
   A. Tibia
   B. Radius
   C. Humerus
   D. Skull
3. Runners with high weekly mileage are at risk of:
   A. Olecranon bursitis
   B. Recurrent lower extremity stress fracture
   C. Pelvis injuries
   D. Prepatellar bursitis
4. Athletes with excessive foot supination tend to experience:
   A. Shin splints
   B. Medial tibial stress syndrome
   C. Stress fracture
   D. None of the above
5. Spondylolysis refers to a stress fracture of the pars interarticularis, usually at L5. Lumbar spondylolysis are more common in:
   A. Adolescent gymnasts
   B. Fast bowlers in cricket
   C. Athletes involved in a contact sport
   D. All of the above
6. Amenorrheic female athletes have increased incidence of:
   A. Stress fractures
   B. Pathological fractures
   C. Comminuted fractures
   D. Traumatic fractures
7. A long-distance runner recovering from a lateral ankle sprain may subconsciously modify their gait, causing increased risk of:

A. Stress fractures of the foot   B. Bursitis
C. Foot drop   D. None of the above

8. Name the common lower limb abnormalities which are linked with stress fractures:
   A. Excessive Q angle   B. Leg length inequality
   C. A and B   D. Knee stiffness

9. In runners, which area of the foot is at the increased risk for a stress fracture in men?
   A. Medial forefoot   B. Hindfoot
   C. Midfoot   D. Lateral forefoot

10. Which foot condition demonstrates the reduced shock-absorbing capacity and is shown to be a risk factor for recurrent lower limb stress fractures in athletes?
    A. Valgus toe   B. Pes cavus
    C. Pes planus   D. B and C

11. Name the stress fracture caused by long or triple jump:
    A. Navicular stress fracture
    B. Metacarpal stress fracture
    C. Femoral stress fracture
    D. None of the above

12. Name the stress fracture caused by running activities:
    A. Tibial stress fracture
    B. Metacarpal stress fracture
    C. Fifth metatarsal stress fracture
    D. A and C

13. Proximal posteromedial cortex tibial stress fractures occur in:
    A. Recreational and competitive runners
    B. Ballet dancers
    C. Basketball players
    D. All of the above

14. The most common area of the foot and ankle which have relatively high incidences of stress fractures is:
    A. Metatarsal   B. Navicular
    C. Talus   D. Calcaneus

15. Name the tarsal stress fracture which results from a heavy heel strike during running or landing?

A. Navicular stress fracture
B. Second metatarsal stress fracture
C. Calcaneus stress fracture
D. Tibial stress fracture

16. _____ is a rare upper extremity stress fracture that primarily affects throwing athletes.
    A. Olecranon stress fracture   B. Navicular stress fracture
    C. Humerus stress fracture   D. Femur stress fracture

17. Which of the following sports person is most susceptible to Olecranon stress fracture?
    A. Football player   B. Baseball player
    C. Runner   D. None of the above

18. In baseball players, olecranon stress fracture occurs from:
    A. Rapid and repetitive varus flexion
    B. Slow and repetitive valgus flexion
    C. Rapid and repetitive valgus extension
    D. Slow and repetitive varus extension

19. Among the following, which stress fracture mostly frequently occurring with an average onset at 12 years of age among the adolescent persons who is a pitcher or catcher role in a throwing sport or throwing a breaking ball?
    A. Clavicular stress fracture   B. Metatarsal stress fracture
    C. Tibial stress fracture   D. Olecranon stress fracture

20. Name the examination maneuver that often reproducibly elicits pain in patients with an olecranon stress fracture:
    A. Snapping extension test   B. Arm bar test
    C. A and B   D. None of the above

21. Anatomic sites for high-risk stress fractures are:
    A. Femoral neck (tension side)
    B. Talar neck
    C. Dorsal tarsal navicular cortex
    D. All of the above

22. Name the fracture representing a fatigue failure of the bone, which occurs with a spectrum of severity of structural injury and characterizes with varying healing potential by location?

A. Stress fracture   B. Pathological fracture
C. Traumatic fracture   D. Comminuted fracture

23. Which of the following sportspersons engage in repetitive impact loading of the lower extremity and is at high risk for developing femoral stress fracture?
    A. Weight lifters   B. Swimmers
    C. Long-distance runners   D. None of the above

24. Considering the nature of the sporting events, which of the following sportspersons is at risk for developing tibial stress fracture?
    A. Cross country runners   B. Track and field runners
    C. Soccer players   D. All of the above

25. _____ is the common midfoot injury that usually occurs in competitive athletes who participate in running or jumping sports.
    A. Calcaneal stress fracture
    B. Patella stress fracture
    C. Fifth metatarsal stress fracture
    D. Femoral neck stress fracture

26. Non-loading activities used in the management of stress fracture to maintain the fitness are:
    A. Cycling   B. Swimming
    C. Rowing   D. All of the above

27. Management of femoral stress fracture include:
    A. Educating of athletes and coaches
    B. Rest and activity modification
    C. Correction of training errors
    D. All of the above

28. The management of stress fractures among athletes include:
    A. Limiting hills and multiple terrains during recovery
    B. Orthotics
    C. Changing shoes
    D. All of the above

29. From the following, identify the critical factors emphasized by the sports physiotherapists to counsel the athletes to prevent stress fractures:

A. Appropriate diet
B. Appropriate training regimen
C. Proper technique and appropriate orthotics
D. All of the above

30. Identify the commonly used electrotherapeutic modalities in the management of stress fracture of foot and ankle among athletes:
    A. Pulsed ultrasound
    B. Extracorporeal shock wave therapy
    C. Bone stimulators
    D. All of the above

31. Which one of the following diagnostic tests would be the most appropriate to identify the stress fracture?
    A. Bone scan
    B. Magnetic resonance imaging
    C. Telethermograph
    D. Ultrasound scan

32. Cleavage fracture appears:
    A. Bright   B. Dull
    C. Difficult to identify   D. None of the above

33. Fracture toughness is measured in terms of:
    A. Strain energy release rate
    B. Stress concentration factor
    C. Both A and B
    D. None

34. Fracture stress (σ) is proportional to:
    A. Crack length   B. 1/crack length
    C. (Crack length)^{½} D. (Crack length)$^{-½}$

35. If the surface crack causing a fracture in a brittle material is made twice as deep, the fracture strength will:
    A. Decrease by a factor of $\sqrt{2}$
    B. Decrease by a factor of 2
    C. Decrease by a factor of 2^2
    D. No change

ANSWERS

1. **D.** Stress fractures occur among sportspersons, such as runners, elite gymnasts, world-class ice skaters, and ballet dancers.
2. **A.** In athletic populations (mainly running and field sports), the classic location has always been the tibia, with much fewer fractures in the femur and other locations, possibly with the exception of ballet dancers.
3. **B.** Once the athlete is running more than 40 miles per week, there is a significant increase in the risk of lower extremity overuse injury, and runners with high weekly mileage are at risk of the recurrent lower extremity stress fracture.
4. **C.** Persons with a supinated foot type, especially runners, may be vulnerable to back, hip, and knee problems. The most severe over-supinators also tend to experience recurrent ankle sprains and/or stress fractures.
5. **D.** Lumbar spondylolysis and spondylolisthesis are more common in sports involving repeated flexion or extension activities, with a high incidence in adolescent gymnasts, fast bowlers in cricket, and athletes involved in a contact sport.
6. **A.** Amenorrheic female athletes have an increased incidence of stress fractures.
7. **A.** A long-distance runner recovering from a lateral ankle sprain may subconsciously modify their gait, causing an increased risk of stress fractures of the foot or other problems through the kinetic chain.
8. **C.** An excessive Q-angle has been shown to be a risk factor for patellofemoral pain syndrome and lower limb stress fractures. Leg length inequality has been shown to be linked with lower extremity injury in runners and specifically stress fractures.
9. **D.** Running flats (flat running shoes) worn by athletes in races and at times in training. The use of these types of shoe has been shown to reduce the contact area between the shoe and the ground, increasing the maximum forces experienced by the athlete beneath the entire foot and specifically the lateral forefoot, which is an area of increased stress fracture risk in men.

10. **D.** Both pes cavus and planus presentations demonstrate reduced shock-absorbing capacity and have been shown to be a risk factor for recurrent lower limb stress fractures in athletes.
11. **A.** Long/triple jump causes navicular stress fractures.
12. **D.** Running causes tibial stress fracture and fifth metatarsal stress fracture.
13. **D.** A higher incidence of proximal posteromedial cortex tibial stress fractures is observed in recreational and competitive runners; ballet dancers and jumping athletes (such as basketball players) more commonly experience stress fractures in the anterior cortex.
14. **A.** Areas of the foot and ankle with relatively high incidences of stress fractures include the metatarsals (most common) and the navicular, although the talus and calcaneus are also vulnerable.
15. **C.** After the navicular, the second most common site for a tarsal stress fracture is calcaneus. This condition is more likely to result from (among other factors) heavy heelstrike during running or landing.
16. **A.** Olecranon stress fractures are a rare upper extremity fracture that primarily affects throwing athletes.
17. **B.** Baseball players are the most susceptible to olecranon stress fracture.
18. **C.** For baseball players, in particular, olecranon stress fracture (OSF) has been attributed to rapid and repetitive valgus extension.
19. **D.** Common risk factors seen in adolescent patients with OSF include an average of 12 years of onset, playing a pitcher or catcher role in a throwing sport, playing more than 100 games a year, or throwing a breaking ball (a type of pitch that increases rotational and angular forces on the elbow), which has been recommended not be thrown before the age of 14 to 16 years, and increased velocity.
20. **C.** There are two focused examination maneuvers that often reproducibly elicit pain in patients with an olecranon stress fracture, i.e., the snapping extension test and the arm bar test.

Chapter 13: Stress Fracture 291

21. **D.** Femoral neck (tension side), patella (tension side), anterior tibial cortex, medial malleolus, talar neck, dorsal tarsal navicular cortex, fifth metatarsal proximal metaphysis, sesamoids of the great toe are the anatomic sites for high-risk stress fractures.
22. **A.** Stress fracture represents a fatigue failure of the bone, occurring with a spectrum of severity of structural injury with healing potential varying by location.
23. **C.** Femoral stress fractures are generally seen in athletes and military recruits who engage in repetitive impact loading of the lower extremity. Long-distance runners, jumpers, dancers, female athletes, and older athletes appear to be at higher risk for developing femoral stress fractures.
24. **D.** Athletes in cross country, track, and field, recreational and competitive running, triathlon, soccer, basketball, and dance are at risk for tibial stress fractures.
25. **C.** Fifth metatarsal fractures are common midfoot injuries among the athletic population, including elite-level athletes. Stress fractures of the fifth metatarsal usually occur in competitive athletes who participate in running or jumping sports.
26. **D.** The management of stress fracture includes non-loading activities that maintain fitness and use as many large muscle groups as possible without overloading the bone. The most common methods of maintaining fitness are cycling, swimming, water running, rowing, and stairmaster. These work-outs should as much as possible mimic the athlete's normal training program in both duration and intensity.
27. **D.** Management of a femoral stress fracture includes educating athletes and coaches, rest and activity modification, and correction of training errors.
28. **D.** Runners who change terrain or run hilly landscapes are more likely to incur stress fractures. Thus, limiting hills and multiple terrains during recovery for future training in individuals susceptible to stress fractures is pertinent. The use of orthotics may be effective for some athletes in reducing lower extremity stressors by increasing shock absorption. Also, decreased shoe shock absorption can be avoided by

changing shoes every six months or 300-500 miles to limit overuse injuries.

29. **D.** Stress fracture prevention focuses on modifying extrinsic risk factors. All athletes should be counseled on an appropriate diet, training regimen, proper technique, conditioning ramp-up, and equipment updates, such as appropriate orthotics.

30. **D.** In managing stress, fracture of foot and ankle among athletes, commonly used modalities include orthotics, bone stimulators, pulsed ultrasound, and extracorporeal shock wave therapy (ESWT).

31. **A.** A bone scan is a diagnostic test that utilizes radioactive isotopes to identify areas of bone that are hypervascular or have an increased rate of bone mineral turnover. Bone scans can demonstrate bone disease or stress fractures with as little as 4-7% bone loss.

32. **A.** Bright: It is a type of crystalline fracture and is associated with low-energy brittle fracture.

33. **C.** Fracture toughness is measured by strain energy release rate and stress concentration factor.

34. **D.** (crack length)$^{-1/2}$: The critical crack length is a term used to describe the defects in materials. It is the length of the crack that grows after the fracture occurs rapidly at the same stress.

35. **A.** Decrease by a factor of $\sqrt{2}$

Basics of Imaging in Sport Injuries for Physical Therapist

CHAPTER 14

1. A 25-year-old male athlete has an injury in the knee due to forceful strain in the patellar tendon. Which one of the following conditions shows changes in the knee joint lateral radiograph?

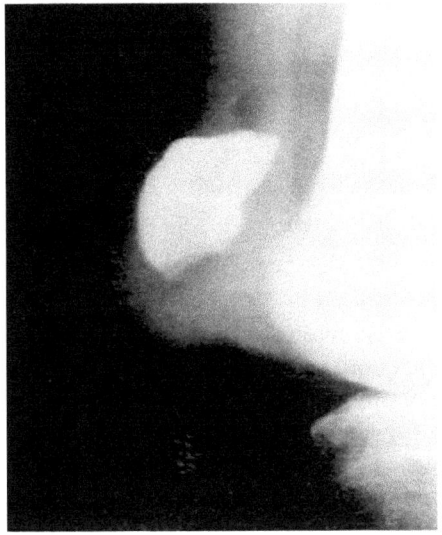

   A. Patella alta
   B. Patellar tilt
   C. Patella baja
   D. Patella fracture

2. A 30-year-old male football player complained of pain and swelling on the left ankle and foot after the injury. Which one of the following conditions confirms the diagnosis in the following MRI (white arrowheads)?

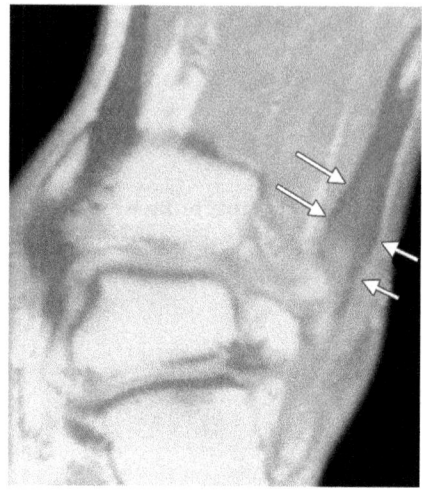

A. Lateral malleolus fracture
B. Ankle dislocation
C. Talar tilt
D. Rupture of the peroneal tendon

3. A 26-year-old male is referred to physical therapy after being diagnosed and treated medically with shoulder dislocation. Which of the following dislocation would be the most typical during the shoulder examination based on the radiological imaging?

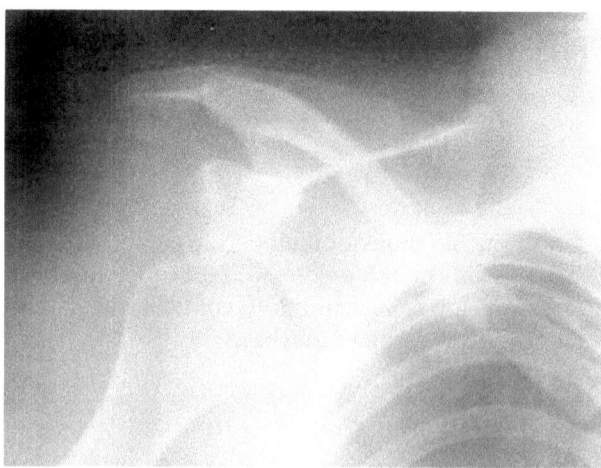

A. Posterior dislocation
B. Subglenoid anterior dislocation
C. Subglenoid inferior dislocation
D. Central dislocation

4. A 60-year-old female with known osteoporosis, and ankle pain after increasing exercise fitness program. Which one of the following diagnosis would be the most typical during the examination of the ankle (white arrow marking) based on the MR imaging?

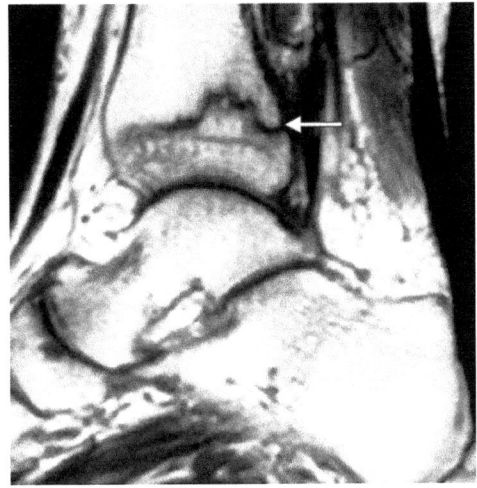

A. High ankle sprain
B. Ankle mortise dislocation
C. Stress fracture in the lower end of the tibia
D. Tibiofibular ligament injury

5. A 35-year-old squash player had an injury in the shoulder joint during the tournament. Examination reveals tenderness on the anterior joint line, limited range of motion, and reduced physical activity. What would be the most appropriate diagnosis you conclude from the following MR image?

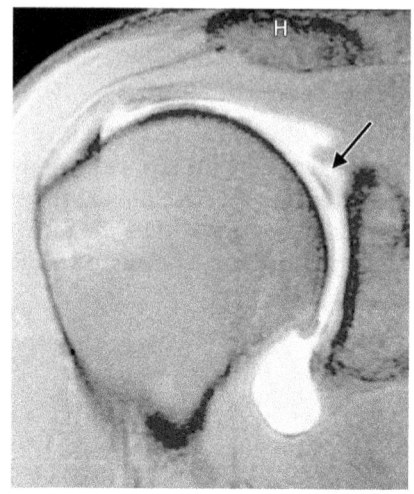

A. SLAP II lesion
B. Subdeltoid bursitis
C. Impingement syndrome
D. Supraspinatus tendinitis

6. A physical therapist discusses the plan of care for a 61-year-old male diagnosed with spinal stenosis with the referring physician. During the discussion the physician shows the therapist a picture of the patient's spine obtained through computed tomography. What color would vertebrae appear when using this imaging technique?

A. Black
B. Light gray
C. Dark gray
D. White

7. A physical therapist obtains an X-ray of a 19-year-old female recently referred to physical therapy following activity. The patient previously participated in competitive gymnastics, further, she states that her back was unable to tolerate the intensity of training. Based on the presented X-ray (Scottie dog decapitated) the therapist would expect the patient's medical diagnosis to be:

Chapter 14: Basics of Imaging in Sport Injuries for Physical Therapist

A. Spondylitis
B. Spondylolysis
C. Spondylolisthesis
D. Spondylectomies

8. A physician completes a physical examination on an 18-year-old male who injured his knee while playing in a soccer contest 2 days ago. The physician's preliminary diagnosis is a grade II anterior cruciate ligament injury with probable meniscal involvement. Which of the following diagnostic tools would be the most appropriate in immediate medical management?
    A. Arthrogram
    B. Computerized tomography
    C. Magnetic resonance imaging
    D. X-rays

9. A physician suspects a stress fracture in a 15-year-old distance runner after completing a physical examination. Assuming the physician's preliminary diagnosis is correct, which of the following diagnostic tests would be the most appropriate to identify the stress fracture?
    A. Bone scan
    B. Magnetic resonance imaging
    C. Telethermograph
    D. Ultrasound scan

10. A physician utilizes diagnostic imaging to show motion in a joint through X-ray. This type of imaging is best termed as:
    A. Computed tomography
    B. Fluoroscopy
    C. Discography
    D. Radionuclide scanning

11. A 25-year-old athlete had a fracture in the right shoulder while falling on the outstretched hand during sprinting. Which of the following structure get affected in the X-ray?

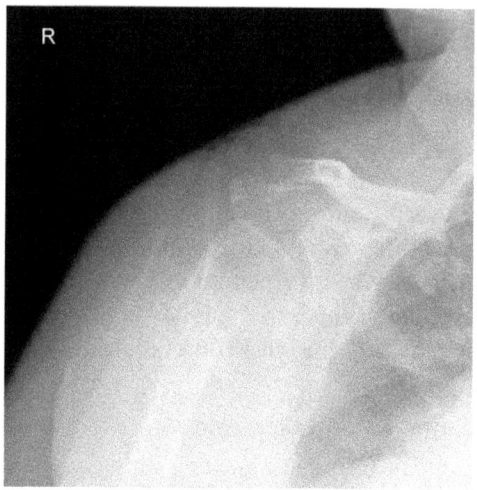

A. Fracture clavicle
B. Fracture acromion
C. Fracture neck of the humerus
D. Shoulder dislocation

12. Which structure can also be assessed with MR imaging in patients who develop flexion contractures of the elbow as a complication of posterior dislocation injury?

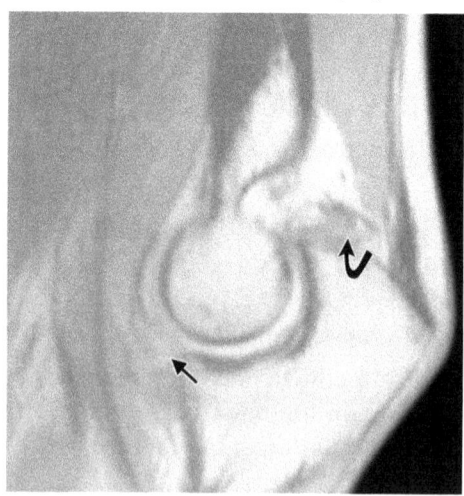

A. Ligaments
B. Bursa
C. Synovial membrane
D. Joint capsule

13. What is the most common complication that can be seen in the rotatory subluxation of the scaphoid in the following radiological findings?

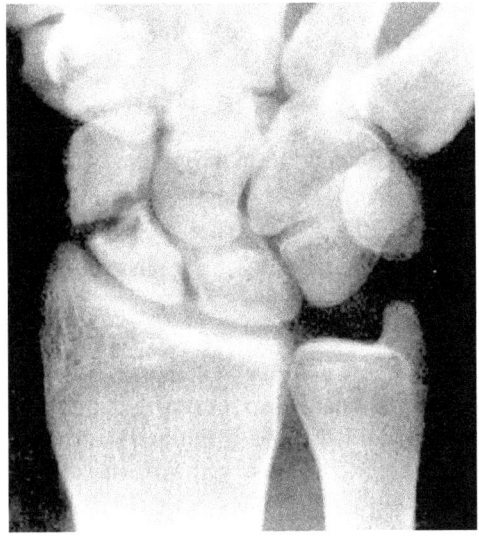

A. Malunion
B. Non-union
C. Avascular necrosis
D. Neuritis

14. A 35-year-old man had a twisting injury on the knee while playing football. On examination, the knee was swollen and an anterior instability was evident during movement. What are the most appropriate features seen in the following X-ray and MR imaging?

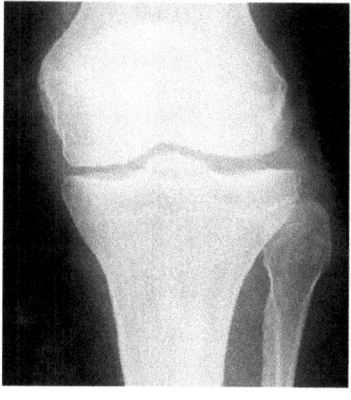
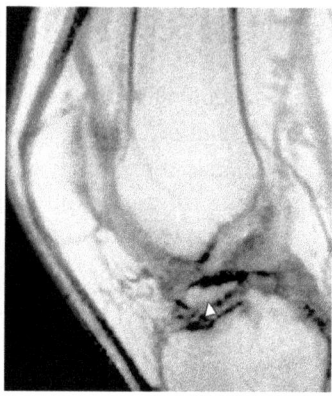

A. Fracture medial tibial condyle and PCL injury
B. Avulsion of the intercondylar eminence and avulsion fracture of the PCL insertion
C. Avulsion of the intercondylar eminence and avulsion fracture of the ACL insertion
D. Fracture neck of fibula and prepatellar bursitis

15. A 25-year-old rugby player had a direct blow injury on his left knee. Physical examination revealed swelling, redness, instability, and limited functional activity. Which one of the following is the most appropriate diagnosis confirmed through MR imaging?

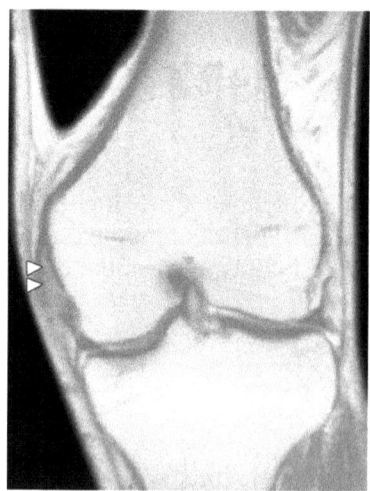

A. Grade II/III MCL tear
B. Grade II/III LCL tear
C. Medial condyle fracture
D. Lateral condyle fracture

16. A 40-year-old tennis player had an injury in the right shoulder. On examination, he finds it difficult to lift the arm overhead and inability to bend the elbow. What would be the most appropriate diagnosis through the radiological examination (black arrowhead)?

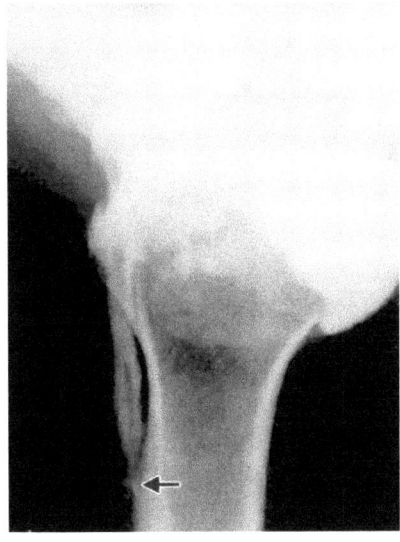

A. Partial tear in the supraspinatus tendon
B. Partial tear in the long head of biceps brachii tendon
C. Supraspinatus tendinitis
D. Fracture neck of the humerus

17. A 23-year-old male had an injury in the elbow while playing squash. The arm is forced into the valgus at the elbow, high compression and shear stresses are created between the radial head and the capitulum. What type of lesion can be identified in the below radiological findings?

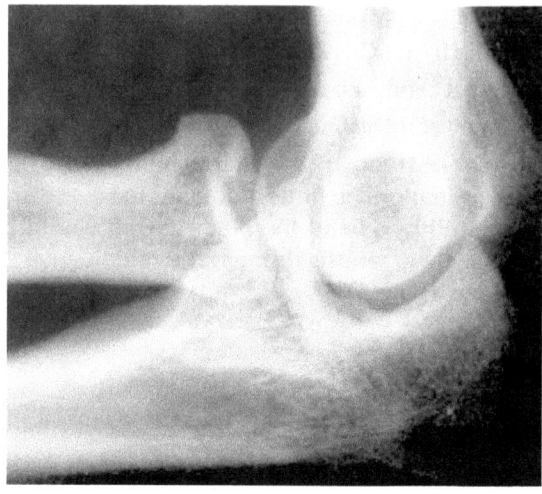

A. Elbow dislocation
B. Avulsion fracture in the capitulum
C. Radial head fracture
D. Radial head dislocation

18. A male adolescent gymnast who fell from the gymnastic apparatus. PA radiograph shows a transverse fracture of the distal ulnar shaft and one more finding in the radius. What are the most appropriate findings seen in the radiological image?

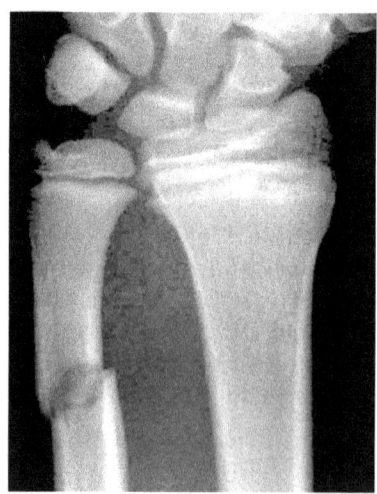

Chapter 14: Basics of Imaging in Sport Injuries for Physical Therapist

A. Stress changes of the digital radius
B. Radiocarpal dislocation
C. Radial styloid process fracture
D. Distal radioulnar joint dislocation

19. A 30-year-old male complaining of knee pain at the medial joint line during running for several weeks. What would be the most appropriate diagnosis concluded through the following sagittal MR image?

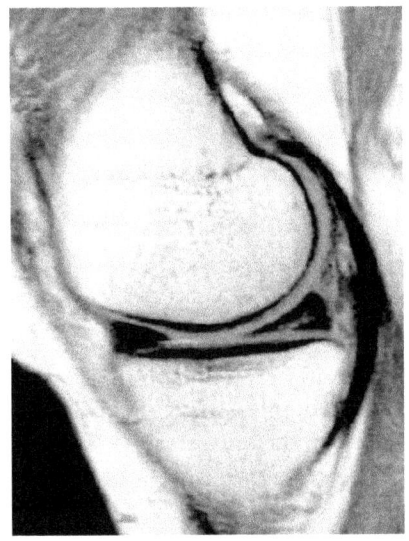

A. Anterior horn of the medial meniscus
B. Posterior horn of the medial meniscus
C. Anterior horn of the lateral meniscus
D. Posterior horn of the medial meniscus

20. A 33-year-old male football player had a twisting injury in the knee. Physical examination shows knee instability and swelling on the joint. What would be the most appropriate diagnosis in the sagittal fat suppressed proton density MR image?

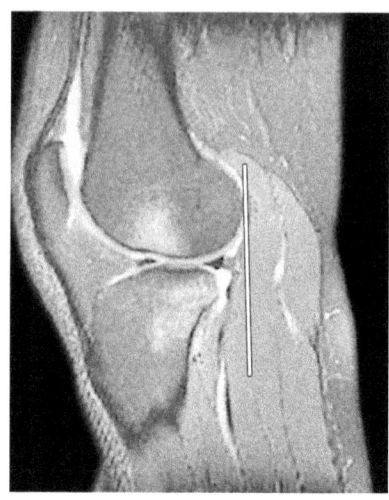

A. Medial collateral ligament tear
B. Lateral collateral ligament tear
C. ACL rupture
D. PCL rupture

21. What is the most common condition seen in runners and is due to impingement of the band against the lateral aspect of the lateral femoral condyle?

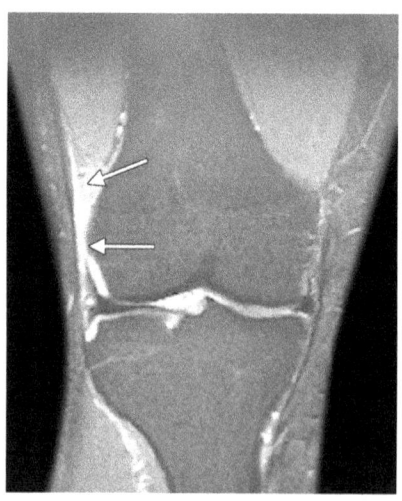

A. Lateral collateral ligament tear
B. Lateral femoral condyle fracture
C. Tensor fascia lata friction
D. Iliotibial band syndrome

22. A 30-year-old athlete had an injury in the posterior aspect of the ankle. On examination, tenderness in the calcaneus, ambulate with limp, unable to run and climbing stairs. What is the most appropriate diagnosis identified in the below MR image?

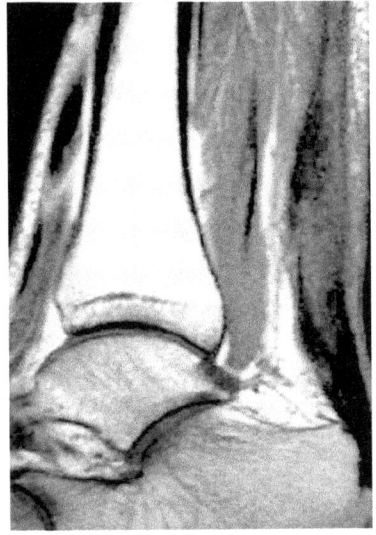

A. Talar tilt
B. Achilles' tendinosis
C. Calcaneal spur
D. Calcaneal fracture

23. A professional footballer sustained an acute left leg injury during a tackle. AP radiograph shows an oblique fracture through the distal diaphysis of the tibia and fibula. From the following radiograph, identify the type of surgery done on the fracture site?

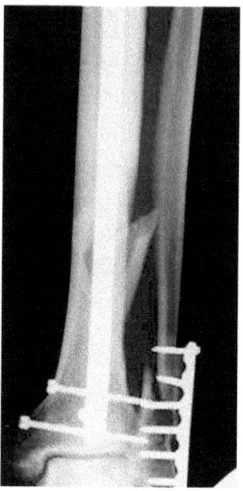

A. Internal and external fixation
B. Plates and cortical screws
C. Intramedullary nail and plate
D. Pins and needles

24. Female marathon runner presenting at major games with continuous anterior tibial pain. A lateral radiograph of the tibia shows anterior cortical thickening and multiple stress fractures. What would be your suggestion to the player as a physical therapist?

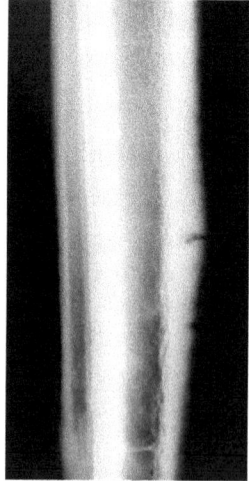

Chapter 14: Basics of Imaging in Sport Injuries for Physical Therapist

A. The athlete had to withdraw from competition
B. The athlete had to continue marathon
C. Advised to go for surgery
D. Exercising before marathon

25. **Distracted hyperflexion injury in a young gymnast shows an abnormality in the plain radiographs of the cervical spine in lateral view. What is the most appropriate diagnosis at C6 and C7 levels?**

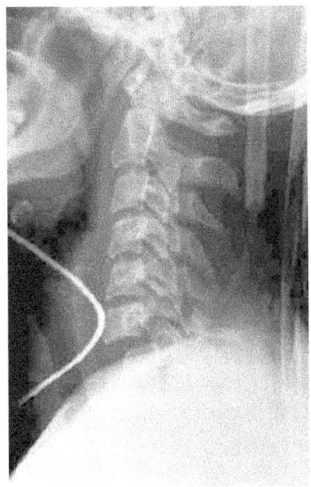

A. Posterior subluxation at C6-C7
B. Anterior subluxation at C6–C7
C. Fracture C6
D. Fracture C7

26. **A 47-year-old recreational squash player, who complained of neck pain and paraesthesia's in both arms after a collision with another player. What would be the most appropriate diagnosis in the MR image?**

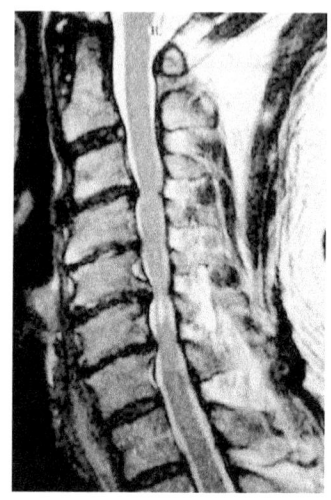

A. Cervical spondylosis
B. Cervical spondylolisthesis
C. Cord contusion secondary to spinal stenosis
D. Bilateral intrafacetal dislocation

27. A 17-year-old dancer is presenting the signs of lumbar disc protrusion. On examination, pain and numbness present on both lower limbs, and the patient has difficulty walking. Which of the following diagnosis appropriate for this patient?

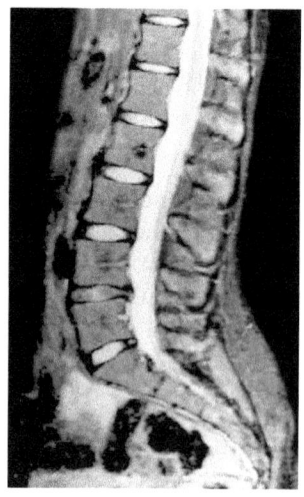

A. L2/L3
B. L3/L4
C. L4/L5
D. L5/S1

28. When an abnormality is typically observed in athletic adolescents during flexion, the anterior part of the disc is pressed under the superior nonfused endplate. What is the most appropriate diagnosis revealed in the radiographic findings?

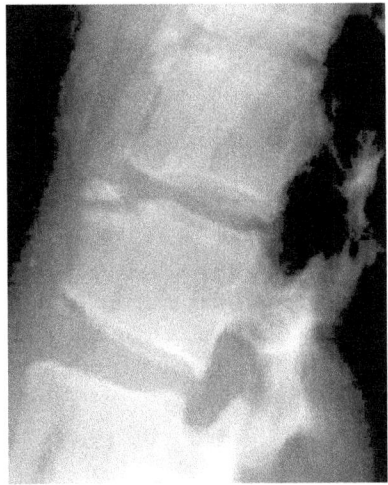

A. Separation of the rim apophyses at multiple levels
B. Vertebral body fractures
C. Spondylolisthesis
D. Limbus vertebra

29. A 45-year-old sprinter had a fall injury in the right pelvic bone. On examination, difficulty in sitting on the chair and ground with marked swelling on the buttock region. What is the appropriate diagnosis from the radiological findings?

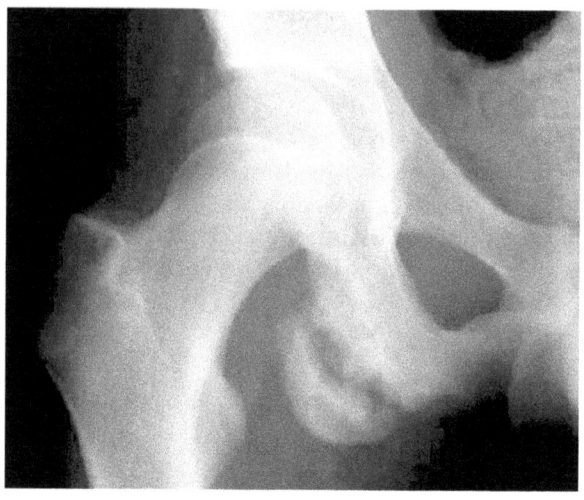

A. Fracture in the ilium
B. Chronic ischial avulsion
C. Fracture femoral neck
D. Hip dislocation

30. A 50-year-old soccer player having pain in the knee for the past 3 months. Physical examination shows crepitus on movement, difficulty in knee bending, and unable to sit on the ground. Which of the following conditions suits the following radiological findings?

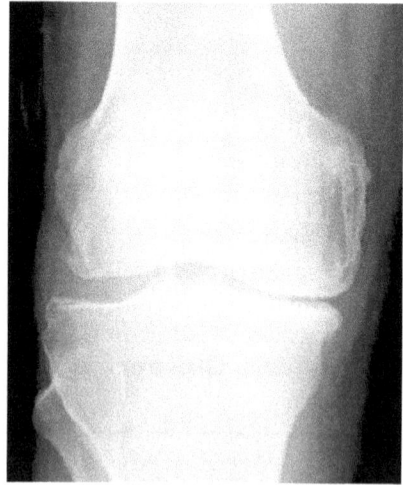

A. Ligament injury
   B. Intercondylar eminence fracture
   C. Knee osteoarthritis
   D. Osteochondritis dissecans
31. A physical therapist reviews a physician's note on an 18-year-old male athlete diagnosed with impingement syndrome. The note indicates standard radiographs were utilized as a part of the examination. Which finding would not be identified using a standard radiograph?
   A. Chronic calcific tendonitis
   B. Acromioclavicular arthritis
   C. Partial thickness tear of the rotator cuff
   D. Unfused acromial apophysis
32. A sports physician examines a 20-year-old male throw-ball player with shoulder pain. As part of the examination the physician orders X-rays. Which medical condition could be confirmed using this type of diagnostic imaging?
   A. Bicipital tendonitis
   B. Calcific tendonitis
   C. Supraspinatus impingement
   D. Subacromial bursitis
33. A physician provides an overview of diagnostic imaging techniques commonly used in clinical practice to a group of physical therapist students. Which imaging technique would not be considered invasive?
   A. Arthrography
   B. Myelography
   C. Discography
   D. Computerized tomography
34. A physician utilizes diagnostic imaging to show motion in a joint through X-ray. This type of imaging is best termed as:
   A. Computed tomography
   B. Fluoroscopy
   C. Discography
   D. Radionuclide scanning
35. A soccer player was diagnosed with an anterior cruciate ligament injury is examined in a physical therapy department. During the examination, the patient asks the physical therapist why the physician would order X-rays after already diagnosing the ligament injury. The primary purpose for ordering the radiographs would be to:

A. Confirm the physician's diagnosis
B. Check for possible meniscal involvement
C. Examine the patient's skeletal maturity
D. Rule out the possibility of a fracture

36. A long-distance runner is presenting with pain in his left foot which occurs gradually. The pain is located towards the middle and front of the foot, and it is made worse by weight-bearing activities, such as walking and running. What do you infer from the following X-ray correlating with those symptoms exhibited by the runner?

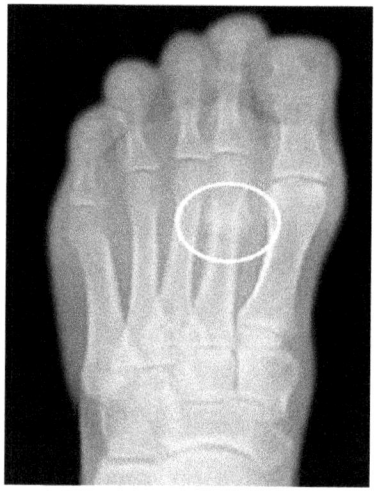

A. Turf toe
B. Second metatarsal stress fracture
C. Inflammation of soft tissue around second metatarsal bone
D. Incomplete fracture of second metatarsal bone

37. Which one of the following modalities are the most sensitive ones to detect stress fractures?
A. X-ray
B. MRI
C. CT scan
D. Bone scintigraphy

38. Following statements are true concerning Kager fat pad, *except*:

A. Fat at within the Kager triangle, which normally appears lucent (fat density) on radiographs.
B. It has relatively well-defined margins.
C. It is also known as the precalcaneal fat pad or preachilles fat pad.
D. The appearance of Kager fat pad is not affected by not affected by thickened tendons and inflammation.

39. A 28-year-old female complains of pain and a pop at the posterior left ankle while doing vertical jumps three weeks ago. She has weak plantar flexion and is unable to stand on her toes with the left foot. Sagittal fat-suppressed T2-weighted MRI images of the ankle is given below. What do you infer from this MRI?

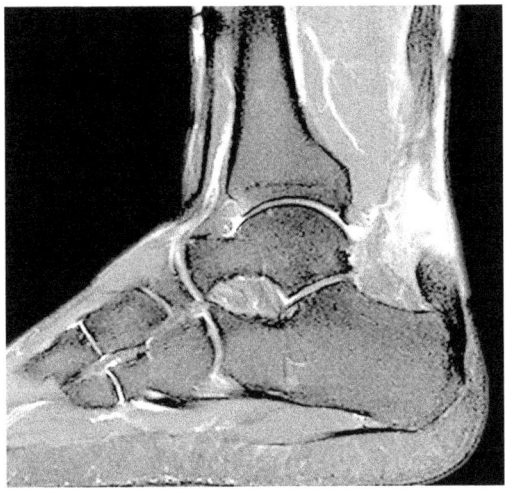

A. Achilles' tendon rupture
B. Ankle joint effusion
C. Retrocalcaneal Bursitis
D. None of the above

40. A 33-year-old recreational swimmer presented with pain in his right shoulder and no history of direct injury. X-ray was taken and it is given below. What's your inference from the X-ray?

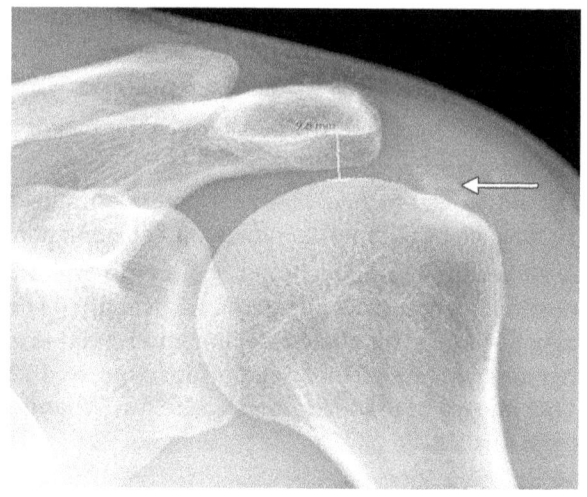

A. Calcific supraspinatus tendinitis
B. Calcific tendonitis of the rotator cuff
C. Glenohumeral joint instability
D. Rupture of acromioclavicular ligament (ACL)

Chapter 14: Basics of Imaging in Sport Injuries for Physical Therapist

ANSWERS

1. **A.** Lateral radiograph of the knee joint showing marked soft tissue swelling and patella alta following rupture of the patella tendon. Rupture of the patellar tendon produces a deficit in active knee extension and usually affects young athletes. Swelling around the patella tendon with obliteration of its normally sharp adjacent fat lines and an abnormally high patella position are characteristic radiographic features.
2. **D.** Rupture of the peroneal tendons with fluid in the "empty" tendon sheath and thickened proximal stump in the coronal Tl W -5E image.
3. **B.** Anteroposterior (AP) radiograph showing a subglenoid anterior dislocation.
4. **C.** Sagittal T1-weighted MR image with tibial stress fracture evident.
5. **A.** SLAP type II lesion: Oblique coronal fat suppressed T1-weighted direct MR arthrogram demonstrates a fragment of the superior labarum separated and inferiorly displaced (arrow).
6. **D.** White: Computed tomography produces cross-sectional images based on X-ray attenuation. Since vertebrae are made of bone and are extremely dense, they appear to be white. Soft tissue structures appear in various shades of gray while cerebrospinal fluid is black.
7. **C.** Spondylolisthesis refers to the forward displacement of one vertebra over another. The X-ray involves spondylolisthesis at the L5-S1 level. Individuals involved in physical activities, such as weightlifting, gymnastics or football are particularly susceptible to this condition. The severity of the spondylolisthesis is classified on a scale of 1–5 based on how much a given vertebral body has slipped forward over the vertebral body beneath it.
8. **D.** X-rays: Immediate medical management should focus on identifying potential complications, such as a fracture. X-rays are a cost-effective diagnostic tool commonly utilized with orthopedic injuries.
9. **A.** A bone scan is a diagnostic test that utilizes radioactive isotopes to identify areas of bone that are hypervascular or have an increased rate of bone mineral turnover. Bone

scans can demonstrate bone disease or stress fractures with as little as 4–7% bone loss.

10. **B.** Fluoroscopy refers to examination by means of a fluoroscope. A fluoroscope allows an examiner to observe the action of joints, organs, or entire systems of the body. The instrument requires a specific body segment to be placed between a fluorescent screen and an X-ray tube. X-rays from the tube pass through the body and project images on the screen.
11. **C.** In this AP radiograph, a fracture of the neck of the humerus is evident. Note the malalignment of the fracture fragments. Also observe the fracture line is less defined, suggesting some early healing.
12. **D.** Flexion contracture 6 months after a posterior subluxation injury of the elbow. A proton density sagittal image in a flexed elbow reveals thickening of the anterior (straight arrow) and posterior (curved arrow) joint capsule compatible with fibrosis that limits full extension of the elbow.
13. **B.** Rotatory subluxation of the scaphoid can be secondary to scaphoid non-union and other causes, i.e., Kienbock's disease.
14. **C.** Chronic avulsion rupture of the ACL. The conventional radiographs in anteroposterior view demonstrate an avulsion of the intercondylar eminence. The sagittal T1-w SE image demonstrates the avulsion fracture of the insertion of the ACL. The displaced intercondylar eminence presents a normal bone marrow signal (arrow head).
15. **A.** MCL tear grade II/III: Coronal T2-w TSE image (TR 3500/TE 99) shows displacement of the proximal MCL from the femur. The proximal MCL is thickened and shows a diffuse signal increase representing torn ligamentous fibers and acute hemorrhage (arrow heads).
16. **B.** Partial tear in the tendon of the long head of the biceps brachii muscle (black arrow).
17. **C.** Radial head fracture better seen on the oblique cranial (25°) profile view. During the acceleration phase, the medial aspect of the elbow is placed under tension and the lateral side is subjected to high compression forces.

18. A. Stress changes of the distal radius and, to a lesser extent, of the distal ulna, adjacent to the growth plates.
19. B. Sagittal PD-WI shows equivocal grade 3 signal in the posterior horn of the medial meniscus.
20. C. Anterior tibial translation as secondary sign of ACL rupture. A line drawn tangential to the lateral femoral condyle passes more than 5 mm from the posterior tibial margin.
21. D. Iliotibial band syndrome: Coronal proton density fat suppressed MRI showing high signal deep to the iliotibial band (arrows).
22. B. Achilles' tendinosis is seen as a heterogeneous signal area of irregular thickening on MRI.
23. C. Intramedullary nail and plate: Professional footballer with acute left leg injury during tackle. AP radiograph shows an oblique fracture through the distal diaphysis of the tibia with external rotation of the distal fragment. The patient underwent intramedullary nailing.
24. A. The athlete had to withdraw from competition.
25. B. The marked anterior displacement of C6 indicates disruption of all ligamentous structures and interfacetal dislocation. This finding is only visible on the lateral view. The cervicothoracic prevertebral soft tissue shadow is widened, indicating the presence of a hematoma secondary to the injury.
26. C. MRI examination with sagittal images show severe narrowing of the spinal canal due to chronic disc herniations and posterior osteophytes. There is a focal intramedullary area of increased signal intensity indicating cord contusion.
27. C. L4/5 disc protrusion on a sagittal TSE T2-weighted MR image
28. A. Conventional radiograph showing typically occurs during the second decade of life after the rim apophysis has formed (7-9 years) and before its fusion with the vertebral body.
29. B. Chronic ischial avulsion in an adolescent male athlete. AP radiograph showing irregularity of the ischial cortex with overgrowth of the avulsed apophysis in the adjacent soft tissues.
30. C. Knee osteoarthritis: AP standard radiograph shows joint space narrowing especially at the medial femorotibial and

patellofemoral compartments, subchondral sclerosis and osteophyte formation.

31. C. Soft tissue structures, such as muscles and tendons do not possess the density necessary to be seen on X-ray.

32. B. Calcific tendonitis is often visible on X-ray due to the relative density of calcium. The greater the density of the tissue, the more visible it will appear on X-ray. The supraspinatus and infraspinatus tendons are common sites for calcific tendonitis at the shoulder.

33. D. Computerized tomography is an imaging technique that uses cross-sectional images based on X-ray attenuation. Computer enhancement allows the imaging to have significantly better contrast resolution when compared to conventional X-rays.

34. B. Fluoroscopy refers to examination by means of a fluoroscope. A fluoroscope allows an examiner to observe the action of joints, organs, or entire systems of the body. The instrument requires a specific body segment to be placed between a fluorescent screen and an X-ray tube. X-rays from the tube pass through the body and project images on the screen.

35. D. Although X-rays can be used to assess skeletal maturity, the primary purpose would be to rule out a fracture.

36. B. A metatarsal stress fracture is a fine fracture in one of the long metatarsal bones in the foot and it can occur through overuse or poor foot biomechanics. In the forefoot, they are most commonly seen within the mid-diaphysis of the second and third metatarsal bones. Stress injuries are classified into fatigue and insufficiency fractures. Fatigue fractures are stress fracture that result from presence of repetitive abnormal stress to a normal bone and commonly seen in athletes and military recruits. Insufficiency fractures are however related to normal stress on abnormal non-tumoral bone commonly seen in osteoporotic patients.

37. B. MRI is a very sensitive modality in detecting abnormalities related to osseous stress response with a spectrum of findings seen. This usually begins with an osseous stress reaction as bone marrow edema on the fluid-sensitive sequences within the medullary cavity without visualization of a hypointense fracture line. As the stresses continue, an irregularly hypointense line abutting the cortex, usually perpendicular to the metatarsal shaft representing the fracture line, is seen. MRI is preferred over bone scintigraphy for the diagnosis of stress fractures because of greater specificity.

38. **D.** Kager fat pad (also known as the precalcaneal fat pad or preAchilles fat pad) refers to the fat within the Kager triangle, which normally appears lucent (fat density) on radiographs and has relatively well-defined margins. Pathologies such as inflammation (e.g., retrocalcaneal bursitis, peritendinitis) and thickened tendons (xanthomatosis, rheumatoid arthritis, gout, ankylosing spondylitis, reactive arthritis) result in loss of the normal margins and increased density in the triangle.

39. **A.** The sagittal image MRI demonstrates a rupture of the Achilles tendon 3.5 cm proximal to the calcaneal attachment with a 2-cm fluid-filled gap (arrow) between the torn ends. The proximal and distal segments of the Achilles tendon are prominently thickened (arrowheads) suggesting underlying Achilles' tendinosis. Edema is demonstrated within the adjacent subcutaneous and pre-Achilles fat.

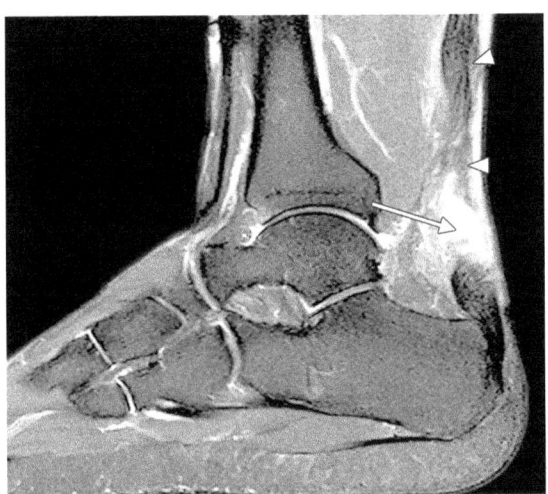

40. **A.** There is calcific deposit in the supraspinatus, close to its humeral insertion and it is typical presentation of calcifying supraspinatus tendinitis due to chronic strain. Further, the acromiohumeral interval was within normal limits (9–10 mm).

Postsurgical Physiotherapy for Sports Injuries

CHAPTER 15

1. Which of the following symptoms cause reflex inhibition of muscle activity that leads to postoperative muscle atrophy after anterior cruciate ligament (ACL) reconstruction of the knee?
   A. Pain and swelling
   B. Muscle laxity
   C. Fever and chills
   D. Depression

2. _____ is commonly used to reduce pain, inflammation, and effusion after ACL reconstruction.
   A. Cryotherapy
   B. Plyometrics
   C. Shortwave diathermy
   D. Progressive resisted exercises

3. Cryotherapy application in ACL reconstruction patients acts through local effects that include:
   A. Reduce fluid extravasation by vasoconstriction
   B. Inhibit afferent nerve conduction that decreases pain and muscle spasm
   C. Prevent cell death by limiting the chemical mediator's release
   D. All of the above

4. Loss of extension is more common after ACL reconstruction and it can result from:
   A. Arthrofibrosis
   B. Inappropriate ACL graft placement or tensioning
   C. Prolonged immobilization
   D. All of the above

5. How does the physiotherapist prevent the motion loss (knee extension) following ACL reconstruction?
   A. Early passive and active range of motion and continuous passive motion (CPM) machine
   B. Early reactivation of the quadriceps by controlling pain and swelling

Chapter 15: Postsurgical Physiotherapy for Sports Injuries

    C. Patellar mobilization techniques to prevent patella tendon shortening or retinacular musculature

    D. All of the above

6. How long is the knee immobilized in a brace locked in full extension during ambulation after ACL reconstruction?
    A. First 6-8 weeks
    B. First 4-6 weeks
    C. First 1-2 weeks
    D. First 6-12 weeks

7. Following ACL reconstruction, the early initiation of muscle training is vital to prevent muscle atrophy and weakness. It can be done through:
    A. Electrical muscle stimulation
    B. Biofeedback [vastus medialis oblique (VMO) biofeedback]
    C. Weight-bearing
    D. All of the above

8. Rehabilitation after ACL reconstruction is focused on the athlete to maintain:
    A. Cardiovascular conditioning
    B. Proprioception
    C. Muscular coordination with appropriate exercise
    D. All of the above

9. What are the aids that used in the functional training of an athlete?
    A. Balance boards
    B. Mini-tramps
    C. Balls
    D. All of the above

10. Criteria for return to sports after ACL reconstruction are:
    A. Full range of motion
    B. Quadriceps strength 85% or more of the contralateral side
    C. No pain and effusion
    D. All of the above

11. Identify the most common complications that occur after ACL reconstruction surgery?
    A. Loss of motion or arthrofibrosis
    B. Patella infera or infrapatellar contracture syndrome
    C. Anterior knee pain
    D. All of the above

12. Name the exercise administered during the immediate postoperative phase (day 1 to 7) according to Wilk accelerated rehabilitation protocol after ACL reconstruction with the central-third patellar tendon?
    A. Leg press
    B. Straight leg raises (four planes)
    C. 30 degrees mini-squats
    D. Lateral step-ups
13. Which of the following exercises are considered to be sport-specific exercises for an athlete who underwent ACL reconstruction?
    A. Wall squats
    B. Cone drills and cariocas
    C. Straight leg raises with brace locked in extension
    D. Isometric quadriceps
14. Mention the exercise advised during the advanced activity phase (weeks 4–7) according to Wilk rehabilitation protocol after arthroscopic partial medial or lateral meniscectomy?
    A. Plyometrics
    B. Running program
    C. Agility drills
    D. All of the above
15. Which of the following conditions are considered paramount in rehabilitation after PCL reconstruction to avoid residual laxity?
    A. Prevention of posterior sag
    B. Anterior knee pain
    C. Hamstring activity
    D. A and C
16. According to the Wilk rehabilitation protocol, what are the criteria for returning to sports after PCL reconstruction with a two-tunnel graft technique?
    A. Full painless ROM
    B. Satisfactory isokinetic test (85% or better)
    C. Functional hop test 85% of the contralateral leg
    D. All of the above
17. The key factors determining the progression of rehabilitation after meniscal repair include:

A. The anatomic site of the tear
   B. Suture fixation
   C. Location of tear
   D. All of the above
18. When does the athlete return to sports if peroneal strength is normal following modified Brostrom ankle ligament reconstruction (Modified Hamilton protocol)?
   A. 4 weeks
   B. 6 weeks
   C. 8-12 weeks
   D. 14-16 weeks
19. What are the criteria for an athlete to return to sports after ankle ligament reconstruction?
   A. Normal peroneal strength
   B. Able to do multiple single-leg hops on the injured side without pain
   C. A and B
   D. None of the above
20. Sensorimotor exercises for an athlete following ACL reconstruction include:
   A. Balance training on a tilt board
   B. Balance training with medicine ball throws
   C. Perturbation training
   D. All of the above
21. What are the exercises focusing on speed, agility, and quickness for return to skiing after ACL reconstruction?
   A. Agility ladder drills
   B. Dot drills and cone drills
   C. Speed circuits
   D. All of the above
22. Criteria for return to sport for an athlete following meniscal repair include:
   A. Less than or equal to 10% deficit quadriceps and hamstring strength isokinetic testing
   B. Less than or equal to 15% deficit lower limb symmetry single-leg hop testing
   C. Full range of knee motion
   D. All of the above
23. Which of the following meniscal repairs needs the maximum degree of protection in the postoperative recovery phase?

A. Radial repair B. Complex repair
C. Incomplete repair D. Central repair

24. Which of the following is not considered to be an early postoperative complication of meniscal repair?
    A. Decrease in knee motion B. Delayed return to running
    C. Quadriceps inhibition D. Hypersensitivity

25. Immediately following PCL reconstruction (i.e., postoperatively), the active contraction of the hamstrings must be evaded to avoid _____ translation of the tibia on the femur, which may cause extreme tensioning of the graft.
    A. Posterior B. Anterior
    C. Lateral D. None of the above

26. Sensorimotor exercises prescribed for an athlete during the final phase of postoperative rehabilitation after ankle LCL repair/reconstruction are:
    A. Standing biomechanical ankle platform system (BAPS) exercise
    B. Single-leg standing balance on a foam mat with perturbation
    C. Single-leg standing balance on wobble board or disc
    D. All of the above

27. In cases of inhibition, neuromuscular electrical stimulation (NMES) was used to facilitate the activation of muscle _____ during the postoperative rehabilitation after Ankle LCL repair/reconstruction.
    A. Peroneus longus B. Peroneus brevis
    C. Tibialis anterior D. All of the above

28. "Shrug sign" following rotator cuff repair in overhead athletes indicates:
    A. Superior displacement of the humerus and compensatory scapular muscle activity
    B. Inferior displacement of the humerus and compensatory elbow muscle activity
    C. Inferior displacement of the humerus and compensatory scapular muscle activity
    D. Superior displacement of the humerus and compensatory elbow muscle activity

Chapter 15: Postsurgical Physiotherapy for Sports Injuries

29. Name the exercise used to restore the dynamic stabilization of the glenohumeral joint and prevent the shrug sign after rotator cuff repair in overhead athletes:
    A. Isometric exercises
    B. Rhythmic stabilization exercises
    C. Progressive resisted exercises
    D. Relaxation exercises

30. Which of the following condition will lead to the superior migration of the humeral head (shrug sign) following rotator cuff repair?
    A. Strong rotator cuff overpowering the weak deltoid
    B. Strong pectoralis overpowering the weak deltoid
    C. Strong deltoid overpowering the weak rotator cuff
    D. None of the above

31. Which of the following motions are prohibited for at least 6 to 8 weeks following rotator cuff repair?
    A. Excessive shoulder extension
    B. Excessive adduction behind the back
    C. Excessive horizontal adduction
    D. All of the above

32. Which of the following muscle's strength is emphasized for re-establishing functional use of the arm following rotator cuff repair?
    A. Shoulder external rotators
    B. Shoulder internal rotators
    C. Shoulder adductors
    D. Shoulder extensors

33. The knee proprioception and kinesthesia are disrupted due to the damage to mechanoreceptors within the collateral ligaments after medial collateral ligament (MCL) injury, which will slow the person's response to perturbations. In such a case, name the exercise that should be started shortly following the patient begins full weight-bearing after MCL repair or reconstruction?
    A. Free exercises
    B. Proprioception exercises
    C. Balance exercises
    D. B and C

34. Which of the following things need to be avoided to prevent stress on the repair/graft after MCL repair or reconstruction?
   A. Resisted hip adduction exercises and external rotation of the tibia
   B. Resisted hip abduction exercises and external rotation of the tibia
   C. Resisted hip adduction exercises and internal rotation of the tibia
   D. Resisted hip extension exercises and internal rotation of the tibia
35. Which of the following criteria is considered as return to sports after subacromial decompression for rotator cuff injuries among athletes?
   A. Partial active range of motion
   B. Altered glenohumeral mechanics
   C. Normal scapulothoracic and glenohumeral mechanics
   D. All of the above
36. During 8–12 weeks after subacromial decompression for rotator cuff injuries, the following movement loss needs to be avoided to prevent the glenohumeral internal rotation deficit and subsequent subacromial impingement among athletes:
   A. Loss of flexion
   B. Loss of internal rotation
   C. Loss of external rotation
   D. Loss of circumduction
37. Following a full-thickness rotator cuff tear, which of the following movement is resisted cautiously if the supraspinatus was surgically repaired:
   A. Internal rotation
   B. Extension
   C. Circumduction
   D. External rotation
38. Following the repair of complete lateral ligament tear at ankle joint, which of the following order of the progression of balance activities should be followed?
   A. Activities first on a balance board, followingly on a soft surface, firm surface, and lastly on a level surface
   B. Activities first on a level surface, followingly on a firm surface, soft surface, and lastly on a balance board
   C. Activities first on a balance board, followingly on a firm surface, level surface, and lastly on a soft surface

D. Activities first on a soft surface, followingly on a level surface, firm surface, and lastly on a balance board

39. What are the means focused in patient education to limit the risk of rerupture of the repaired Achilles tendon?
    A. Warming up before strenuous activity
    B. Daily stretching
    C. A and B
    D. Immobilization

40. Following the lateral ligament repair, which of the following muscle need to be strengthened particularly for the dynamic stability of the ankle?
    A. Evertors
    B. Invertors
    C. Plantar flexors
    D. Adductors

41. A 23-year-old male diagnosed with a medial meniscus injury of his right knee is referred to physical therapy following arthroscopic surgery. During the examination, the physical therapist identifies a decreased range of motion in the involved knee. This objective finding is best termed as:
    A. Pathology
    B. Impairment
    C. Functional limitation
    D. Disability

42. A physical therapist treats a snow skier who injured his thumb approximately three weeks ago while skiing and underwent surgical repair of the ulnar collateral ligament of the thumb. Which of the following would be the most realistic postoperative time frame for the patient to resume unrestricted activity?
    A. 6 weeks
    B. 12 weeks
    C. 18 weeks
    D. 24 weeks

43. A 29-year-old male is forced to contemplate knee surgery after spraining the anterior cruciate ligament while playing soccer. Which situation would provide the most direct support for an anterior cruciate ligament reconstruction?
    A. Grade III ACL and grade I PCL injury
    B. Grade III ACL sprain with a lateral meniscus tear
    C. Grade II ACL sprain with a medial meniscus tear
    D. Functional instability

44. An examination of a soccer player's four-week status post-arthroscopic medial meniscectomy reveals a limitation in the knee flexion range of motion. Which mobilization technique would be the most beneficial to increase knee flexion?
   A. Anterior glide of the tibia
   B. Superior glide of the patella
   C. Posterior glide of the tibia
   D. Anterior glide of the fibula head
45. A physical therapist conducts a preoperative training session for a middle-aged recreational tennis player for surgery to repair a large rotator cuff tear. During the preoperative training session, the patient inquiries about the amount of time before he can return to recreational activities, such as tennis and golf. The most appropriate time frame is:
   A. 6-8 weeks   B. 12-14 weeks
   C. 24-28 weeks   D. 36-40 weeks
46. A 32-year-old ice hockey player rehabilitating from knee surgery exhibits significant weakness in the involved extremity. During the most recent therapy session, the patient was able to complete an independent straight leg raise. What muscle is emphasized in the exercise?
   A. Vastus medialis
   B. Rectus femoris
   C. Vastus lateralis
   D. Sartorius
47. A physical therapist develops a plan of care for a collegiate sports person who underwent knee surgery. As part of a postoperative care plan, the therapist elects to utilize a continuous passive motion machine. Which treatment objective would not be addressed using this intervention?
   A. Increase vascular dynamics
   B. Prevent muscle atrophy
   C. Prevent contractures
   D. Decrease pain
48. A recreational football player scheduled for posterior cruciate ligament reconstruction in two weeks is examined in the physical therapy department. The patient has diminished

quadriceps strength and walks with a noticeable limp. The involved knee has mild edema and 15-degree flexion contracture. The most appropriate treatment priority is:

A. Improve quadriceps strength
B. Improve the fluidity of gait
C. Reduce edema
D. Improve range of motion

49. A patient who underwent an anterior cruciate ligament reconstruction using a patellar tendon autograft is examined on the eighth postoperative day in the physical therapy department. Which of the following exercises would be the most appropriate based on the patient's postoperative status?

A. Limited range isokinetics at 30° per second
B. Unilateral leg press
C. Mini-squats in standing
D. Active knee extension in a short sitting

50. A physical therapist designs an exercise program consisting of closed-chain activities for a jockey player rehabilitating from a medial meniscus repair. An appropriate closed-chain exercise to include in the rehabilitation program is:

A. Submaximal velocity spectrum isokinetic exercise
B. Bilateral mini-squats in standing
C. Short-arc terminal knee extension
D. Prone leg curls with a two-pound cuff weight

ANSWERS

1. **A.** Pain and swelling are common after any surgical procedure. Because they cause reflex inhibition of muscle activity and thus postoperative muscle atrophy, it is essential to control these problems quickly to facilitate an early range of motion and strengthening activities.
2. **A.** Cryotherapy is commonly used to reduce pain, inflammation, and effusion after ACL reconstruction.
3. **D.** Cryotherapy acts through local effects, causing vasoconstriction, which reduces fluid extravasation; inhibiting afferent nerve conduction, decreasing pain and muscle spasm; and preventing cell death, limiting the release of chemical mediators of pain, inflammation, and edema.
4. **D.** Loss of motion is perhaps the most common complication after ACL reconstruction. Loss of extension is more common than loss of flexion and is poorly tolerated. Loss of extension can result in arthrofibrosis, infrapatellar contracture syndrome, inappropriate ACL graft placement or tensioning, acute surgery on a swollen inflamed knee, prolonged immobilization, and a poorly supervised or poorly designed rehabilitation program.
5. **D.** Physiotherapists can do the following things to prevent motion loss after ACL reconstruction. Those are an early passive and active range of motion and continuous passive motion (CPM) machine, early reactivation of the quadriceps by controlling pain and swelling, and patellar mobilization techniques to prevent patella tendon shortening or retinacular musculature.
6. **B.** It is recommended to maintain the knee in a brace locked in full extension during ambulation for the first 4 to 6 weeks after surgery to limit the forces transmitted through the extensor mechanism and to protect the extensor mechanism if the patient slips or falls.
7. **D.** The early initiation of muscle training is crucial to prevent muscle atrophy and weakness. Electrical muscle stimulation may be helpful to initiate muscle activation in patients who are unable to overcome reflex inhibition voluntarily. Biofeedback (such as VMO biofeedback) can be used to

Chapter 15: Postsurgical Physiotherapy for Sports Injuries

enhance the force of muscular contraction. Weight-bearing has also been shown to be beneficial in promoting muscle reactivation.

8. **D.** Rehabilitation after ACL reconstruction is focused on the whole athlete to maintain cardiovascular conditioning, proprioception, and muscular coordination with appropriate exercises and activities that are gradually phased into the rehabilitation program.

9. **D.** In functional training, the use of aids includes balance boards, mini-tramps, steps, balls, and the pool adds variety, breaks up the "routine" of therapy, and maintains patient motivation.

10. **D.** Criteria for return to sports after ACL reconstruction are Full ROM, KT-l000 side-to-side difference <3 mm, quadriceps strength 85% or more of contralateral side, hamstring strength 100% of contralateral side, hamstring-to-quadriceps strength ratio 70% or greater, functional testing battery 85% or greater compared with the contralateral side, no effusion, and no pain or other symptoms.

11. **D.** Complications after ACL reconstruction include loss of motion or arthrofibrosis, patella infera or infrapatellar contracture syndrome, and anterior knee pain.

12. **C.** Exercises administered during the immediate postoperative phase (Day 1 to 7) according to Wilk accelerated rehabilitation protocol after ACL reconstruction with central-third patellar tendon are ankle pumps, Overpressure into full passive knee extension, active and passive knee flexion (90° by day 5), SLR (flexion, abduction, adduction), Quadriceps isometric setting, hamstring stretches, closed-kinetic chain exercises, 30° mini-squats, weight shifts.

13. **B.** Sport-specific exercises for an athlete following ACL reconstruction include cone drills, side shuffles, grapevine drills, cariocas, sudden start/stops, 45° cutting maneuvers, 90° cutting maneuvers, and combinations of agility drills.

14. **D.** According to the Wilk accelerated rehabilitation protocol after arthroscopic partial medial or lateral meniscectomy, exercises advised during the advanced activity phase (weeks 4-7) include plyometrics, running program, agility drills.

15. D. In rehabilitation after PCL reconstruction, prevention of posterior sag and hamstring activity are considered paramount to avoid residual laxity.

16. D. Criteria for return to sports after PCL reconstruction with a two-tunnel graft technique according to the Wilk rehabilitation protocol include full, nonpainful ROM, satisfactory isokinetic test (85% or better), satisfactory KT 2,000 test, functional hop test 85% of the contralateral leg, satisfactory clinical examination by the physician.

17. D. Key factors in determining progression of rehabilitation after the meniscal repair include the anatomic site of the tear, suture fixation (too vigorous rehabilitation can lead to failure), location of tear (anterior or posterior), and other pathology (PCL, MCL, or ACL injury).

18. C. Following modified Brostrom ankle ligament reconstruction (modified Hamilton protocol), the patient can return to dancing or sport if peroneal strength is normal by 8–12 weeks.

19. C. After ankle ligament reconstruction, the return to sports or dancing is allowed when peroneal strength is normal, and the patient can perform multiple single-leg hops on the injured side without pain.

20. D. Sensorimotor exercises for an athlete following ACL reconstruction include: balance training on a tilt board, balance training with medicine ball throws, and perturbation training.

21. D. Training for speed, agility, and quickness include, agility ladder drills, dot drills, cone drills, speed circuits during return to skiing after ACL reconstruction.

22. D. Criteria for return to sport for an athlete following meniscus repair include no knee joint pain or swelling, full range of knee motion, less than or equal to 10% deficit quadriceps and hamstrings strength isokinetic testing, less than or equal to 15% deficit lower limb symmetry single-leg hop testing, successful completion running and functional training, complete trial of function by returning to the sport, monitor for overuse symptoms, and patient education for re-evaluation if any future knee problems occur.

23. **A.** Radial meniscal repair needs the maximum degree of protection in the postoperative recovery phase.
24. **B.** During the immediate postoperative period, the therapist should monitor for posteromedial or infrapatellar burning, posteromedial tenderness along the distal pes anserine tendons, tenderness of Hunter's canal along the medial thigh, hypersensitivity to light pressure or temperature change, abnormal pain response, quadriceps shutdown, and inability to achieve knee motion goals. Hence, delayed return to running is not considered to be an early postoperative complication of meniscal repair.
25. **A.** Immediately following PCL reconstruction (i.e., postoperatively), the hamstrings' active contraction must be evaded to avoid posterior translation of the tibia on the femur, which may cause extreme tensioning of the graft.
26. **D.** Sensorimotor exercises prescribed for an athlete during the final phase of postoperative rehabilitation after ankle LCL repair/reconstruction are standing biomechanical ankle platform system (BAPS) exercise, single-leg standing balance on a foam mat with perturbation, and single-leg standing balance on wobble board or disc.
27. **D.** In case of inhibition, neuromuscular electrical stimulation (NMES) was used to facilitate the activation of muscles, such as peroneus longus, peroneus brevis, and tibialis anterior during the postoperative rehabilitation after Ankle LCL repair/reconstruction.
28. **A.** Rhythmic stabilization exercises (in the supine position) are begun at 10-14 days postoperative (type 2 protocol) to restore the dynamic stabilization of the GH joint through cocontraction of the surrounding musculature. These exercises are designed to prevent and treat the "shrug" sign (superior displacement of the humerus and compensatory scapular muscle activity).
29. **B.** Rhythmic stabilization exercises (in the supine position) are begun at 10-14 days postoperative (type 2 protocol) to restore the dynamic stabilization of the GH joint through cocontraction of the surrounding musculature. These exercises are designed to prevent and treat the "shrug" sign.

Negative ulnar variance means, the ulna is, on average 9 mm shorter than the radius.

30. C. The shrug sign occurs with a strong deltoid muscle overpowering the weakened rotator cuff, causing the humeral head to migrate superiorly.

31. D. In rehabilitation after rotator cuff repair, motions, such as excessive shoulder extension, adduction behind the back, and horizontal adduction are prohibited for at least 6 to 8 weeks.

32. A. Following rotator cuff repair, emphasis is on external rotation strength because this strength is critical in re-establishing functional use of the arm.

33. D. The knee proprioception and kinesthesia are disrupted due to the damage to mechanoreceptors within the collateral ligaments after medial collateral ligament (MCL) injury. It will slow the person's response to perturbations. In such case, balance and proprioception exercises should be started shortly following the patient begins full weight-bearing after MCL repair or reconstruction (Phase II weeks 2-4 postoperatively).

34. A. During Phase III (weeks 4-8 postoperatively) of postoperative rehabilitation after MCL repair or reconstruction, the patient should continue to avoid resisted hip adduction exercises and external rotation of the tibia to avoid stress on the repair/graft.

35. C. General criteria for returning to sports after subacromial decompression for rotator cuff injuries among athletes include: normal scapulothoracic and glenohumeral mechanics, full active range of motion, and normal strength to manual muscle testing.

36. B. Athletes who maintain proper scapulothoracic mechanics have significantly less injury. Avoiding loss of motion, particularly internal rotation, can prevent the occurrence of glenohumeral internal rotation deficit (GIRD) and subsequent impingement.

37. D. If the supraspinatus was repaired following the full-thickness rotator cuff tear, proceed cautiously when resisting external rotation.

38. **B.** Initiate proprioceptive/balance training at about 6 weeks postoperatively or when the patient is able to bear full weight on the operated lower extremity without ankle pain. Emphasize a progression of bilateral to unilateral balance activities first on a level, firm surface, then on a soft surface, such as dense foam, and then on a balance board.
39. **C.** Following the repair of the acute Achilles tendon, patient education focuses on ways to reduce the risk of rerupture of the repaired tendon, such as warming up before strenuous activity and daily stretching.
40. **A.** After surgical repair of the lateral ligaments, improving the strength of the evertors is particularly important for the dynamic stability of the ankle.
41. **B.** An impairment is defined as a loss or abnormality of physiological, psychological or anatomic structure or function.
42. **B.** Surgical repair of the ulnar collateral ligament of the thumb requires a pin to be inserted into the metacarpophalangeal joint of the thumb. The pin may remain in place for 3-6 weeks followed by the application of a wrist and thumb splint. Progressive strengthening typically commences at eight weeks and a return to unrestricted activity may occur at approximately 12 weeks.
43. **D.** Many individuals are able to continue to function at high levels despite a variety of ligamentous and meniscal injuries, therefore functional instability provides the most direct support for an anterior cruciate ligament reconstruction.
44. **C.** The tibiofemoral articulation consists of a concave tibial plateau articulating with the convex femoral condyles. A posterior glide of the tibia on the femur is indicated to increase knee flexion.
45. **C.** The majority of rotator cuff tears occur in individuals greater than 40 years of age with a history of recurrent shoulder symptoms. A large tear is typically considered between 3-5 cm in diameter and most often requires 24-28 weeks of rehabilitation before a patient is allowed to return to full activity without restrictions.
46. **B.** Performing a straight leg raise requires dynamic hip flexion and an isometric contraction of the quadriceps. The rectus

femoris is the prime mover during the straight leg raise exercise. The muscle is a component of the quadriceps femoris muscle group and is innervated by the femoral nerve.

47. **B.** Muscle atrophy would not be prevented using a continuous passive motion machine since the device incorporates only a passive range of motion and does not require any form of muscle contraction.

48. **D.** A physical therapist should work with the patient to restore normal range of motion in the involved knee prior to surgery. By improving range of motion, the patient will likely be able to improve the fluidity of gait and diminish abnormal loading of the patellofemoral joint.

49. **C.** A mini-squat is a closed chain exercise typically performed in standing that enables the patient to vary the force through the involved extremity by simply shifting their weight. This exercise significantly limits the amount of knee flexion and as a result does not place a great deal of stress through the reconstructed knee.

50. **B.** Closed-chain activities require the distal segment to be in contact with the ground or some other surface.

Robotics in Sports Rehabilitation

CHAPTER 16

1. The first robotic device designed specifically for rehabilitation was launched in which year?
   A. 1990
   B. 1992
   C. 1994
   D. 1996
2. Which one of the following statements are true concerning the term 'Robotics'?
   A. The application of electronic, computerized control systems to mechanical devices designed to perform human functions.
   B. A mechanical device that is capable of performing a variety of complex human tasks on command or through programming in advance.
   C. A rehabilitation devise that aimed at facilitating the recovery of impaired sensory, motor, and cognitive skills.
   D. All of the above
3. Robots are commonly used in sports to fulfill the following goals, *expect*:
   A. Helping in providing sport training
   B. Substituting humans during training
   C. Participating in competition against human
   D. Replacing a player in the real sport event
4. The key focus of the rehabilitation robotics aimed at facilitating the recovery of impaired:
   A. Sensory skills
   B. Motor skills
   C. Cognitive skills
   D. All of the above
5. Most robotic devices used in clinical settings are active or interactive, and they may also act passively. Considering the interface of the device with the user and its structure, identify the most appropriate robotic devices used for upper limb rehabilitation:

A. End-effector devices B. Exoskeletal devices
C. Both options A and B D. None of the above

6. According to their treatment approaches, rehabilitation robotics are classified into two types. Identify the most accurate option from the following:
   A. Continuous passive movement (CPM) approach
   B. Active-assisted movement approach
   C. Both A and C
   D. Exoskeleton robotic approach

7. Rehabilitation robots are designed based on the active-assisted movement approach and found to be superior than robots designed to work on the basis of continuous passive movement (CPM) approach. Choose the most accurate reason from the following options:
   A. Require voluntary effort from the patient and provide significant motor improvement
   B. Requires no volunteer effort from the patient where the limb is moved by the robots
   C. Reduces muscle tone, which eventually improves the mobility of muscles, joints and tendons
   D. All of the above

8. Which one of the following statements are true concerning exoskeleton robots?
   A. Unable calculate the required torque for each joint and control the limb movements
   B. Require a larger working environment
   C. Not feasible for bilateral rehabilitation
   D. All of the above

9. Which of the following types of robots primarily employs bilateral therapy where the impaired limb copies the movement of the functional limb, which gives the user full control of the affected limb?
   A. The Gait-Trainer GT 1
   B. Mirror image movement enabler (MIME)
   C. MIT-MANUS
   D. None of the above

10. To build robots for application within the sport, the sports biomechanist needs data on mechanical sports performance, especially to investigate the movement of sportspersons and sports equipment. Which one of the following parameters should be taken into account for implementing the mechanisms of robots in sports?
    A. Kinematic data on displacement, velocity and acceleration
    B. Dynamic data on force, moments of force and force impulses
    C. Both A and B
    D. None of the above
11. A type of robot that can help a player by acting as a trainer and practice partner from a beginner's level through intermediate to an advanced player is:
    A. BumperNets Robo-pong
    B. The Jada badminton robot
    C. MIT-MANUS
    D. Mirror image movement enabler (MIME)
12. Humanoid robots are also called as:
    A. Anthropomorphic robots
    B. Partly anthropomorphic robots
    C. Nonanthropomorphic robots
    D. All of the above
13. Communication between humans and robots are accomplished through which one of the following ways:
    A. Gesture and face mimicry
    B. Auditory cues
    C. Chemical cues
    D. All of the above
14. The clinical gold standard for the assessment of musculoskeletal performance is:
    A. Manual muscle testing
    B. Isokinetic dynamometers
    C. Functional muscle testing
    D. Isometric dynamometry
15. An end effector robotic device used for shoulder and elbow neurorehabilitation is:

A. The Mirror Image Movement Enabler (MIME)
B. SUEFUL-7 exoskeleton
C. Assisted Rehabilitation and Measurement (ARM) guide
D. NEUROExos

16. Identify the most appropriate physical activity of machines that can participate in a sport like competition to win:
    A. Robo-sport
    B. Sport play machine
    C. Simulation of motion
    D. Mobile machines

17. Which one of the following fields can offer many interesting devices to sportspeople to enhance sports performance?
    A. Medical
    B. Engineering
    C. Sciences
    D. Mathematics

18. Which one of the following tools is used by biomechanists to measure the loads and movements of competitors during the training sessions?
    A. Balance board
    B. Wobble board
    C. Cameras and sensors attached to sport equipment
    D. Biomarkers

19. What is the robot version of the World Cup (football/soccer) and the (self-proclaimed) most important robot contest in the world?
    A. Humanoid Cup
    B. Honda's ASIMO Cup
    C. Robonaut Cup
    D. RoboCup

20. Which of the rehabilitation robotics provides the patient with the minimal robotic assistance to move their weakened limbs along desired patterns, in a similar manner to "active-assisted" exercises performed by physical therapists?
    A. Challenge-based control
    B. Haptic stimulation
    C. Assistive control
    D. Contact coaching

21. What refers to controllers that provide resistance to the participant's limb movements during exercise, requiring specific patterns of force generation or increasing the size of movement errors?
    A. Challenge-based control
    B. Active-assisted control
    C. Assistive control
    D. Noncontact coaching

22. Which one of the following methods is specifically used to practice ADL movements in a virtual environment since it offers flexibility, convenience, and safety compared to performing actions in a physical environment?
    A. Assistive control
    B. Haptic simulation
    C. Impedance based
    D. Counter-balance based
23. Which type of robotics is a relatively new subdiscipline of health care and clinical science that bridges established features of robot-assisted rehabilitation?
    A. Telehealth care
    B. Telemedicine
    C. Clinical trial
    D. Telerehabilitation robotics
24. The robot that repeats the same motions according to recorded information is called as:
    A. Fixed sequence robot
    B. Variable sequence robot
    C. Playback robot
    D. Numerical control robot
25. Which of the following is not a functionality of robotics?
    A. Re-programmability
    B. Multifunctionality
    C. Efficient performance
    D. Responsibility
26. Which of the following terms refers to the use of compressed gasses to drive (power) the robot device?
    A. Pneumatic
    B. Hydraulic
    C. Piezoelectric
    D. Photosensitive
27. The basic components of robot are:
    A. The mechanical linkage
    B. Sensors and controllers
    C. User interface and power conversion unit
    D. All of the above
28. Which of the following IS NOT one of the advantages associated with a robotics implementation program?
    A. Low costs for hardware and software
    B. Robots work continuously around the clock
    C. Quality of manufactured goods can be improved
    D. Reduced company cost for worker fringe benefits

29. Which of the robotic tools is used in rehabilitation settings to lengthen muscles through repeated precise and direct pressure to the soft tissue?
   A. Therbo robotic arm
   B. Continuous passive motion arm
   C. Machine arm
   D. Active assisted movement arm
30. Which one of the systems having mutual adaptation is a key mechanism to be considered in the control of rehabilitation mechatronic systems?
   A. Mechanical equipment
   B. Human-robot
   C. Dynamics
   D. Biomechatronic

ANSWERS

1. **C.** The first robot, MIT-MANUS was designed at the Burke Rehabilitation Hospital, White Plains, NY in the year 1994 for managing stroke patients.
2. **D.**
3. **D.**
4. **D.** Rehabilitation robotics specifically focuses on systems—devices, exercise scenarios, and control strategies—aimed at facilitating the recovery of impaired sensory, motor, and cognitive skills.
5. **C.** Based on the interface of the robotic device with the user, it may be classified as end-effector devices or exoskeletal devices and are used for upper limb rehabilitation.
6. **C.** Rehabilitation robots can be classified into two types, according to their treatment approaches. The first approach is continuous passive movement (CPM), and it requires no volunteer effort performed by the patient where the limb is controlled and moved by the robots. The second approach is active-assisted movement, where the robot needs a signal from the patient to perform the movement. This signal could be an electromyogram (EMG) and follows the patient's intention to move the limb.
7. **A.** Rehabilitation robots with active-assisted movement require voluntary effort from the patient and, consequently, provide significant motor improvement compared to CPM rehabilitation. Therefore, most of the current researchers focus on active-assisted rehabilitation using robots.
8. **C.** Exoskeleton robots are characterized by encapsulating the limb with a splint or bionic structure. Exoskeleton robots calculate the required torque for each joint and control the limb movements. Compared with end-effector robots, exoskeletons require a smaller working environment and comprise the limb joint axes as they provide a precise movement. Further, exoskeleton robots are not feasible for bilateral rehabilitation, as the right limb exoskeleton cannot be used for the left limb, and eventually, it is expensive to design right and left exoskeleton robots to perform bilateral rehabilitation training.

9. **B.** Mirror image movement enabler (MIME) and a few other exoskeletons employ bilateral therapy, refers to the mirroring principle in performing rehabilitation.
10. **C.**
11. **A.** BumperNets Robo-pong is a robot that can help a player as a trainer and practice partner from a beginner's level through intermediate to an advanced player. There is an option of ball recycling, where the robot reuses the balls, it receives from the player. The head of the robot, which serves balls, can move left and right to get balls from different sides of the table.
12. **A.** Humanoid robots, also called anthropomorphic robots are of great concern among scientists and engineers. They are essential components in supporting society, and they play a role in personal use. They would coexist with humans and provide support, such as assistance for housework and care of the aged and the physically disabled.
13. **D.**
14. **B.** Isokinetic dynamometers (IDs) are devices that measure joint moment while maintaining a constant joint velocity or rather a constant angular velocity of the machine's lever against which muscle action occurs. The ID movements are two-dimensional and rotational around a joint. The way for creating a moment may be hydraulic, frictional, or electro-magnetic, and the angle moment curves between these systems may differ considerably.
15. **A.** The Mirror Image Movement Enabler (MIME) is a 6 degrees of freedom (DOF) end effector robotic device for shoulder and elbow neurorehabilitation. It is equipped with a 6-axis force sensor that allows for unilateral and bilateral training.
16. **A.** Robo-Sport for its excellent user interface, ease of programming, and quick play.
17. **B.** Within sport engineering there are products devoted to: (a) the body, (b) movable products, (c) immovable products, and (d) information technology.
18. **C.** The great advantage of sports biomechanics is the possibility of measuring the loads and movements of competitors, not only during training sessions but especially during competitions. Biomechanists using different cameras and

Chapter 16: Robotics in Sports Rehabilitation

sensors attached to sports equipment and sometimes to a sportsperson's body can monitor sports performance in a real competition.
19. D. RoboCup has several different classifications for robots, which include small-sized, middle-sized, four-legged robots and humanoids.
20. A. Assistive control rehabilitation robotics provides such control that allows promoting user's active involvement.
21. A. Challenge-base control is so-called "error-amplification" strategies.
22. B. Haptic simulation has great potential to improve medical training. A haptic device is a mechanical input/output device that enables users to interact with virtual environments by adding the sense of touch, enhancing the learning quality.
23. D. Telerehabilitation robotics: It is the delivery of rehabilitation services over telecommunication networks and the internet. Tele healthcare to provide efficacious services at a distance using information and communication technologies.
24. C. Playback robot: A robot that repeats the same sequence of motions in all its operations, and is first instructed by an operator who puts it through this sequence.
25. D. Responsibility: Essentially robots carry out three functions—sense, think and act.
26. A. Pneumatic robots are different from robots with hydraulic systems or electric motors. They receive locomotion from compressed air rather than from electrical-mechanical energy or hydraulic fluid, valves, and circuits. Controls are the amount of air being supplied to the robot or the air-powered tool.
27. D. All of the above
28. A. Low costs for hardware and software
29. A. Therbo robotic arm has been purported to improve range of motion, muscle endurance, muscle flexibility, and circulation.
30. B. Robots have to synchronously adapt to the intended motion of the user, who in turn should be allowed to exploit robotic physical support with an active participation and a training activity for the improvement of the residual motor functions.

CHAPTER 17

Sports Nutrition

1. Which of the following proteins has an amino acid profile more similar to the body's needs?
   A. Egg
   B. Wheat
   C. Rice
   D. Soy

2. Following are the essential amino acids which are obtained through dietary substance, *except*:
   A. Lysine
   B. Tryptophan
   C. Leucine
   D. Glycine

3. Which of the following best explains the requirements for increased protein intake by athletes?
   A. Decreased protein oxidation during aerobic exercise
   B. Increased need for tissue repair
   C. Restriction of calorie to lose weight
   D. The quality of protein consumed

4. Which of the following food substances is having the highest glycemic index?
   A. Apple juice
   B. Carrots
   C. Grape fruit juice
   D. Orange

5. Which of the following has the greatest influence on an athlete's dietary carbohydrate requirements?
   A. Resting blood sugar levels
   B. Current average daily fat intake
   C. Duration and frequency of exercise
   D. Body size and body fat percentage

6. The type of cholesterol which is increased by exercise and weight loss that protect against heart disease is known as:
   A. High-density lipoprotein
   B. Low-density lipoprotein
   C. Both A and B
   D. None of the above

7. Which of the following best describes dietary fat consumption?
   A. It should never be higher than 40% of total calories.
   B. Its restriction can be harmful to health and performance.
   C. It is not an essential nutrient.
   D. It should be less than 15% of total calories for healthy subjects.
8. Which of the following may indicate a need for an athlete to supplement his or her diet with vitamins?
   A. No dairy product consumption
   B. No green leafy vegetable consumption
   C. Frequent fast-food intake
   D. Chronically insufficient caloric intake
9. While monitoring hydration status of an athlete, each pound of weight lost during practice is equal to how much of fluid loss:
   A. 0.50 L
   B. 0.75 L
   C. 1.0 L
   D. 1.5 L
10. What is the ideal time recommended for an athlete who often participates in contact sports and high risk of injury to take precompetition meal?
    A. 12 hours before competition
    B. 30 minutes before competition
    C. 3-4 hours prior to the event
    D. Immediately before the event
11. Which of the following is true regarding dietary supplements?
    A. Their safety is guaranteed.
    B. They must be approved by government agencies prior to being sold.
    C. They must be effective to be sold.
    D. They may not be advertised as food replacements.
12. All of the following describe caffeine's role in improving athlete performance, *except*:
    A. Delayed fatigue
    B. Glycogen sparing
    C. Increased alertness
    D. Decreased urine production

13. Greater than normal intake of vitamin D results in:
    A. Improved aerobic performance
    B. Weight gain
    C. Excessive calcium deposition
    D. Increased 1RM strength
14. Which of the following substances has been shown by multiple research studies to improve performance?
    A. Androstenedione
    B. Creatine
    C. L-carnitine
    D. Chromium
15. Which of the following is the best reason for endurance athlete to avoid erythropoietin use?
    A. The athlete's hematocrit may decrease.
    B. It may cause the heart to fail.
    C. Resistance to infectious disease may be impaired.
    D. It may reduce the ability of blood to carry oxygen.
16. A 75 kg male wrestler with 10% body fat wishes to achieve an optimum of 5% body fat. How many kilograms that the wrestler has to lose to achieve 5% of body fat?
    A. 3.50 kg   B. 4 kg
    C. 3.75 kg   D. 4.25 kg
17. The purpose or aim of providing carbohydrate loading diet to an athlete is:
    A. To decrease the muscle glycogen level of exercising muscle
    B. To increase the muscle glycogen level of exercising muscle
    C. To supply energy for shorter period of time
    D. To allow the athlete to participate more intensely
18. How many vital nutrients exist in the foods and beverages required for growth, repairing tissues, regulating the body processes and preventing infections?
    A. Four   B. Five
    C. Six   D. Seven
19. The high energy that is released as a result of breaking down of absorbed nutrients during the metabolic pathways for the formation of energy within the cells is:

A. Adenosine tetraphosphate
B. Adenosine triphosphate
C. Phosphate triadenosine
D. None of the above

20. **How the dietary reference intakes are expressed?**
    A. Recommended Dietetic Allocation (RDAs)
    B. Recommendation for Dietary Allowances (RDAs)
    C. Recommended Daily Allowances (RDAs)
    D. Recommended Dietary Allowances (RDAs)

21. **Why should an athlete interpret the ingredients of food in the food labels on the food packages?**
    A. Enables to ensure the quality of nutrition and to avoid food additives which is allergic/intolerant
    B. Enables to understand the fiber content when instructed to increase fiber intake
    C. Enables to ensure that the athletes opt for low calorie, and healthy food
    D. All of the above

22. **Whether it is possible to generalize the dietary plan of sports personals, i.e., "one-size-fits-all" meal plan:**
    A. Yes
    B. No
    C. Cannot judge
    D. Based on the situation

23. **After digestion and absorption, the dietary proteins are broken down into the basic building blocks of the body called:**
    A. Fatty acid
    B. Lactic acid
    C. Amino acid
    D. None of the above

24. **The reason for considering bioenergetics and logistics while planning sports nutrition is because:**
    A. The calorific requirement of different sports items varies between each other
    B. The energy level varies during the intermittent exertion throughout the sporting event
    C. The logistics if training and competitions differs between each other
    D. All of the above

25. Which macronutrient is called the "master fuel" which is required for the optimal sports performance?
    A. Protein
    B. Fat
    C. Carbohydrate
    D. All of the above
26. How much is the recommended daily carbohydrate intake for a competitive athlete with a training frequency of 5–6 days per week and a moderate training intensity with a training duration of 1 to 2 hours a day?
    A. 3–6 g per kg body weight
    B. 6–8 g per kg body weight
    C. 8–10 g per kg body weight
    D. 10–12 g per kg body weight
27. In addition to the desired quality and quantity of carbohydrates, protein, and fat, why the fruit and vegetable food group are best options for athletes?
    A. It provides fiber (soluble and insoluble).
    B. It provides vitamin C, potassium and beta carotene.
    C. It provides antioxidants and provides few calories.
    D. All of the above
28. What diet is preferable for an athlete 24 hours before going for intense training or competition?
    A. Protein rich diet
    B. Carbohydrate rich diet
    C. Fat rich diet
    D. All of the above
29. An athlete who consumes an unbalanced diet is more prone to the lack of which one of the following nutrients:
    A. Fat
    B. Macronutrients
    C. Micronutrients
    D. None of the above
30. Muscle glycogen replenishment of athletes is required for continuous physical excursion. What rate of carbohydrate intake is needed post-exertion or a sport to maximize glycogen synthesis?

A. 1.0–1.5 g/kg body weight every 2 hours for six hours post exercise
B. 2.0–2.5 g/kg body weight every 2 hours for six hours post exercise
C. 3.0–3.5 g/kg body weight every 2 hours for six hours post exercise
D. None of the above

31. The daily recommended dietary fat intake of an athlete is:
    A. 10–25% of total calories
    B. 20–35% of total calories
    C. 30–45% of total calories
    D. None of the above

32. What will be the outcome of a diet which is too low in fat, combined with low calorie and protein?
    A. Negative energy balance
    B. Weight loss
    C. Fatigue
    D. All of the above

33. It is recommended to have fat intake of 30–35% from total calories. How to calculate the percentage of calories from fat to make a healthy food choice?
    A. (Calories from fat ÷ total calories) × 100
    B. (Total calories ÷ fat) × 100
    C. (Total fat + protein ÷ calories) × 100
    D. None of the above

34. What cholesterol is known as good cholesterol or a scavenger?
    A. Low-density lipoprotein (LDL)
    B. High-density lipoprotein (HDL)
    C. Total cholesterol
    D. All of the above

35. Which one of the following combinations contains complementing proteins?
    A. Soy and grains
    B. Legumes and grains
    C. Legumes, nuts and soy
    D. All of the above

36. What is the latest daily protein recommendation for strength athletes?
    A. 1.4–2.0 g/kg body weight
    B. 1 g/kg body weight
    C. 2 g/kg body weight
    D. None of the above

37. Consumption of excess protein is harmful. Hence, how much is the daily recommended level of protein consumption?
   A. Should not exceed 20% of total calories from protein
   B. Should not exceed 30% of total calories from protein
   C. Should not exceed 35% of total calories from protein
   D. None of the above

38. Which B complex vitamin plays a major role in energy production and for maintaining a healthy nervous system?
   A. Thiamin (B_1)
   B. Riboflavin (B_2)
   C. Niacin (B_3)
   D. A and C

39. Vitamin C generally promotes health and boosts immune system. Why the vitamin C is more important for athletes?
   A. It is critical for the formation of collagen
   B. For wound healing and act as antioxidant
   C. It enhances iron absorption
   D. All of the above

40. Which of the following are the major minerals required for the body in amounts greater than 100 mg per day?
   A. Calcium and phosphorous
   B. Magnesium and sodium
   C. Chloride, potassium and sulfur
   D. All of the above

41. Regular calcium intake help build and strengthen the bone, and it plays a crucial role in many body functions. Which food is a rich source of calcium?
   A. Dairy products-milk, yogurt, cheese, etc.
   B. Egg, soy products
   C. Green leafy vegetables
   D. All of the above

42. What are the consequences of dehydration in athletes?
   A. Increase in body temperature, fatigue and muscle cramps
   B. Heat cramps, heat stroke, heat exhaustion
   C. Optimal sports performance
   D. A and B

ANSWERS

1. **A.** High quality protein includes proteins of animal origin of those in eggs, meat, fish, poultry and dairy products. High quality protein, high biological value and complete protein are synonymous terms used to describe the amino acid pattern of the proteins that is similar to the body's needs.

2. **D.** Glycine is a nonessential amino acid synthesized by the human body and they do not need to be consumed in the diet.

3. **B.** Protein requirements are increased by both aerobic endurance training and strength training. For aerobic endurance athletes, the underlying mechanism could include tissue repair and the use of the branched-chain amino acids for auxiliary fuel, whereas for strength and power athletes, the mechanisms are probably tissue repair and the maintenance of a positive nitrogen balance so that the hypertrophy stimulus is minimized.

4. **B.** The foods such as carrots are digested quickly and rapidly, raises blood glucose (and insulin), have a high glycemic index value.

5. **C.** The frequency and duration of exercise training are the important factors to be considered when determining recommendations for carbohydrate intake.

6. **A.** High levels of HDL protect against heart disease and HDL can be increased by exercise and weight loss. In patients with heart disease and high total cholesterol levels, a low fat diet and exercise can decrease total cholesterol and decrease the ratio of total cholesterol to HDL cholesterol.

7. **B.** Reducing dietary fat to 10% of total calories may actually worsen lipid profiles. Diets extremely low in fat (less than 15% of total calories) may decrease testosterone production, thus decreasing metabolism and muscle development, which is harmful to health and performance.

8. **D.** Training couples with low energy intake or a diet deficient in certain vitamins and minerals could cause performance decrements, which in turn necessitates a need for an athlete to supplement his or her diet with vitamins.

9. **A.** Each pound (0.45 kg) lost during practice represents 1pt (0.5L) of fluid loss which must be replaced before next practice.
10. **C.** The most common recommendation is to eat 3 to 4 hours prior to the event to avoid becoming nauseated or uncomfortable during competition.
11. **D.** Dietary supplements are highly refined products that would not be confused with a food. It must also be intended for ingestion and cannot be advertised for use as conventional food or as the sole item of a meal or diet.
12. **D.** The principle drawback to caffeine use is a potential diuretic effect, which would be expected to occur most prominently in non-habitual users, theoretically producing a range of effects from inconvenience to performance—threatening dehydration.
13. **C.** Doses exceeding 10 times the recommended daily allowances can produce excessive calcium deposition and weight loss.
14. **B.** Caffeine and creatine are two of the few dietary supplements that are known to be effective in enhancing specific types of athletic performance for some individuals.
15. **B.**
16. **C.** Weight loss formula

   a. $\dfrac{\text{Percentage body}}{100} \times \dfrac{\text{Fat weight in kg}}{1} = \text{Total kg fat}$

   $\dfrac{10}{100} \times 75 = 7.5$ kg of body fat

   b. $\dfrac{\text{Percentage of body fat to lose}}{\text{Actual percentage body fat}} \times \text{kg fat} = \text{kg to lose}$

   $\dfrac{5}{10} \times 7.5 = 3.75$ kg of lose

17. **B.** The aim of carbohydrate loading diet is to increase the muscle glycogen levels of the existing muscle, so there is more glycogen available to supply energy for a longer period of time.
18. **C.** Six nutrients: This includes carbohydrates, proteins, fat, minerals, vitamins, and water. The body cannot endogenously generate as per the daily requirement; hence this must be supplied through the diet.

Chapter 17: Sports Nutrition   355

19. **B.** Adenosine triphosphate or ATP, is the body's direct energy source trapped within the nutrients that are released at the end of metabolic pathways. For an athlete's physical performance, spontaneous and continuous supply of ATP is required, without which the muscles would not generate force.

20. **D.** Recommended dietary allowances (RDAs) are formed in 1941 by the United States National Academy of Sciences. The nutritionists use RDAs to plan a balanced diet for individuals and communities.

21. **D.** The quality of food products can be assessed from the food labels where the ingredients are listed in descending order of predominance in the product.

22. **B.** The dietary requirement of each sports personnel varies; hence one cannot generalize the dietary plan of an athlete. Individual to individual, the mean plan varies depending upon the intensity of training and the hydration schedule. However, the basic concepts can be adopted universally.

23. **C.** Amino acids are the building blocks of the body. After digestion of protein and its absorption at the small intestine, the protease and peptidase enzymes act upon the protein to break the protein chain into smaller units called amino acids, which are then absorbed into the bloodstream.

24. **D.** The energy requirement of a football player having intermittent exertion for more than an hour is entirely different from that of a rower, who needs continuous thrust with an activity period of less than 10-20 minutes. Similarly, the energy utilization of a sprinter with short, intense effort is different from that of a marathon runner having sustained moderate effort. Besides, the logistics of training and competition also vary. Eating and drinking is possible in biking, but a swimmer in the open water cannot have fluid and energy intake and sports.

25. **C.** Even though fat is rich in calories, carbohydrates are the primary source of energy supply. Higher the intensity of aerobic physical excretion (like sprinting), there is a greater body dependency on carbohydrates. An adequate supply of carbohydrates spares muscle tissue because a low carbohydrate supply will lead to muscle protein breakdown.

26. **B.** It is 6–8 g per k body weight for a moderate type of athlete. The calorific requirement from carbohydrates always depends on the intensity of athletic activity (light, moderate to high intensity), how many days of training per week, how long he/she trains, etc.
27. **D.** Fruits and vegetables nourish the body with vitamins, minerals and with both soluble and insoluble fiber. It is advisable to include a variety of fruits and vegetables into the dietary plan.
28. **B.** Carbohydrate-rich diet: In the hours leading up (24 hours before the event) for intense training or competition, the athlete should have a high carbohydrate load, which will help increase the muscle glycogen, a storehouse of quick energy. The quick release of energy maximizes the energy levels leading to better athletic performance.
29. **C.** Micronutrients: At the time when the athletes undergo intense training and competition, chances of imbalanced dietary intake are common. They often consume refined carbohydrates, which are deficient in micronutrients like vitamins, including B_6, and minerals, like zinc, magnesium, and selenium. Hence, it is recommended to measure the micronutrient level of those athletes who consume an unbalanced diet.
30. **A.** The muscle and liver glycogen should be replenished soon after draining during exercise. It can take 20 hours or more even if the athlete consumes 60% of total calories from carbohydrates. However, slow replenishment is acceptable for recreational athletes, but multiple workouts per day need fast glycogen replenishment for continuous high-intensity workouts.
31. **B.** Generally, the studies reported that the athletes consume an average fat intake of 35%. However, the consumption varies from person to person and depends on the type of sports activities. Though, the recommended dietary fat allowance is from 20 to 35% of total calories.
32. **D.** A diet of an athlete that is too low in fat, calories, and protein will lead to negative energy balance, and its implications will be counterproductive, resulting in low physical performance.

Chapter 17: Sports Nutrition

33. **A.** For better health, it is advisable to consume a fat intake of less than or equal to 30–35% of total calories. The percentage calories from fat can be calculated by dividing calories taken from fat divided by total calories and then make it into a percentage by multiplying the result by 100.

34. **B.** Irrespective of the physical status, it is undesirable to have high blood cholesterol, a combination of HDL, LDL, and triglycerides. The HDL plays the role of picking up cholesterol from the bloodstream and arteries to the liver, where it is transformed as bile and excretes from the system. Hence called good cholesterol or known as a scavenger. Therefore, a sportsperson should be selective in the diet and choose low cholesterol food.

35. **D.** An incomplete protein source lacks certain essential amino acids, known as the limiting amino acids. Hence, consuming a variety of protein sources or a combination of two or more protein sources will complement each other, and the limiting amino acids will compensate.

36. **A.** The latest research on the protein requirement of sports personals indicates a higher protein requirement, while the established protein requirement of an average person is 0.8 g/kg body weight. Though the current protein recommendations of athletes are 1.4 to 2 g/kg, some research recommends the upper limit as 2.5 g/kg body weight.

37. **C.** Adequate amount of protein is required for the athletes for their optimal performance. However, long-term excess consumption above 35% of total calories from protein will create an adverse effect on the kidneys, ultimately increasing the workload and stress of kidneys to eliminate urea, which is an end product of protein metabolism. It also leads to dehydration and an increase in the excretion of calcium from the bones.

38. **D.** Thiamin (B_1) and Niacin (B_3) are an integral component in the energy production mechanism and it helps develop, and maintain a healthy nervous system. The studies also demonstrated that athletes who consume low thiamin had diminished exercise endurance.

39. **D.** Vitamin C is required for the formation of collagen (tendons, ligaments, cartilage, teeth, and bone). Collagen

is an important component of wound healing to form scar tissues. It also boosts the immune system and improves iron absorption, thereby preventing iron deficiency anemia. It also acts as an antioxidant that prevents heart disease, and it averts oxidative damage during intense exercise.

40. **D.** Minerals are integral components of bodily functions, keeping athletes healthy and strong, but the requirement is in milligrams or micrograms. Of which, some minerals are required by the body in greater amounts, above 100 mg/day; such minerals are called major minerals.

41. **D.** High calcium intake will help build and strengthen the bone and is critical for many body functions. Dairy products, eggs, and green leafy vegetables are rich sources. Calcium supplements are required for athletes who are in low-calorie food, but the supply of more than 500 mg is not absorbed well if taken together.

42. **C.** If the athlete cannot maintain the water balance, it will affect his/her performance. There are two stages of water imbalance, dehydration (less than normal) and hyperhydration (higher than normal). Both the stages are not good for optimal performance. Dehydration leads to the low blood supply to the muscles and low cardiac output, resulting in faster fatigue and muscle cramps.

CHAPTER 18

Sports Psychology

1. During the closing seconds of a basketball game, an athlete's team is down by one point and he has been awarded two free throw shots. The player is apprehensive about the outcome of the game. Which of the following best describes the athlete's situation?
   A. He is experiencing trait anxiety
   B. He is experiencing state anxiety
   C. He is in control of his arousal
   D. His anxiety will improve his performance

2. The type of anxiety experienced by the athlete would proportionately reduce his performance requiring high amount of information processing is known as:
   A. Somatic anxiety   B. Cognitive anxiety
   C. Trait anxiety   D. Psychic arousal

3. Which of the following is more important to achieve an ideal performance state?
   A. Fear of failure
   B. Analyzing performance
   C. Personal control
   D. Broad focus on the activity and the environment

4. An athlete's desire to perform to his/her potential is an example of:
   A. Motive to avoid failure   B. Achievement motivation
   C. Intrinsic motivation   D. Dissociation

5. A cognitive psychological skill in which the athlete uses all the senses to create a mental experience of an athletic performance is known as:
   A. Mental imagery   B. Self-efficacy
   C. Mental efficacy   D. Eustress

6. For the high school football team, if any player squats two times his bodyweight, his name is displayed on the wall. This is an example of:

- A. Negative reinforcement
- B. Positive reinforcement
- C. Negative punishment
- D. Positive punishment

7. A somatopsychic technique by which psychological and physical arousal are self-regulated through the control of skeletal muscle tension is knows as:
   - A. Autogenic training
   - B. Counter conditioning
   - C. Systematic desensitization
   - D. Progressive muscular relaxation

8. An Olympic weightlifter attempting a personal record is able to ignore the audience to concentrate solely on his performance. Which of the following abilities is the athlete most likely using to perform the lift?
   - A. Somatic anxiety
   - B. Successive approximation
   - C. Dissociation
   - D. Selective attention

9. How does an athlete's amount or latitude of optimal arousal change with limited skill and ability of the activity?
   - A. It increases
   - B. It decreases
   - C. It has no effect
   - D. Performance improve with greater arousal

10. Prior to performing the long jump, an athlete reviews and concentrates on the technique required to jump as far as possible. Which of the following strategies is the athlete using to prepare for the jump?
    - A. Reliance of experience
    - B. Association
    - C. Trait anxiety
    - D. Focusing on task-relevant cues

11. Which of the following is NOT a primary role of a sports psychologist?
    - A. Consultant
    - B. Teacher
    - C. Strength and conditioning coach
    - D. Researcher

Chapter 18: Sports Psychology

12. An athlete in gymnastics is diagnosed with anorexia nervosa. Which of the following specialists might be asked to help treat this emotional disorder?
    A. Pedagogical Sports psychologist
    B. Educational sports psychologist
    C. Clinical sports psychologist
    D. Experimental kinesiologist

13. Sports psychology is accepted as what form of "science" in academic circles?
    A. Hard science
    B. Social science
    C. Educational science
    D. Soft science

14. As sports and exercise psychologists, there is an ethical responsibility to protect an athlete's welfare. Which of the following is NOT one of the six general ethical principles espoused by the AAASP (American Association for the Advancement of Applied Sport Psychology)?
    A. Winning
    B. Competence
    C. Respect for People's Rights and Dignity
    D. Integrity

15. Sports psychologists commonly are found in which of the following settings?
    A. National and Olympic Teams
    B. All are common settings
    C. Universities and Colleges
    D. Professional Sports Teams

16. Sports psychology uses the scientific method to bridge science and practice and build a knowledge base that can foster improved athletic performance in athletes. Which of the following is NOT a component of the scientific method?
    A. Systematic approach and empirical observation
    B. Critical analysis and rigorous evaluation
    C. Guesswork and quasi-experimental designs
    D. Experimental controls and objective evidence gathering

17. As part of their training, sports psychologists usually have to take classes in many different areas. Which of the following subjects might a student have to study to become a certified sports psychologist?
    A. All are common classes in sports psychology curriculums
    B. Abnormal Psychology and Developmental Psychology
    C. Biomechanics and Counselling Psychology
    D. Motor Development and Exercise Physiology
18. The following are some of the psychological approaches adopted by sports psychologists for service delivery:
    A. Team therapy, coach therapy, and substitute therapy
    B. Environment-centered, external focused, and irrational behavior therapy
    C. Person-centered, psychoanalytic, and rational-emotive behavior therapy
    D. Listening therapy, vision therapy and linguistic therapy
19. A sport psychologist's competencies include:
    A. Emotional intelligence quotient, height and authority
    B. Client welfare, professional relationships and assessment techniques
    C. Confidence, frustration, tolerance and networking ability
    D. Personality, confidence, and intelligent quotient
20. Sport psychology consultants triangulate their assessment techniques by:
    A. Talking to the interviewing the athlete, asking the athlete to complete psychometric assessments and interviewing the athlete's coach
    B. Athlete's coach, talking to the athlete's teammates and talking to the athlete's parents
    C. Observing the athlete, watching the athlete and making videos of the athlete
    D. Talking to the athlete, listening to the athlete and watching the athlete

ANSWERS

1. **B.** State anxiety is a subjective experience of apprehension and uncertainty accompanied by elevated autonomic and voluntary neural outflow and increased endocrine activity. The impact of state anxiety on athletic performance may positive, negative or indifferent depending on athlete's skill level, personality and complexity of task to be performed.

2. **B.** Cognitive anxiety is a psychological state-involving task-irrelevant mental processes that are negative in nature, flood attention and can deter performance proportionately, especially activities requiring high amounts of information processing.

3. **C.** The most important in achieving ideal performance state is that, the athlete's trust in their skill and conditioning level and just "let it happen" without interference from negative associative process in the cerebral cortex.

4. **C.** Intrinsic motivation is defined as a desire to be competent and self-determining. With intrinsic motivation, the athlete is the self-starter because of his or her love of game.

5. **A.** Mental imagery is a cognitive skill in which the athlete simulates reality by mentally rehearsing a movement, imaging visual, auditory, kinesthetic olfactory factory and even exertional cues.

6. **B.** Positive reinforcement is the act of increasing the probability of occurrence of a given behavior by following it with or presenting an action, object or event such as praise, decals on the helmets or prizes and awards.

7. **D.** Progressive muscular relaxation technique is employed by the athletes to achieve an appropriate level of psychic vigor and physiological arousal before performance. In this technique, by going through a series of alternate muscular tension and relaxing phases, the athlete learns to become aware of somatic tension and thereby to control it. Theoretically, the technique exerts its effect by means of a process termed reciprocal inhibition, stating that a relaxed body will promote a relaxed mind.

8. **D.** Selective attention is the ability to inhibit awareness of some stimuli in order to process others and it suppresses

task-irrelevant cues (e.g., people on side lines) in order to process the task-relevant cues in the limited attentional space.

9. **B.** An athlete's skill level can increase the latitude of optimal arousal. The more skill an athlete has developed, the better he or she performs during states of greater or less than optimal arousal. Increase in arousal beyond the optimal level resulted in gradual, proportionate declines in performance.

10. **D.** Task-relevant cue strategy can reduce distractions, which often deter optimal effort. Such focusing strategies can promote mental consistency during the preparatory state, which in turn, can promote physical consistency—the hallmark of a skilled athlete.

11. **C.** Strength and conditioning coach: While many coaches use sports psychology skills and techniques to help their athletes, professional sports psychologists usually teach college classes, conduct research, or provide psychological skills training to athletes.

12. **C.** Clinical sports psychologist: There are two primary specialties in sports psychology: clinical sports psychology and educational sports psychology. A clinical sports psychologist is usually licensed by a state board to treat athlete who have severe emotional disorders. Depression, eating disorders, and substance abuse are examples of issues a clinical sports psychologist might work with.

13. **B.** Social science: Sport and exercise psychology is recognized as a social science much like sociology, anthropology, developmental psychology, and social work. Researcher's study how athletes interact with their environment and how sports-specific behaviors are shaped over time and contexts.

14. **A.** Winning: The remaining three guidelines and general principles include: professional and scientific responsibility, concern for welfare of others, and social responsibility. These guidelines are based upon the American Psychological Association's 1992 ethical standards and promotes a protection of basic human fundamental rights.

15. **B.** All are common settings. Applied sports psychologists are experiencing a growth of career opportunities within a wide variety of different sports-exercise settings. Some

Chapter 18: Sports Psychology

sports psychologists have even moved successfully into the business sector. Lane4 Management Group is an example of a global consulting group initiated by a sports psychologist and a British Olympic swimmer.

16. **C.** Guesswork and quasi-experimental designs. Sport psychology is an accepted science and thus is subject to the scientific method in directing a systematic collection of evidence to build a knowledge base. Objective evidence collected must be open to external evaluation, observation, and testing.

17. **A.** All are common classes in sports psychology curriculums. Other classes that are common requirements in sports psychology curricula include: motor learning, kinesiology, sports medicine, sports pedagogy, clinical psychology, experimental psychology, personality psychology, and nutrition.

18. **C.** Psychological approaches adopted by sport psychologists include person-centered, psychoanalytic, and rational-emotive behavior therapy.

19. **B.** A sport psychologist's competencies include: client welfare, professional relationships and assessment techniques.

20. **A.** Sport psychology consultants triangulate their assessments by interviewing the athlete, asking the athlete to complete psychometric assessments and interviewing the athlete's coach.

Bibliography

LIST OF TEXTBOOKS

1. Anderson MK, Gail P, Parr GP, Hall SJ. Foundations of athletic training prevention, assessment, and management, 4th edition. Wolters Kluwer Health/Lippincott Williams & Wilkins; 2009.
2. Andrews JR, Harrelson GL, Wilk KE. Physical rehabilitation of the injured athlete, 4th edition. Saunders (Elsevier); 2012.
3. Baechle TR. Essentials of strength training and conditioning. Human Kinetics; 1994.
4. Booher JM, Thibodeau GA. Athletic injury assessment. McGraw-Hill; 2000.
5. Brotzman SB, Manske RC. Clinical orthopaedic rehabilitation: An evidence-based approach, 3rd edition. Mosby (Elsevier); 2011.
6. Brotzman SB, Wilk KE. Clinical orthopaedic rehabilitation, 2nd edition. Mosby; 2003.
7. Canavan P. Rehabilitation in sports medicine. Appleton & Lange; 1998.
8. Chen MYM, Pope TL, Ott DJ. Basic radiology. McGraw-Hill Medical; 2011.
9. Colombo R, Sanguineti V. Rehabilitation robotics technology and application. Academic Press (Elsevier); 2018.
10. Comfort P, Abrahamson E. Sports rehabilitation and injury prevention. Wiley-Blackwell; 2010.
11. Das S. A manual on clinical surgey. 7th edition. Dr S Das; 2008.
12. Doral MN. Sports injuries: Prevention, diagnosis, treatment and rehabilitation. Springer-Verlag Berlin Heidelberg; 2012.
13. Driskell J, Wolinsky I. Nutritional assessment of athletes, 2nd edition. CRC Press; 2011.
14. Dutton M. Dutton's orthopaedic examination, evaluation, and intervention, 3rd edition. McGraw-Hill Education Medical; 2012.
15. Ebnezar J. Textbook of Orthopedics, 4th edition. Jaypee Brothers Medical Publishers (P) Ltd.; 2010.
16. Evans RC. Illustrated essentials in orthopaedic physical assessment. Mosby; 1994.
17. Fink HH, Mikesky AE. Practical applications in sports nutrition, 4th edition. Jones & Bartlett Learning; 2015.

18. Garrett WE, Speer KP, Kirkendall DT. Principles and practice of orthopaedic sports medicine. Lippincott Williams & Wilkins; 2000.
19. Guermazi A, Roemer FW, Crema MD. Imaging in sports-specific musculoskeletal injuries. Springer International Publishing; 2016.
20. Harries M, Williams C, Stanish WD, Micheli LJ. Oxford textbook of sports medicine. Oxford University Press; 1996.
21. Irvin R, Iversen D, Roy S. Sports medicine: prevention, management & rehabilitation of athletic injuries. Pearson; 1999
22. Joshi J, Kotwal P. Essentials of orthopaedics and applied physiotherapy, 3rd edition. RELX India Pvt. Ltd (Elsevier); 2017.
23. Kanosue K, Ogawa T, Fukano M, Fukubayashi T. Sports Injuries and Prevention. Springer Japan; 2015.
24. Kirkaldy-Wills WH, Bernard TN. Managing low back pain. Churchill Livingstone; 1999.
25. Kisner C, Colby LA. Therapeutic exercise foundations and technique, 6th edition. FA Davis company; 2012.
26. Kulkarni GS, Babhulkar S. Textbook of orthopedics and trauma, 3rd edition. Jaypee Brothers Medical Publishers (P) Ltd.; 2015.
27. Levangie PK, Norkin CC. Joint structure and function: a comprehensive analysis. FA Davis Company; 2011.
28. Magee DJ. Orthopaedic physical assessment, 6th edition. Saunders (Elsevier); 2013.
29. Malone TR, Mc Poil T, Nitz AJ. Orthopaedic and sports therapy. Mosby; 1996.
30. Masciocchi C. Radiological imaging of sports injuries. Springer-Verlag Berlin Heidelberg; 1998.
31. Miller LT, Kaeding CC. Stress fractures in athletes: Diagnosis and management. Springer International Publishing; 2015.
32. Nicholas JA. Upper extremity in sports medicine. Mosby; 1994.
33. O' Sullivan S, Schmitz T J. Physical rehabilitation: Assessment and treatment. FA Davis Co.; 1994.
34. Prentice WE. Rehabilitation techniques for sports medicine and athletic training, 5th edition. McGraw-Hill; 2011.
35. Puffer JC. 20 Common problems in sports medicine. McGraw-Hill Education Medical; 2001.
36. Reid DC. Sports injury assessment and rehabilitation. Churchill Livingstone; 1991.
37. Reider B, Davies GJ, Provencher M. Orthopaedic rehabilitation of the athlete: Getting back in the game. Saunders (Elsevier); 2015.
38. Reider B. Sports medicine: The school-age athlete. W B Saunders; 1996.

39. Robert C, Schenck RC. Athletic training and sports medicine. Jones & Barlett Publishers; 1999.
40. Rocon E, Pons JL. Exoskeletons in rehabilitation robotics-tremor suppression. Springer-Verlag Berlin Heidelberg; 2011.
41. Scuderi GR, McCann P, Bruno PJ. Sports medicine: Principles of primary care. Mosby; 1996.
42. Solomon L, Warwick D, Nayagam S. Apley's system of orthopaedics and fractures. Hodder Education Publishers; 2001.
43. Sueki D, Brechter J. Orthopedic rehabilitation clinical advisor. Mosby (Elsevier); 2010.
44. Torg JS, Welsh RP, Shephard R J. Current therapy in sports medicine, 2nd edition. BC Decker Inc.; 1989.
45. Vanhoenacker FM, Maas M, Gielen JL, Faletti C, Baert AL. Imaging of orthopedic sports injuries. Springer; 2007.
46. Ward K. Routledge handbook of sports therapy, injury assessment and rehabilitation. Routledge; 2016.
47. Zeisig E, Fahlstrom M. Lateral and medial elbow tendinopathies. In: Doral MN, Karlsson J (Eds.), Sports injuries: Prevention, diagnosis, treatment and rehabilitation. Springer-Verlag Berlin/Heidelberg; 2015. pp. 587-92.

LIST OF JOURNALS

1. Bennell K, Brukner P. Preventing and managing stress fractures in athletes. Physiotherapy in Sport. 2005;6:171-80.
2. Chmielewski TL, Myer GD, Kauffman D, Tillman SM. Plyometric exercise in the rehabilitation of athletes: physiological responses and clinical application. Journal of Orthopaedic Sports Physical Therapy. 2006; 36(5): 308-19.
3. Erdmann WS. Problems of sport biomechanics and robotics. International Journal of Advanced Robotic Systems. 2013;10:123. https://doi.org/10.5772/52499.
4. Grief DN, Emerson CP, Allegra P, Shallop BJ, Kaplan LD. Olecranon stress fracture. Clinics in Sports Medicine. 2020;39(3):575-88.
5. Kahanov L, Eberman LE, Games KE, Wasik M. Diagnosis, treatment, and rehabilitation of stress fractures in the lower extremity in runners. Open Access Journal of Sports Medicine. 2015; 6: 87-95.
6. Kaiser PB, Guss D, DiGiovanni CW. Stress fractures of the foot and ankle in athletes. Foot Ankle Orthopaedics. 2018. https://doi.org/10.1177/2473011418790078.

7. Laut J, Porfiri M, Raghavan P. The present and future of robotic technology in rehabilitation. Current Physical Medicine and Rehabilitation Reports. 2016; 4(4):312-9.
8. Lee AT, Lee-Robinson AL. The prevalence of medial epicondylitis among patients with c6 and c7 radiculopathy. Sports Health. 2010;2(4), 334-6.
9. Qassim HM, Hasan WZW. A review on upper limb rehabilitation robots. Applied Sciences. 2002; 10(19): 6976.
10. Terrell SL, Allen CR, Lynch J. Robotic rehabilitation treatment influences power and active straight leg raise performance in division II female athletes. Journal of Athletic Enhancement. 2017; 6: 4. 10.4172/2324-9080.1000271.
11. Toigo M, Fluck M, Riener R, Klamroth-MarganskaV. Robot-assisted assessment of muscle strength. Journal of Neuro Engineering and Rehabilitation. 2017;14:10. https://doi.org/10.1186/s12984-017-0314-2.
12. Valado CT, Loterio F, Cardoso V, Bastos T, Frizera-Neto A, Carelli R. Robotics as a tool for physiotherapy and rehabilitation sessions. IFAC-Papers Online. 2015;48(19):148-153.
13. Wilk KE, Arrigo CA. Rehabilitation of elbow injuries. Clinics in Sports Medicine. 2020; 39(3): 687-715.
14. Zhang M, Davies TC, Xie S. Effectiveness of robot-assisted therapy on ankle rehabilitation: A systematic review. Journal of Neuro Engineering and Rehabilitation. 2013;10:30. http://www.jneuroengrehab.com/content/10/1/30.

www.ingramcontent.com/pod-product-compliance
Ingram Content Group UK Ltd.
Pitfield, Milton Keynes, MK11 3LW, UK
UKHW021832140426
521711PUK000211B/1406

EU GSPR Authorised Representative
Logos Europe, 9 rue Nicolas Poussin
1700, La Rochelle, France
Phone: +33 (0) 6 67 93 73 78
E-mail: contact@logoseurope.eu